THE CHILDHOOD OBESITY EPIDEMIC
WHY ARE OUR CHILDREN OBESE— AND WHAT CAN WE DO ABOUT IT?

THE CHILDHOOD OBESITY EPIDEMIC

WHY ARE OUR CHILDREN OBESE—
AND WHAT CAN WE DO ABOUT IT?

Edited by
Peter D. Vash, MD, MPH

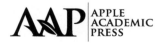

Apple Academic Press Inc.
3333 Mistwell Crescent
Oakville, ON L6L 0A2
Canada

Apple Academic Press Inc.
9 Spinnaker Way
Waretown, NJ 08758
USA

©2015 by Apple Academic Press, Inc.
Exclusive worldwide distribution by CRC Press, a member of Taylor & Francis Group

No claim to original U.S. Government works
Printed in the United States of America on acid-free paper

International Standard Book Number-13: 978-1-77188-102-9 (Hardcover)

This book contains information obtained from authentic and highly regarded sources. Reprinted material is quoted with permission and sources are indicated. Copyright for individual articles remains with the authors as indicated. A wide variety of references are listed. Reasonable efforts have been made to publish reliable data and information, but the authors, editors, and the publisher cannot assume responsibility for the validity of all materials or the consequences of their use. The authors, editors, and the publisher have attempted to trace the copyright holders of all material reproduced in this publication and apologize to copyright holders if permission to publish in this form has not been obtained. If any copyright material has not been acknowledged, please write and let us know so we may rectify in any future reprint.

Trademark Notice: Registered trademark of products or corporate names are used only for explanation and identification without intent to infringe.

Library of Congress Control Number: 2014952128

Library and Archives Canada Cataloguing in Publication

The childhood obesity epidemic: why are our children obese--and what can we do about it? / edited by Peter D. Vash, MD, MPH.

Includes bibliographical references and index.
ISBN 978-1-77188-102-9 (bound)
1. Obesity in children. 2. Obesity in children--Prevention.
3. Obesity in children--Treatment. I. Vash, Peter D., editor

RJ399.C6C45 2015   618.92'398   C2014-906650-3

Apple Academic Press also publishes its books in a variety of electronic formats. Some content that appears in print may not be available in electronic format. For information about Apple Academic Press products, visit our website at **www.appleacademicpress.com** and the CRC Press website at **www.crcpress.com**

ABOUT THE EDITOR

PETER D. VASH, MD, MPH

Peter D. Vash, MD, MPH, FACE, Assistant Clinical Professor of Medicine at UCLA. Medical Center and Fellow of the American Association of Clinical Endocrinologists, is a board-certified internist specializing in endocrinology and metabolism and a Diplomat in Obesity Medicine. He is the past president of the American Society of Bariatric Physicians, and served on the Board of the North American Society for the Study of Obesity (NASSO). Dr. Vash works in private practice with patients suffering from obesity and eating disorders, and has lectured extensively nationally and internationally, on the medical management and treatment of obesity. He has been an invited expert witness to speak before a Senate sub committee and the FTC. concerning medical weight-loss issues and the safety and impact of commercial weight-loss programs. He has written four books—*The Fat to Muscle Diet, The Dieter's Dictionary, A Matter of Fat: A Physician's Program*, and *Lose It and Keep It Off.* He has served on the board of *Shape Magazine*, writing numerous articles regarding health, fitness and weight problems. Dr. Vash has worked closely in consultation with the media (TV, radio, print), aiding them with information and explanations of issues regarding obesity and eating disorders. He is currently the Executive Medical Director of the Lindora Medical Clinics, the largest and oldest medical weight-loss clinic in Southern California.

CONTENTS

Acknowledgment and How to Cite... *ix*
List of Contributors... *xi*
Introduction...*xvii*

Part I: Prevalence

1. **A Multilevel Approach to Estimating Small Area Childhood Obesity Prevalence at the Census Block-Group Level**........................... 3
   Xingyou Zhang, Stephen Onufrak, James B. Holt, and Janet B. Croft

2. **Unexpected Plateauing of Childhood Obesity Rates in Developed Countries** 21
   Martin Wabitsch, Anja Moss, and Katrin Kromeyer-Hauschild

3. **Prevalence, Disparities, and Trends in Obesity and Severe Obesity Among Students in the Philadelphia, Pennsylvania, School District, 2006–2010** 29
   Jessica M. Robbins, Giridhar Mallya, Marcia Polansky, and Donald F. Schwarz

Part II: What Makes Our Children Obese and Overweight?

4. **Physical Activity, Screen Time and Obesity Status in a Nationally Representative Sample of Maltese Youth with International Comparisons** 45
   Andrew Decelis, Russell Jago, and Kenneth R. Fox

5. **Impulsivity, "Advergames," and Food Intake** 69
   Frans Folkvord, Doeschka J. Anschütz, Chantal Nederkoorn, Henk Westerik, and Moniek Buijzen

6. **Assessing Causality in the Association between Child Adiposity and Physical Activity Levels: A Mendelian Randomization Analysis**.. 83
   Rebecca C. Richmond, George Davey Smith, Andy R. Ness, Marcel den Hoed, George McMahon, and Nicholas J. Timpson

7. Associations Between Eating Frequency, Adiposity, Diet, and Activity in 9–10-Year-Old Healthy-Weight and Centrally Obese Children 109

   Amy Jennings, Aedín Cassidy, Esther M. F. van Sluijs, Simon J. Griffin, and Ailsa A. Welch

8. Role of Developmental Overnutrition in Pediatric Obesity and Type 2 Diabetes 127

   Dana Dabelea and Curtis S. Harrod

Part III: What Can We Do to End the Epidemic?

9. Protecting Children from Harmful Food Marketing: Options for Local Government to Make a Difference 145

   Jennifer L. Harris and Samantha K. Graff

10. Life Course Impact of School-Based Promotion of Healthy Eating and Active Living to Prevent Childhood Obesity 157

    Bach Xuan Tran, Arto Ohinmaa, Stefan Kuhle, Jeffrey A. Johnson, and Paul J. Veugelers

11. Modeling Social Transmission Dynamics of Unhealthy Behaviors for Evaluating Prevention and Treatment Interventions on Childhood Obesity 175

    Leah M. Frerichs, Ozgur M. Araz, and Terry T–K Huang

12. Effects of an Intervention Aimed at Reducing the Intake of Sugar-Sweetened Beverages in Primary School Children: A Controlled Trial 211

    Vivian M. van de Gaar, Wilma Jansen, Amy van Grieken, Gerard J. J. M. Borsboom, Stef Kremers, and Hein Raat

13. Listening to the Experts: Is There a Place for Food Taxation in the Fight Against Obesity in Early Childhood? 235

    Erin Pitt, Elizabeth Kendall, Andrew P. Hills, and Tracy Comans

14. The Costs and Cost-Effectiveness of a School-Based Comprehensive Intervention Study on Childhood Obesity in China 255

    Liping Meng, Haiquan Xu, Ailing Liu, Joop van Raaij, Wanda Bemelmans, Xiaoqi Hu, Qian Zhang, Songming Du, Hongyun Fang, Jun Ma, Guifa Xu, Ying Li, Hongwei Guo, Lin Du, and Guansheng Ma

Author Notes 277

Index 285

ACKNOWLEDGMENT AND HOW TO CITE

The editor and publisher thank each of the authors who contributed to this book, whether by granting their permission individually or by releasing their research as open source articles or under a license that permits free use, provided that attribution is made. The chapters in this book were previously published in various places in various formats. To cite the work contained in this book and to view the individual permissions, please refer to the citation at the beginning of each chapter. Each chapter was read individually and carefully selected by the editor; the result is a book that provides a nuanced study of child obesity. The chapters included examine the following topics:

- Before tackling any problem, it is vital to understand the scope of the problem. When it comes to assessing the number of children who are obese or overweight, traditional surveys are impractical for a variety of reasons. Chapter 1 provides a valid alternative for estimating the prevalence of this condition.
- Positive indications that interventions are effective in the fight against obesity should not be cause for complacency. Instead, the evidence in Chapter 2 should encourage and empower individuals, clinicians, school districts, and policy-makers to continue their efforts in the ongoing battle against childhood obesity.
- Although Chapter 3 focuses on only one North American city, the findings can be generalized: first, that obesity interventions do have power to bring about positive and significant change; and second, that the problem continues to be enormous, meaning that ongoing research and intervention in this field is vital.
- Common sense tells us that there is a connection between the time children spend in front of a television, their level of physical activity, and their tendency to be obese. Chapter 4 draws conclusions from an investigative study based in a nation that has one of the highest childhood obesity levels in the world, with results that should provide direction to schools around the world.
- What makes some children more susceptible to unhealthy lifestyle habits than others? The authors' research in Chapter 5 indicates a connection between impulsivity, junk food, and child-targeted advertisements. With as many as 5 percent of all children being diagnosed as having ADHD, it be-

- hooves us to be aware of ways in which this demographic may be particularly vulnerable to lifestyle habits that often lead to obesity.
- Again, few of us would claim to be surprised that there is a connection between obesity and physical activity levels. Chapter 6, however, investigates the connection from the reverse, exposing the "vicious circle" nature of the relationship. Children who are less physically active are more prone to adiposity, but unfortunately the reverse is also true: children who are obese are less likely to be physically active, thus compounding the problem.
- Children (as well as adults) are often encouraged to "graze" throughout the day. The research in Chapter 7 indicates that while frequent eating may be healthy for children who are already at healthy weights, it offers no help to the child who is already obese.
- Chapter 8 explores the transgenerational cycle of obesity and diabetes. The findings of this article have important implications for public health policy, as well as future research directions.
- Childhood obesity is a multifaceted problem that must be attacked from multiple directions. One of the most obvious is to change the messages our children receive about food. Given that corporations are unlikely to readily change their advertising practices, governments must get involved. The policy options outlined in Chapter 9 empower local communities to take action.
- Like the previous article, the Canadian study in Chapter 10 underlines the importance of school-based obesity intervention.
- The research in Chapter 11 takes a different slant from the previous two, suggesting that parental interventions may have the most successful results when combating childhood obesity. The various studies' combined message indicates that a multi-pronged approach might be most effective.
- Underlining the conclusion made above, Chapter 12 looks at a small yet powerful intervention: simply replacing children's sugary juice drinks with water.
- Unfortunately, we cannot simply pass a taxation law and get rid of childhood obesity. Chapter 13 argues that although some products may lend themselves to being effectively taxed—such as sugar-sweetened beverages—others do not. However, since sugary beverages is play so key a role in childhood obesity, governments might do well to seek out practical ways to discourage its consumption.
- When tackling the problem of childhood obesity, we want to get the most "bang for our buck." The Chinese study in Chapter 14 demonstrates the effectiveness of comprehensive interventions that tackle both diet and physical activity.

LIST OF CONTRIBUTORS

Doeschka J. Anschütz
Behavioural Science Institute, Radboud University, Nijmegen, Netherlands

Ozgur M. Araz
College of Public Health, University of Nebraska Medical Center, Omaha, Nebraska, United States of America

Wanda Bemelmans
National Institute for Public Health and the Environment, Bilthoven, The Netherlands

Gerard J.J.M. Borsboom
Department of Public Health, Erasmus University Medical Centre, Rotterdam, 3000, CA, the Netherlands

Moniek Buijzen
Behavioural Science Institute, Radboud University, Nijmegen, Netherlands

Aedín Cassidy
Department of Nutrition, Norwich Medical School, University of East Anglia, Norwich, UK

Tracy Comans
Population and Social Health Research Program, Griffith Health Institute, Griffith University, Logan Campus, University Drive, Meadowbrook 4131, QLD, Australia

Janet B. Croft
Centers for Disease Control and Prevention, Atlanta, Georgia

Dana Dabelea
Department of Epidemiology, Colorado School of Public Health, University of Colorado Denver, Aurora, Colorado, USA

Andrew Decelis
Institute for Physical Education and Sport, University Sports Complex, University of Malta, Msida, MSD2080, Malta and Centre for Exercise, Nutrition and Health Sciences, School for Policy Studies, University of Bristol, 8, Priory Road, Bristol BS8 1TZ, UK

Marcel den Hoed
Molecular Epidemiology and Science for Life Laboratory, Department of Medical Sciences, Uppsala University, Uppsala, Sweden

Lin Du
Guangzhou Center For Disease Control And Prevention, Guangdong Province, China

Songming Du
National Institute for Nutrition and Food Safety, Chinese Center for Disease Control and Prevention, Beijing, China

Yifan Duan
National Institute For Nutrition And Food Safety, Chinese Center For Disease Control And Prevention, Beijing, China

Hongyun Fang
National Institute For Nutrition And Food Safety, Chinese Center For Disease Control And Prevention, Beijing, China

Frans Folkvord
Behavioural Science Institute, Radboud University, Nijmegen, Netherlands

Kenneth R. Fox
Centre for Exercise, Nutrition and Health Sciences, School for Policy Studies, University of Bristol, 8, Priory Road, Bristol BS8 1TZ, UK

Leah M. Frerichs
College of Public Health, University of Nebraska Medical Center, Omaha, Nebraska, United States of America

Samantha K. Graff
Public Health Law & Policy, Oakland, California

Simon J. Griffin
Centre of Excellence in Diet and Activity Research, MRC Epidemiology Unit, Cambridge, UK

Hongwei Guo
School Of Public Health, Fudan University, Shanghai, China

Linan Hao
National Institute For Nutrition And Food Safety, Chinese Center For Disease Control And Prevention, Beijing, China

Jennifer L. Harris
Rudd Center for Food Policy and Obesity, Yale University, New Haven, CT, USA

Curtis S. Harrod
Department of Epidemiology, Colorado School of Public Health, University of Colorado Denver, Aurora, Colorado, USA

Andrew P. Hills
Griffith Health Institute, Griffith University and Mater Research Institute – The University of Queensland, Raymond Terrace, South Brisbane 4101, QLD, Australia

James B. Holt
Centers for Disease Control and Prevention, Atlanta, Georgia

Xiaoqi Hu
National Institute For Nutrition And Food Safety, Chinese Center For Disease Control And Prevention, Beijing, China

Terry T. K. Huang
College of Public Health, University of Nebraska Medical Center, Omaha, Nebraska, United States of America

Russell Jago
Centre for Exercise, Nutrition and Health Sciences, School for Policy Studies, University of Bristol, 8, Priory Road, Bristol BS8 1TZ, UK

Wilma Jansen
Department of Social Development, City of Rotterdam, Rotterdam, 3000 BA, the Netherlands

Amy Jennings
Department of Nutrition, Norwich Medical School, University of East Anglia, Norwich, UK

Jeffrey A. Johnson
School of Public Health, University of Alberta, Edmonton, Alberta, Canada

Elizabeth Kendall
Centre of National Research on Disability and Rehabilitation, Population and Social Health Research Program, Griffith Health Institute, Griffith University, Logan Campus, University Drive, Meadowbrook 4131, QLD, Australia

Stef Kremers
Department of Health Sciences, University Maastricht, Maastricht, MD, the Netherlands

Katrin Kromeyer-Hauschild
Institute of Human Genetics, Jena University Hospital, Friedrich-Schiller-University Jena, Kollegiengasse 10, D-07740 Jena, Germany

Stefan Kuhle
Department of Pediatrics, Obstetrics & Gynecology, Dalhousie University, Halifax, NS, Canada

Tingyu Li
Chongqing Children's Hospital, Chongqing, China

Yanping Li
National Institute For Nutrition And Food Safety, Chinese Center For Disease Control And Prevention, Beijing, China and

Ying Li
Public Health College, Harbin Medical University, Heilongjiang Province, China

Ailing Liu
National Institute For Nutrition And Food Safety, Chinese Center For Disease Control And Prevention, Beijing, China

Guansheng Ma
National Institute For Nutrition And Food Safety, Chinese Center For Disease Control And Prevention, Beijing, China

Jun Ma
Institute Of Children And Adolescent Health, Peking University Health Science Center, Beijing, China and Beijing University Health Science Center, Beijing, China

Giridhar Mallya
Philadelphia Department of Public Health, Philadelphia, Pennsylvania

George McMahon
MRC Integrative Epidemiology Unit, School of Social and Community Medicine, University of Bristol, Bristol, United Kingdom

Liping Meng
National Institute for Nutrition and Food Safety, Chinese Center for Disease Control and Prevention, Beijing, China

Anja Moss
Division of Pediatric Endocrinology and Diabetes, Interdisciplinary Obesity Unit, Department of Pediatrics and Adolescent Medicine, Ulm University, Eythstr. 24, D-89073 Ulm, Germany

List of Contributors

Chantal Nederkoorn
Department of Psychology and Neuroscience, Maastricht University, Maastricht, Netherlands

Andy R. Ness
Department of Oral and Dental Science, University of Bristol, Bristol, United Kingdom

Arto Ohinmaa
School of Public Health, University of Alberta, Edmonton, Alberta, Canada

Stephen Onufrak
Centers for Disease Control and Prevention, Atlanta, Georgia

Erin Pitt
Population and Social Health Research Program, Griffith Health Institute, Griffith University, Logan Campus, University Drive, Meadowbrook 4131, QLD, Australia

Marcia Polansky
Drexel University School of Public Health, Philadelphia, Pennsylvania.

Hein Raat
Department of Public Health, Erasmus University Medical Centre, Rotterdam, 3000, CA, the Netherlands

Rebecca C. Richmond
MRC Integrative Epidemiology Unit, School of Social and Community Medicine, University of Bristol, Bristol, United Kingdom

Jessica M. Robbins
Philadelphia Department of Public Health, AHS, 500 S Broad St, Philadelphia, PA 19146

Donald F. Schwarz
Philadelphia Department of Public Health, Philadelphia, Pennsylvania

Xianwen Shang
National Institute For Nutrition And Food Safety, Chinese Center For Disease Control And Prevention, Beijing, China

George Davey Smith
MRC Integrative Epidemiology Unit, School of Social and Community Medicine, University of Bristol, Bristol, United Kingdom

Nicholas J. Timpson
MRC Integrative Epidemiology Unit, School of Social and Community Medicine, University of Bristol, Bristol, United Kingdom

Bach Xuan Tran
School of Public Health, University of Alberta, Edmonton, Alberta, Canada

Vivian M. van de Gaar
Department of Public Health, Erasmus University Medical Centre, Rotterdam, 3000, CA, the Netherlands

Amy van Grieken
Department of Public Health, Erasmus University Medical Centre, Rotterdam, 3000, CA, the Netherlands

Joop van Raaij
National Institute for Public Health and the Environment, Bilthoven, The Netherlands

Esther M.F. van Sluijs
Centre of Excellence in Diet and Activity Research, MRC Epidemiology Unit, Cambridge, UK

Paul J. Veugelers
School of Public Health, University of Alberta, Edmonton, Alberta, Canada

Martin Wabitsch
Division of Pediatric Endocrinology and Diabetes, Interdisciplinary Obesity Unit, Department of Pediatrics and Adolescent Medicine, Ulm University, Eythstr. 24, D-89073 Ulm, Germany

Ailsa A. Welch
Department of Nutrition, Norwich Medical School, University of East Anglia, Norwich, UK

Henk Westerik
Behavioural Science Institute, Radboud University, Nijmegen, Netherlands

Guifa Xu
Department Of Public Health, Shandong University, Shandong Province, China

Haiquan Xu
National Institute For Nutrition And Food Safety, Chinese Center For Disease Control And Prevention, Beijing, China

Qian Zhang
National Institute For Nutrition And Food Safety, Chinese Center For Disease Control And Prevention, Beijing, China

Xingyou Zhang
Centers for Disease Control and Prevention, Atlanta, Georgia

INTRODUCTION

Childhood obesity, a serious and escalating medical condition that affects children in developed and underdeveloped countries alike, has significant potential comorbidities and increased risk for numerous chronic diseases. Its prevalence has more that tripled in the last 30 years, and at present more than 30 percent of American children are overweight or obese.

The cause for the increased rates of childhood obesity is a complex mix of environmental, genetic, medical, and bio-psychosocial factors. It is a medical condition that progresses over time to become a medical disease, one that is frustrating for both children and their families, as well as for their health care providers. It has become a condition that is difficult to prevent and disappointing to treat—and yet relentless in its ability to reduce an individual's health and quality of life, while at the same time, increasing the cost of health-care services to society. Unfortunately, to make the situation still more grave, it's a situation from which few obese children will be able to outgrow.

This urgent crisis, addressed in this compendium of research articles, must be more clearly understood. Researchers, clinicians, and ordinary people alike are faced with the challenge of building a broader and more practical comprehension of what causes childhood obesity, what its consequences are, and what can be done to prevent and/or treat it. This research contained in this volume provide the reader with a rich, diverse, and probing examination of what forces influence the epidemic of childhood obesity and what can be done to end it.

Peter Vash, MD, MPh

Traditional survey methods for obtaining nationwide small-area estimates (SAEs) of childhood obesity are costly. In Chapter 1, Zhang and colleagues applied a geocoded national health survey in a multilevel modeling framework to estimate prevalence of childhood obesity at the census block-group level. The authors constructed a multilevel logistic regression model to evaluate the influence of individual demographic characteristics, zip code, county, and state on the childhood obesity measures from the 2007 National Survey of Children's Health. The obesity risk for a child in each census block group was then estimated on the basis of this multilevel model. They compared direct survey and model-based SAEs to evaluate the model specification. Multilevel models in this study explained about 60% of state-level variances associated with childhood obesity, 82.8% to 86.5% of county-level, and 93.1% of zip code-level. The 95% confidence intervals of block- group level SAEs have a wide range (0.795-20.0), a low median of 2.02, and a mean of 2.12. The model-based SAEs of childhood obesity prevalence ranged from 2.3% to 54.7% with a median of 16.0% at the block-group level. The geographic variances among census block groups, counties, and states demonstrate that locale may be as significant as individual characteristics such as race/ethnicity in the development of the childhood obesity epidemic. The estimates provide data to identify priority areas for local health programs and to establish feasible local intervention goals. Model-based SAEs of population health outcomes could be a tool of public health assessment and surveillance.

Surveys performed in the past 10 to 15 years show a yet unexplained stabilization or decline in prevalence rates of childhood obesity in developed countries. The projected continuous increase in obesity prevalence throughout future decades seems not to occur at present. Apparently, saturation has been reached, which might be related to societal adjustments. In Chapter 2, Wabitsch and colleagues postulate a cumulative effect of public health programs for obesity prevention resulting, for example, in an increase in physical activity, and a decline in television viewing and in the consumption of sugar-sweetened soft drinks by children. Effective public health programs are urgently needed for developing countries, where obesity rates in children still continued to increase during the past decade.

Epidemic increases in obesity negatively affect the health of US children, individually and at the population level. Although surveillance of childhood obesity at the local level is challenging, height and weight data routinely collected by school districts are valuable and often underused public health resources. In Chapter 3, Robbins and colleagues analyzed data from the School District of Philadelphia for 4 school years (2006–2007 through 2009–2010) to assess the prevalence of and trends in obesity and severe obesity among public school children. The prevalence of obesity decreased from 21.5% in 2006–2007 to 20.5% in 2009–2010, and the prevalence of severe obesity decreased from 8.5% to 7.9%. Both obesity and severe obesity were more common among students in grades 6 through 8 than among children in lower grades or among high school students. Hispanic boys and African American girls had the highest prevalence of obesity and severe obesity; Asian girls had much lower rates of obesity and severe obesity than any other group. Although obesity and severe obesity declined during the 4-year period in almost all demographic groups, the decreases were generally smaller in the groups with the highest prevalence, including high school students, Hispanic males, and African American females. Although these data suggest that the epidemic of childhood obesity may have begun to recede in Philadelphia, unacceptably high rates of obesity and severe obesity continue to threaten the health and futures of many school children.

There is some evidence that physical activity (PA), sedentary time and screen time (ST) are associated with childhood obesity, but research is inconclusive and studies are mainly based on self-reported data. The literature is dominated by data from North American countries and there is a shortage of objective data from Malta which has one of the highest prevalences of childhood obesity in the world. The aims of Decelis and colleagues in Chapter 4 were to assess the PA levels and ST patterns of Maltese boys and girls and how they compared with children in other countries while also examining differences in PA and ST by weight status. A nationally representative sample of 1126 Maltese boys and girls aged 10–11 years, of which 811 provided complete data. Physical activity was assessed using accelerometry, and ST by questionnaire. Body mass index (BMI) was computed from measured height and weight. Only 39% of boys and 10% of girls met the recommendation of one hour of daily MVPA. Comparison with international data indicated that mean MVPA (58.1 min for boys; 41.7 min for girls) was higher than in North America and Australia, but lower than in England. Girls were less active than boys at all measured times and spent less time in ST. A quarter of the children exceeded guidelines of two hours of TV on weekends, and double the amount on weekdays. Obese children were less active than normal weight children on weekdays and on weekends, reaching significance during the period after school, and they spent more time in ST than their normal weight counterparts. A low percentage of Maltese 10–11 year olds, particularly girls, reached the recommended levels of daily MVPA and spent large amounts of time engaged in screen time. Obese children were less active than non-obese children. As children spend most of their waking time at school and that activity during this time is less than one third of the daily requirements, aiming to increase MVPA at school for all Maltese children is likely to be an important strategy to promote MVPA. Targeting less active and obese children is important.

Previous studies have focused on the effect of food advertisements on the caloric intake of children. However, the role of individual susceptibility in this effect is unclear. In Chapter 5, the aim of Folkvord and colleagues was to examine the role of impulsivity in the effect of advergames that promote energy-dense snacks on children's snack intake. First, impulsivity scores were assessed with a computer task. Then a randomized between-subject design was conducted with 261 children aged 7 to 10 years who played an advergame promoting either energy-dense snacks or nonfood products. As an extra manipulation, half of the children in each condition were rewarded for refraining from eating, the other half were not. Children could eat freely while playing the game. Food intake was measured. The children then completed questionnaire measures, and were weighed and measured. Overall, playing an advergame containing food cues increased general caloric intake. Furthermore, rewarding children to refrain from eating decreased their caloric intake. Finally, rewarding impulsive children to refrain from eating had no influence when they were playing an advergame promoting energy-dense snacks, whereas it did lead to reduced intake among low impulsive children and children who played nonfood advergames. Playing an advergame promoting energy-dense snacks contributes to increased caloric intake in children. The advergame promoting energy-dense snacks overruled the inhibition task to refrain from eating among impulsive children, making it more difficult for them to refrain from eating. The findings suggest that impulsivity plays an important role in susceptibility to food advertisements.

Cross-sectional studies have shown that objectively measured physical activity is associated with childhood adiposity, and a strong inverse dose–response association with body mass index (BMI) has been found. However, few studies have explored the extent to which this association reflects reverse causation. In Chapter 6, Richmond and colleagues aimed to determine whether childhood adiposity causally influences levels of physical activity using genetic variants reliably associated with adiposity to estimate causal effects. The Avon Longitudinal Study of Parents and Children collected data on objectively assessed activity levels of 4,296 children at age 11 y with recorded BMI and genotypic data. The authors used 32 established genetic correlates of BMI combined in a weighted allelic score as an instrumental variable for adiposity to estimate the causal effect of adiposity on activity In observational analysis, a 3.3 kg/m^2 (one standard deviation) higher BMI was associated with 22.3 (95% CI, 17.0, 27.6) movement counts/min less total physical activity ($p = 1.6 \times 10^{-16}$), 2.6 (2.1, 3.1) min/d less moderate-to-vigorous-intensity activity ($p = 3.7 \times 10^{-29}$), and 3.5 (1.5, 5.5) min/d more sedentary time ($p = 5.0 \times 10^{-4}$). In Mendelian randomization analyses, the same difference in BMI was associated with 32.4 (0.9, 63.9) movement counts/min less total physical activity ($p = 0.04$) (~5.3% of the mean counts/minute), 2.8 (0.1, 5.5) min/d less moderate-to-vigorous-intensity activity ($p = 0.04$), and 13.2 (1.3, 25.2) min/d more sedentary time ($p = 0.03$). There was no strong evidence for a difference between variable estimates from observational estimates. Similar results were obtained using fat mass index. Low power and poor instrumentation of activity limited causal analysis of the influence of physical activity on BMI. The results suggest that increased adiposity causes a reduction in physical activity in children and support research into the targeting of BMI in efforts to increase childhood activity levels. Importantly, this does not exclude lower physical activity also leading to increased adiposity, i.e., bidirectional causation.

The rising prevalence of childhood obesity is a key public health issue worldwide. Increased eating frequency (EF) is one aspect of diet that has been beneficially associated with obesity, although the mechanisms are unclear. The aims of Jennings and colleagues in Chapter 7 were to determine whether increased EF was associated with improved adiposity in children, and if this was due to differences in dietary and activity behaviors. Cross-sectional data from 1,700 children aged 9–10 year were analyzed to examine the associations between EF, as estimated from diet diaries, measures of adiposity, and activity measured by accelerometer. Analyses were stratified by obesity status using waist-to-height ratio to define obesity as it has been shown to be a good predictor of adverse health outcomes. Mean EF was 4.3 occasions/day and after adjustment for underreporting, energy intake (EI), and activity significant relative mean differences of −2.4% for body weight ($P = 0.001$), −1.0% for BMI ($P = 0.020$), −33% for BMI z-score ($P = 0.014$), and −0.6% for waist circumference ($P = 0.031$) per increase in eating occasion were found in healthy-weight but not centrally obese children. Differences between the extreme quartiles of EF were observed for total fat intake at breakfast (−18%, $P < 0.001$), fruit and vegetables from snacks (201% healthy-weight and 209% centrally obese children, $P < 0.01$), and for healthy-weight children, vigorous activity (4%, $P = 0.003$). Increased EF was favorably associated with adiposity, diet quality, and activity behaviors in healthy-weight but not centrally obese children. Future obesity interventions should consider the mediating role of diet quality and activity in the relationship between EF and adiposity in children.

Childhood obesity continues to be a significant public health burden. Empirical evidence has begun to identify intrauterine and postnatal pathways that increase the likelihood of excess adiposity and increased risk of type 2 diabetes among offspring. In Chapter 8, Dabelea and Harrod present the evidence supporting a transgenerational vicious cycle that increases obesity and diabetes in offspring and contributes substantially to the increases in obesity and type 2 diabetes observed over the past several decades. The public health impact of these findings is discussed and future research opportunities are outlined.

The obesity epidemic cannot be reversed without substantial improvements in the food marketing environment that surrounds children. Food marketing targeted to children almost exclusively promotes calorie-dense, nutrient-poor foods and takes advantage of children's vulnerability to persuasive messages. Increasing scientific evidence reveals potentially profound effects of food marketing on children's lifelong eating behaviors and health. Much of this marketing occurs in nationwide media (eg, television, the Internet), but companies also directly target children in their own communities through the use of billboards and through local environments such as stores, restaurants, and schools. Given the harmful effect of this marketing environment on children's health and the industry's reluctance to make necessary changes to its food marketing practices, government at all levels has an obligation to act. Chapter 9, by Harris and Graff, focuses on policy options for municipalities that are seeking ways to limit harmful food marketing at the community level.

The Alberta Project Promoting active Living and healthy Eating in Schools (APPLE Schools) is a comprehensive school health program that is proven feasible and effective in preventing obesity among school aged children. To support decision making on expanding this program, evidence on its long-term health and economic impacts is particularly critical. In Chapter 10, Tran and colleagues estimate the life course impact of the APPLE Schools programs in terms of future body weights and avoided health care costs. The authors modeled growth rates of body mass index (BMI) using longitudinal data from the National Population Health Survey collected between 1996–2008. These growth rate characteristics were used to project BMI trajectories for students that attended APPLE Schools and for students who attended control schools (141 randomly selected schools) in the Canadian province of Alberta. Throughout the life course, the prevalence of overweight (including obesity) was 1.2% to 2.8% (1.7 on average) less among students attending APPLE Schools relative to their peers attending control schools. The life course prevalence of obesity was 0.4% to 1.4% (0.8% on average) less among APPLE Schools students. If the APPLE Schools program were to be scaled up, the potential cost savings would be $33 to 82 million per year for the province of Alberta, or $150 to 330 million per year for Canada. These projected health and economic benefits seem to support broader implementation of school-based health promotion programs.

Research evidence indicates that obesity has spread through social networks, but lever points for interventions based on overlapping networks are not well studied. In Chapter 11, the objective of Frerichs and colleagues was to construct and parameterize a system dynamics model of the social transmission of behaviors through adult and youth influence in order to explore hypotheses and identify plausible lever points for future childhood obesity intervention research. The objectives of this study were:

(1) to assess the sensitivity of childhood overweight and obesity prevalence to peer and adult social transmission rates, and (2) to test the effect of combinations of prevention and treatment interventions on the prevalence of childhood overweight and obesity. To address the first objective, the authors conducted two-way sensitivity analyses of adult-to-child and child-to-child social transmission in relation to childhood overweight and obesity prevalence. For the second objective, alternative combinations of prevention and treatment interventions were tested by varying model parameters of social transmission and weight loss behavior rates. The results indicated child overweight and obesity prevalence might be slightly more sensitive to the same relative change in the adult-to-child compared to the child-to-child social transmission rate. In the simulations, alternatives with treatment alone, compared to prevention alone, reduced the prevalence of childhood overweight and obesity more after 10 years (1.2–1.8% and 0.2–1.0% greater reduction when targeted at children and adults respectively). Also, as the impact of adult interventions on children was increased, the rank of six alternatives that included adults became better (i.e., resulting in lower 10 year childhood overweight and obesity prevalence) than alternatives that only involved children. The findings imply that social transmission dynamics should be considered when designing both prevention and treatment intervention approaches. Finally, targeting adults may be more efficient, and research should strengthen and expand adult-focused interventions that have a high residual impact on children.

Since sugar-sweetened beverages (SSB) may contribute to the development of overweight in children, effective interventions to reduce their consumption are needed. In Chapter 12, van de Gaar and colleagues evaluated the effect of a combined school- and community-based intervention aimed at reducing children's SSB consumption by promoting the intake of water. Favourable intervention effects on children's SSB consumption were hypothesized. In 2011-2012, a controlled trial was conducted among four primary schools, comprising 1288 children aged 6-12 years who lived in multi-ethnic, socially deprived neighbourhoods in Rotterdam, the Netherlands. Intervention schools adopted the "water campaign," an intervention developed using social marketing. Control schools continued with their regular health promotion programme. Primary outcome was children's SSB consumption, measured using parent and child questionnaires and through observations at school, both at baseline and after one year of intervention. Significant positive intervention effects were found for average SSB consumption (B -0.19 litres, 95% CI -0.28;-0.10; parent report), average SSB servings (B -0.54 servings, 95% CI -0.82;-0.26; parent report) and bringing SSB to school (OR 0.51, 95% CI 0.36;0.72; observation report). This study supports the effectiveness of the water campaign intervention in reducing children's SSB consumption. Further studies are needed to replicate our findings.

Childhood obesity is a global public health problem as a result of poor eating and activity behaviours. Periodically, taxation has been proposed as a strategy to modify food purchasing behaviour, and once again, there is growing interest in the feasibility of this approach towards obesity prevention. Chapter 13, by Pitt and colleagues, examines the outcomes of an expert panel that was convened to obtain consensus on 1) which foods are most problematic in terms of obesity if consumed during early childhood and 2) which foods would be amenable to taxation as a strategy to reduce consumption. A nominal group technique was facilitated with a panel of 12 Australian experts including nutrition professionals, academics and clinicians with an interest in childhood obesity. In addition to routine ranking analysis, transcripts were explored using thematic analysis to reveal the collective beliefs of the experts. The panel reached consensus about the types of foods that were problematic in terms of their consumption and contribution to early childhood obesity which included prepared foods consumed outside the home, high protein infant formula products and sugar-sweetened beverages. However of these food and beverage items, the panel only deemed sugar-sweetened beverages and infant formula to be potentially amenable to taxation. They also highlighted the importance of subsidizing fresh fruit and vegetables, whole and unprocessed foods and hence topic complexities resulted in panel discussion being extended beyond the central notion of taxation. The panel identified several food groups that contributed to early childhood obesity but noted that these foods were not equally amenable to taxation. Results of this research should be considered during decision making and planning regarding population policy and regulation to reduce childhood obesity in the very early years.

The dramatic rise of overweight and obesity among Chinese children has greatly affected the social economic development. However, no information on the cost-effectiveness of interventions in China is available. The objective of Chapter 14 is to evaluate the cost and the cost-effectiveness of a comprehensive intervention program for childhood obesity. Meng and colleagues hypothesized the integrated intervention which combined nutrition education and physical activity (PA) is more cost-effective than the same intensity of single intervention. A multi-center randomized controlled trial conducted in six large cities during 2009-2010. A total of 8301 primary school students were categorized into five groups and followed one academic year. Nutrition intervention, PA intervention and their shared common control group were located in Beijing. The combined intervention and its' control group were located in other 5 cities. In nutrition education group, 'nutrition and health classes' were given 6 times for the students, 2 times for the parents and 4 times for the teachers and health workers. "Happy 10" was carried out twice per day in PA group. The comprehensive intervention was a combination of nutrition and PA interventions. BMI and BAZ increment was 0.65 kg/m^2 (SE 0.09) and 0.01 (SE 0.11) in the combined intervention, respectively, significantly lower than that in its' control group (0.82±0.09 for BMI, 0.10±0.11 for BAZ). No significant difference were found neither in BMI nor in BAZ change between the PA intervention and its' control, which is the same case in the nutrition intervention. The single intervention has a relative lower intervention costs compared with the combined intervention. Labor costs in Guangzhou, Shanghai and Jinan was higher compared to other cities. The cost-effectiveness ratio was $120.3 for BMI and $249.3 for BAZ in combined intervention, respectively. The school-based integrated obesity intervention program was cost-effectiveness for children in urban China.

PART I

PREVALENCE

CHAPTER 1

A MULTILEVEL APPROACH TO ESTIMATING SMALL AREA CHILDHOOD OBESITY PREVALENCE AT THE CENSUS BLOCK-GROUP LEVEL

XINGYOU ZHANG, STEPHEN ONUFRAK, JAMES B. HOLT, AND JANET B. CROFT

1.1 INTRODUCTION

The prevalence of childhood obesity tripled during the last 3 decades in the United States (1); data for 2009 through 2010, showed that 16.9% (approximately 12.0 million) of US children aged 2 to 19 years were obese (2). Besides disparities in childhood obesity among various racial/ethnic groups (2–4), research shows significant disparities by geographic area: by state (5), city (6), and community (7). Small-area data can reveal wide disparities in obesity outcomes and facilitate community-based initiatives for obesity prevention (8). Having reliable data for each community or small area allows state, county, and local decision makers and health pro-

---

Reprinted with permission from the CDC. Zhang X, Onufrak S, Holt JB, Croft JB. Preventing Chronic Disease *10 (2013). http://dx.doi.org/10.5888/pcd10.120252.*

fessionals to tailor programs for preventing childhood obesity to conditions and factors that affect their community (9), identify priority areas for action, and optimize the use of limited resources.

Local public health practitioners often lack small-area data on childhood obesity. National health surveys, such as the National Health and Nutrition Examination Survey (NHANES) (www.cdc.gov/NCHS/nhanes.htm), the National Survey of Children's Health (NSCH) (www.cdc.gov/nchs/slaits/nsch.htm), and the Youth Risk Behavior Survey (YRBS) were designed to provide data on national or state childhood obesity. Direct estimates of obesity rates in small areas or communities cannot be calculated on the basis of data gathered through these surveys. Use of the surveillance methods for obtaining national (ie, large-area) data to obtain small-area data on childhood obesity is prohibitively expensive.

There are, however, cost-effective methods of generating health-related data, particularly on obesity, for small-area populations (10–12). Recently, considerable research has been done on multilevel, model-based, small-area estimation methods (10,13–15). These methods can produce data on variations in the multilevel influence of local social and physical environments on health outcomes among people in small areas by using various demographic characteristics (eg, age, sex, race/ethnicity). Another advantage is that model-based small-area estimation methods borrow information from both individual-level data within the survey sample and from area-level covariates external to the original sample, and they tend to generate smoothed estimates with better precision (16). Malec et al constructed a 2-stage hierarchical model with NHANES III to generate state-level prevalence estimates of adult overweight (11). Li et al used Massachusetts Behavioral Risk Factor Surveillance System (BRFSS) data to generate multilevel model-based zip code-level estimates to prioritize communities for obesity prevention (10). More recently, Congdon extended this framework for multilevel small-area estimation modeling by using BRFSS data with county-level covariates and predicted heart disease prevalence estimates for zip code tabulation area levels (13). We used a similar approach in this study to construct a multilevel model with county- and zip code-level covariates using NSCH 2007; we then predicted census block-group level small-area estimates (SAEs) of childhood obesity by combining the estimated model parameters and block-group level covariates with population counts for children, by age, sex, and race/ethnicity.

The objectives of our study were to 1) identify and evaluate individual and geographic factors that influence childhood obesity; 2) use multilevel small-area estimation methods to generate cost-effective data on the prevalence of childhood obesity at the block-group level for the United States; and 3) characterize the geographic disparities in childhood obesity by block groups, counties, and states.

1.2 METHODS

1.2.1 STUDY POPULATION

The 2007 NSCH, a household landline–telephone-based interview survey stratified by state, has 91,642 completed interviews for children aged 0 to 17 years, with a minimum of 1,700 per state. The 2003 NSCH suggested that parent- or guardian-reported weight and height for children aged 0-9 years were not valid (17). We therefore included in this study only the 44,906 children aged 10 to 17 years with a validated obesity outcome; these children were from 2,618 counties and 13,291 zip codes in 50 states and the District of Columbia. The sample sizes for states range from 736 (Nevada) to 947 (North Dakota) with a median of 876 (Vermont) and a mean of 865. This geographic diversity in the sampled local communities (zip codes and counties) provides a solid basis on which to evaluate geographic effects on childhood obesity.

1.2.2 INDIVIDUAL DATA

We obtained individual data on the study children's age, sex, race/ethnicity, and obesity status from the 2007 NSCH. A child was considered obese if his or her body mass index (kg/m^2) was equal to or greater than the sex- and age-specific 95th percentile on the Centers for Disease Control and Prevention (CDC) 2000 growth charts (18). Age was categorized into

2 groups (10–14 y, 15–17 y) to match the age groups in block-group population data. Racial/ethnic categories were white, black, Asian, Hispanic, American Indian/Alaska Native, Native Hawaiian/Pacific Islander, multiracial, and other race.

1.2.3 GEOGRAPHIC AREA DATA

Geographic area variables were block group, zip code, and county. We obtained the population count for children by sex, age, and race/ethnicity at the block-group level from 2010 ESRI Demographics (ESRI, Redlands, California). We also obtained median household income from ESRI for block groups, zip code areas, and counties, and we divided income into 8 levels. Lifestyle and urbanization levels (by block-group and zip code) were obtained from the 2010 ESRI Tapestry Segmentation dataset (19). The ESRI segmentation methodology incorporates sociodemographic, geographic, and physical features (eg, population density, city size, metropolitan status, proximity to economic and social centers) into community lifestyle and urbanization classifications. We used a 2006 National Center for Health Statistics (NCHS) 6-level urban-rural classification scheme for counties (20).

1.2.4 MULTILEVEL MODEL DEVELOPMENT AND ESTIMATION

Multilevel logistic regression models were constructed to evaluate the influence of individual child covariates and area-level covariates on a child's obesity status in the NSCH. The full multilevel model was as follows:

NSCH child obesity status (yes or no) = sex + age + race/ethnicity (individual level) + median household income + lifestyle classifications + urbanization levels (zip-code level) + median household income + urban-rural (county-level) + random effects (state- and county-levels)

Zip-code level and county-level measures were included because neighborhood social and built environments and residential area (rural or urban) have been significantly associated with childhood obesity (21,22). We included zip code median household income and lifestyle classifications and urbanization levels to quantify local effects on childhood obesity. County median household income and urban-rural status were included to assess a regional effect on childhood obesity beyond neighborhood. State-level random effects represent the statewide social, economic, and political influences on childhood obesity. The multilevel logistic models were implemented in SAS 9.2 GLIMMIX (SAS Institute, Cary, North Carolina) by using maximum likelihood with the Laplace approximation estimation method.

To generate SAEs of childhood obesity prevalence at the block-group level, we estimated the obesity risk for a child calculated on the basis of age group, sex, and race/ethnicity for each block group from the 2010 ESRI Demographics data (19) by using the following predictive model:

A child's predicted obesity risk = sex + age + race/ethnicity (individual-level) + median household income + lifestyle classifications + urbanization levels (block-group level) + median household income + urban-rural (county-level) + random effects (state-level)

The regression coefficients of block-group level covariates were adopted from those at the zip code level with an assumption that the block group and zip code-level influences on childhood obesity are at similar scales. Thus, each subpopulation of children defined by sex, age group, and race/ethnicity in each block group has its own obesity risk. The predicted number of obese children in each block group can be estimated by multiplying the predicted obesity risk by the number of children in the subpopulation. The overall model-based childhood obesity SAE in a block group is the population-weighted average of the sex-, age-, and racial/ethnic-specific SAEs for all the subpopulation groups within it. A Monte Carlo simulation approach was used to generate 95% confidence intervals (CIs) for all block group-predicted prevalence estimates of childhood obesity (23). The simulation was based on regression coefficients and their standard errors from the prevalence model on the basis of NSCH survey data, and 1,000 childhood obesity-prevalence SAEs were generated for each age-, sex-, and racial/ethnic-specific population for each block group.

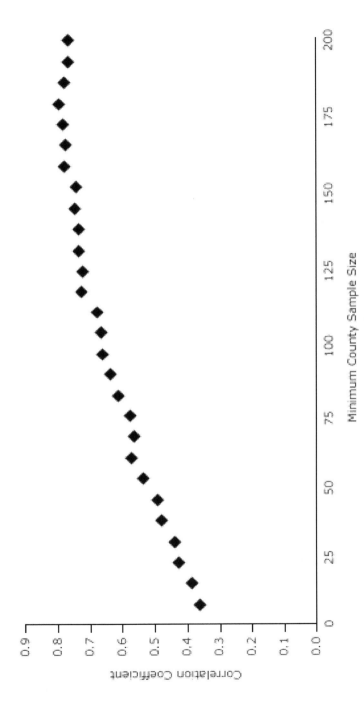

FIGURE 1: The relationship between correlation coefficients of model-based and direct survey estimates and minimum county sample size. The figure shows an increasing positive relationship between the correlation coefficients of model-based and direct survey estimates and the minimum county sample sizes. As the minimum county sample size increases, the correlation between model-based and direct survey estimates also increases. The correlation reaches approximately 0.90 and levels off once the minimum county sample size reaches 150.

1.2.5 EVALUATION OF MODEL-BASED SAES

Direct survey estimates, such as those from NSCH, are often treated as the benchmark to evaluate and compare with model-based SAEs, to identify potential bias of model-based estimates, and to evaluate model specification (24). Although it would be ideal to compare SAEs at the block-group level, this comparison was not possible because NSCH cannot generate reliable block-group level estimates directly. However, we aggregated block-group level SAEs to county, state, and national levels and then compared them with NSCH direct survey estimates.

We evaluated model specification in 3 ways. First, we compared national-level direct survey and model-based estimates of childhood obesity prevalence for each age, sex, and race/ethnicity group to assess consistency between them. Second, we compared 40 state-specific model-based estimates with direct survey estimates available from both NSCH and YRBS because these surveys were designed to provide reliable state-level childhood obesity prevalence. Finally, we compared county-level, model-based SAEs with direct survey estimates for counties with data on at least 30 children and for which the ratio of standard errors to means was less than 0.3 (a reliability measure of survey estimation commonly used by the Centers for Disease Control and Prevention [CDC]) (25); we compared the estimates by using paired t-tests.

1.3 RESULTS

1.3.1 MULTILEVEL MODEL ADEQUACY AND SELECTION

We fitted 4 different multilevel logistic models with 1) state random effects, 2) county random effects, 3) both state and county random effects, and 4) zip-code random effects. No generally accepted criterion exists to evaluate the adequacy of multilevel models for small area estimation. We followed the recommendation that a multilevel model should explain at least 40% between area-level variance for the outcome measure of interest to justify model adequacy (26). Compared with their null models, the

4 full models in this study explained 59.8% (state random effect model) to 93.1% (zip code random effect model) area-level variances associated with childhood obesity (Table 1).

For the full models, variance estimates at both zip code and county levels were not significant; only state-level variance estimates were significant (Table 1). We selected the full model with both state and county random effects having the smallest Akaike information criterion (27) for our small-area estimation.

We analyzed the details of the variables and the signs and significances of their regression coefficients in the full multilevel model with state- and county-level random effects (Table 2). After controlling for individual age, sex, race/ethnicity, and zip code-level median household income and lifestyle, we found that county-level median household income and rural–urban status were not significantly associated with childhood obesity. Zip-code urbanization levels were not significant. Therefore, county-level variables and zip code urbanization levels were excluded in the final multilevel model to predict risk for childhood obesity in a neighborhood.

1.3.2 COMPARISON BETWEEN MODEL-BASED AND DIRECT SURVEY ESTIMATES

The national model-based childhood obesity estimate of 16.8% obesity among children aged 10 to 17 years was a nonsignificant 0.4 percentage points higher than the estimate based on direct survey (16.4%, <2.5% difference). At the state level, the observed childhood obesity prevalence ranged from 9.6% (Oregon) to 21.9% (Mississippi). Compared with these direct state-level estimates, the model-based estimates for each state fell within the 95% confidence intervals (CIs). The differences between state-specific direct survey estimates and model-based estimates ranged from −1.48 percentage points (West Virginia) to 1.73 percentage points (District of Columbia) with a median of 0.16 percentage points (Georgia). Paired t-tests showed no significant difference between direct-survey and model-based estimates. Finally, when we compared state-level model-based estimates for children aged 15 to 17 years with the observed prevalence of obesity found by YRBS for schoolchildren in grades 9 through 12, the average model-based SAEs of obesity prevalence for states with YRBS estimates was 12.6% compared with 12.2% for YRBS. A paired t test showed no significant difference between these 2 sets of estimates.

At the county level, the model-based estimates are consistent with direct survey estimates. We plotted the relationship between model-based estimates and direct survey estimates for counties with a minimum sample size of 15. When the minimum sample size is exceeded for county-level direct survey estimates, the correlation between model-based and direct survey estimates increases substantially. When the minimum sample size nears 100, the correlation coefficients between model-based and direct survey estimates are consistently 0.7 or greater (Figure 1). By using our data suppression rules, we obtained 103 reliable county-level, direct-observed NSCH prevalence estimates. Although 12 model-based predicted SAEs were significantly higher or lower than their direct survey estimates, the median difference in county levels between model-based SAEs and direct-observed NSCH estimates was near zero (<0.0045 percentage points), and the first and third quartile differences were 1.38 and −1.98 percentage points, respectively.

1.3.3 SAES OF CHILDHOOD OBESITY PREVALENCE FROM PREDICTIVE MODEL

We calculated the summary statistics of the confidence intervals (95% CIs) and coefficient of variation (CV) of model-based childhood obesity estimates at block-group, county, and state levels (Table 3). The 95% CIs for the block-group level have a large range (0.80%–20.0%), but their median is 2.02% and mean is 2.12% (Table 3). For block groups with large numbers of children, the 95% CIs are expected to be smaller. The CVs for block-group estimates have a range of 0.07% to 0.58%, a median of 0.14%, and a mean of 0.14%. Therefore, in most cases, model-based block-group estimates may be appropriate for ranking childhood obesity prevalence among communities. Model-based county and state SAEs are reliable.

The model-based national childhood obesity prevalence estimate was 16.8% on the basis of the 2010 ESRI Demographics population aged 10 to 17 years. The model-based SAEs of prevalence of childhood obesity ranged from 10.2% (Oregon) to 21.8% (District of Columbia) with a median of 14.9% at state level; from 7.2% to 31.9% with a median of 18.4% at the county level; and from 3.3% to 43.7% with a median of 16.8% at the block-group level. The overall geographic patterns of SAEs at the block-group level (Figure 2) show that obesity prevalence was higher in 1) large metropolitan areas such as New York, Los Angeles, and Chicago; 2) Southeastern and Midwestern rural areas; 3) along the US-Mexican border in Texas and California; and 4) in some local tribal areas in western and northern states.

1.4 DISCUSSION

We applied a multilevel modeling framework that incorporated demographic and geographic influences to estimate childhood obesity prevalence at local levels across the United States. Although SAEs of obesity prevalence among adults have been studied (10–12), to our knowledge, this is the first study of SAEs of obesity prevalence among children.

1.4.1 THE USE OF MODEL-BASED SAES IN CHILDHOOD OBESITY

Multilevel statistical modeling is an alternative approach to generating reliable SAEs; this model combines NSCH data with data from NCHS and other sources. But the estimates derived from the model must be used with caution for 2 reasons: first, the model-based estimates are the expected prevalence of childhood obesity for block groups given the demographic characteristics of the children in the population and their community's socioeconomic status and lifestyle. These estimates are not; therefore, they could be very different from the actual prevalence of childhood obesity in a community. Second, we are not able to validate block-group level estimates, either internally or externally. In some cases, these estimates could be significantly biased.

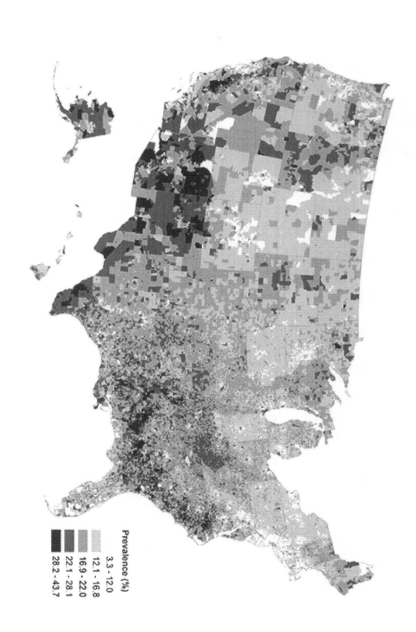

FIGURE 2: Model-Based Childhood Obesity Prevalence Estimates by Block Group in the United States, 2010.

1.4.2 NATIONAL HEALTH SURVEYS FOR SAES IN CHILDHOOD OBESITY PREVALENCE

Although the sample populations of national health surveys usually are adequately representative demographically, they often lack sufficient geographic diversity to evaluate geographic effects on childhood obesity, especially for SAEs. NHANES aims to provide reliable national measures of obesity prevalence; however, it has limited geographic coverage because little more than 1.0% of 3,141 US counties are sampled (28). The BRFSS sampled all states and most counties, and its data have been used to generate county-level and zip-code level obesity prevalence for adults via model-SAE methods (10,12). However, BRFSS, like the National Health Interview Survey, has no obesity estimates for children. YRBS, a school-based survey, does have student-reported obesity measures but focuses on adolescents in grades 9 through 12; the schools surveyed are located in only 2% of US counties in 40 states, and the survey does not include obesity data for some large states such as California. Thus, the YRBS sampling framework has limited demographic and geographic coverage of children. We chose NSCH data for our analysis because it offers geographic diversity similar to that of BRFSS and validated obesity measures for the sampled children aged 10 to 17 years.

1.4.3 LIMITATIONS

Our study had limitations. First, our study assumed that neighborhood influences on childhood obesity were similar at zip-code and block-group levels. On average, block groups are smaller geographic units than zip code areas, and this difference could cause some inference bias associated with the effects of modifiable area unit problems on the relationship between childhood obesity and neighborhood characteristics (29). The variance between areas increases when area size decreases (from state, county, to zip code) (Table 1). So we could expect greater variation in childhood obesity prevalence between block groups. We are examining this cross-level inference bias in a further study. Second, the NSCH 2007 relied on height and weight measurements reported by a parent or guardian. Parent-reported measures and directly measured height and weight for children yielded similar obesity estimates for children aged 9 to 11 years (30). No study has assessed the parent-reported bias for children aged 12 to 17 years. NSCH estimates of obesity prevalence for children aged 14 to 17 did not differ significantly from the YRBS estimates based on self-reported height and weights among adolescents in grades 9 through 12; this finding suggests that the bias due to parental report may not be significantly different from bias due to self-reports by adolescents. Another potential limitation is that childhood obesity may be associated with more neighborhood factors than just those in our multilevel model. Neighborhood grocery stores and restaurants and safety issues related to physical activity may also contribute to childhood obesity. Future multilevel SAE models of childhood obesity should take these community factors into account.

TABLE 1: Proportion of Area-Level Variance for Childhood Obesity in Null Models Explained by Fixed Effects in Full Multilevel Models, by Type of Geographic Area

Logistic Model Level	Random Effects	Between-Area Variance (Null Model)[a]	SE	Between Area Variance (Full Model)[b]	SE	% Area-Level Variance Explained
I	Zip code	0.1950	0.03	0.0134	0.02	93.1
II	State	0.0530	0.01	0.0213	0.01	59.8
III	County	0.0928	0.02	0.0160	0.01	82.8
IV	State	0.0526	0.01	0.0211	0.01	60.0
	County (state)[c]	0.0456	0.01	0.0061	0.01	86.5

Abbreviation: SE, standard error. [a]Null models are the models with random effects only. [b] Full models are the models with random effects as well as fixed effects including age, sex, race/ethnicity, zip code level median household income, lifestyle and urbanity, and county level urban-rural status and median household income. [c]Model IV has 2 random effects, state and county, which are nested in state.

TABLE 2: Regression Coefficients of Model Covariates for Estimating Predicted Risk for Childhood Obesity

Effect	Coefficients	SE	P Value
Variable	−3.4529	0.15	<.001
Age, y			
10-14	0.4117	0.03	<.001
15-17			Reference
Sex			
Male	0.5753	0.03	<.001
Female			Reference
Race			
White			Reference
Black	0.6804	0.05478	<.001
Hispanic	0.5697	0.05	<.001
Asian	−0.1188	0.1714	.49
American Indian/Alaska Native	0.7070	0.14	<.001
Hawaii Native/Pacific Islander	0.7325	0.25	.003
Multiracial	0.1655	0.12	.16
Other races	0.0220	0.12	.85
Zip code, median household income, $			
1st octile (≤36,388)	0.8478	0.11	<.001
2nd octile (36,389–42,730)	0.7535	0.11	<.001
3rd octile (42,731–47,927)	0.6750	0.10	<.001
4th octile (47,928–53,351)	0.7204	0.10	<.001
5th octile (53,352–60,371)	0.5944	0.10	<.001
6th octile (60,372–68,513)	0.4319	0.08	<.001
7th octile (68,514–81,395)	0.3410	0.08	<.001
8th octile (≥81,396)			Reference
Zip code, lifestyles (19)			
High Society	0.3810	0.12	.002
Upscale Avenues	0.3063	0.12	.01
Metropolis	0.3515	0.12	.005
Solo Acts			Reference
Senior Styles	0.2716	0.13	.03
Scholars and Patriots	−0.1758	0.17	.29
High Hopes	0.3312	0.11	.003

TABLE 2: *Cont.*

Effect	Coefficients	SE	P Value
Global Roots	0.4404	0.11	<.0001
Family Portrait	0.4092	0.12	.001
Traditional Living	0.3541	0.11	.001
Factories and Farms	0.4768	0.13	<.001
American Quilt	0.3711	0.13	.004
Zip code, urbanization[a]			
Principal Urban Centers I			Reference
Principal Urban Centers II	0.0574	0.12	.63
Metro Cities I	−0.0739	0.11	.51
Metro Cities II	0.1325	0.11	.21
Urban Outskirts I	0.0561	0.11	.61
Urban Outskirts II	0.1739	0.13	.18
Suburban Periphery I	−0.0788	0.11	.49
Suburban Periphery II	0.0746	0.12	.53
Small Towns	0.1453	0.14	.29
Rural I	0.0458	0.13	.72
Rural II	0.2242	0.14	.11
County, median annual household income, $			
1st (≤40,647)	−0.1670	0.12	.15
2nd (40,648–46,323)	−0.1919	0.11	.08
3rd (46,324–51,075)	−0.1783	0.10	.09
4th (51,076–54,755)	−0.1616	0.10	.12
5th (54,756–57,898)	−0.0259	0.10	.81
6th (57,890–63,046)	−0.0455	0.10	.64
7th (63,047–76,686)	0.0031	0.09	.97
8th octile (≥76,687)			Reference
County National Survey of Children's Health rural-urban status (20)			
Central metro	Reference		
Fringe metro	0.0027	0.07	.97
Medium metro	0.0118	0.06	.83
Small metro	−0.0168	0.07	.80
Micropolitan	−0.0136	0.07	.84
Noncore rural	−0.0526	0.08	.51

[a] *Urbanization groupings are from ESRI (19).*

TABLE 3: Summary Statistics of 95% Confidence Intervals and Coefficient of Variation of Childhood Obesity Estimates at Block Group, County, and State Levels

Geographic Unit	N	Minimum	1st Quartile	Median	3rd Quartile	Maximum	Mean	Inter-quartile Range
95% CI								
Block group	216,206	0.80	3.57	4.57	5.66	20.04	4.71	2.09
County	3,142	0.09	0.78	1.27	1.89	7.70	1.47	1.10
State	51a	0.04	0.07	0.10	0.17	0.44	0.13	0.10
Coefficient of variation								
Block group	216,206	0.07	0.12	0.14	0.16	0.58	0.14	0.04
County	3,142	<0.01	0.02	0.03	0.05	0.19	0.04	0.03
State	51	<0.01	<0.01	<0.01	0.01	0.01	<0.01	<0.01

Abbreviation: CI, confidence interval. a District of Columbia included in state count.

1.5 CONCLUSION

Our study results show the effects of applying a multilevel, small-area modeling framework to NSCH data when zip code and county identifiers are used to estimate the prevalence of childhood obesity at the block-group level. The disparities among block groups, counties, and states show that "place of residence" may be as significant a contributor to the obesity epidemic among children as are individual characteristics such as race/ethnicity. Our estimates are useful for local public health programs when they set priorities and establish intervention goals (10). Health care systems and school- and community-based intervention programs to prevent childhood obesity will be more effective and efficient if they consider that local geographic factors contribute to local rates of obesity and need to be taken into account when intervention programs to reduce obesity are being designed. Model-based, small-area estimates of a population's health status could be an important tool of public health assessment and surveillance (16).

REFERENCES

1. Ogden C, Carroll M. Prevalence of obesity among children and adolescents: United States, trends 1963–1965 through 2007–2008. Hyattsville (MD): National Center for Health Statistics; 2010.
2. Ogden CL, Carroll MD, Kit BK, Flegal KM. Prevalence of obesity and trends in body mass index among US children and adolescents, 1999-2010. JAMA 2012;307(5):483–90.
3. Ogden CL, Carroll MD, Curtin LR, McDowell MA, Tabak CJ, Flegal KM. Prevalence of overweight and obesity in the United States, 1999-2004. JAMA 2006;295(13):1549–55.
4. Singh GK, Siahpush M, Kogan MD. Rising social inequalities in US childhood obesity, 2003-2007. Ann Epidemiol 2010;20(1):40–52.
5. Singh GK, Kogan MD, van Dyck PC. Changes in state-specific childhood obesity and overweight prevalence in the United States from 2003 to 2007. Arch Pediatr Adolesc Med 2010;164(7):598–607.
6. Centers for Disease Control and Prevention. Obesity, dietary behavior, & physical activity fact sheets. Atlanta (GA); 2011 http://www.cdc.gov/healthyyouth/yrbs/factsheets/obesity.htm. Accessed March 6, 2012.
7. Margellos-Anast H, Shah AM, Whitman S. Prevalence of obesity among children in six Chicago communities: findings from a health survey. Public Health Rep 2008;123(2):117–25.
8. Khan LK, Sobush K, Keener D, Goodman K, Lowry A, Kakietek J, et al. Recommended community strategies and measurements to prevent obesity in the United States. MMWR Recomm Rep 2009;58(RR-7):1–26.
9. Bethell C, Simpson L, Stumbo S, Carle AC, Gombojav N. National, state, and local disparities in childhood obesity. Health Aff (Millwood) 2010;29(3):347–56.
10. Li W, Kelsey JL, Zhang Z, Lemon SC, Mezgebu S, Boddie-Willis C, et al. Small-area estimation and prioritizing communities for obesity control in Massachusetts. Am J Public Health 2009;99(3):511–9.
11. Malec D, Davis WW, Cao X. Model-based small area estimates of overweight prevalence using sample selection adjustment. Stat Med 1999;18(23):3189–200.
12. Zhang Z, Zhang L, Penman A, May W. Using small-area estimation method to calculate county-level prevalence of obesity in Mississippi, 2007-2009. Prev Chronic Dis 2011;8(4):A85.
13. Congdon P. A multilevel model for cardiovascular disease prevalence in the US and its application to micro area prevalence estimates. Int J Health Geogr 2009;8:6.
14. Li W, Land T, Zhang Z, Keithly L, Kelsey JL. Small-area estimation and prioritizing communities for tobacco control efforts in Massachusetts. Am J Public Health 2009;99(3):470–9.
15. Twigg L, Moon G, Jones K. Predicting small-area health-related behaviour: a comparison of smoking and drinking indicators. Soc Sci Med 2000;50(7-8):1109–20.
16. Srebotnjak T, Mokdad AH, Murray CJ. A novel framework for validating and applying standardized small area measurement strategies. Popul Health Metr 2010;8:26.

17. Blumberg SJ, Foster EB, Frasier AM, Satorius J, Skalland BJ, Nysse-Carris KL, et al. National Center for Health Statistics; 2009.
18. Kuczmarski RJ, Ogden CL, Guo SS, Grummer-Strawn LM, Flegal KM, Mei Z, et al. 2000 CDC growth charts for the United States: methods and development. Vital Health Stat11; 2002(246):1-190.
19. ESRI. Tapestry segmentation reference guide. Redlands (CA): Environmental Systems Research Institute; 2011. http://www.esri.com/library/brochures/pdfs/tapestry-segmentation.pdf
20. Ingram DD, Franco SJ. NCHS urban-rural classification scheme for counties. Hyattsville (MD): National Center for Health Statistics, Centers for Disease Control and Prevention; 2012.
21. Singh GK, Kogan MD, Van Dyck PC, Siahpush M. Racial/ethnic, socioeconomic, and behavioral determinants of childhood and adolescent obesity in the United States: analyzing independent and joint associations. Ann Epidemiol 2008;18(9):682–95.
22. Singh GK, Siahpush M, Kogan MD. Neighborhood socioeconomic conditions, built environments, and childhood obesity. Health Aff (Millwood) 2010;29(3):503–12.
23. Robert CP, Casella G. Monte Carlo statistical methods. 2nd edition. Springer Texts in Statistics. New York (NY): Springer; 2004.
24. Scarborough P, Allender S, Rayner M, Goldacre M. Validation of model-based estimates (synthetic estimates) of the prevalence of risk factors for coronary heart disease for wards in England. Health Place 2009;15(2):596–605.
25. Klein RJ, Proctor SE, Boudreault MA, Turczyn KM. Healthy People 2010 criteria for data suppression. Statistical Notes, no 24. Hyattsville (MD): National Center for Health Statistics; 2002.
26. Pickering K, Scholes S, Bajekal M. Synthetic estimation of healthy lifestyles indicators: stage 3 report. London (UK): National Centre for Social Research; 2005.
27. Akaike H. Citation Classic — a new look at the statistical-model identification. Cc/Eng Tech Appl Sci 1981(51):22-22.
28. Centers for Disease Control and Prevention, National Center for Health Statistics. National Health and Nutrition Examination Survey 2007-2008: overview. Hyattsville (MD): US Department of Health and Human Services; 2007. http://www.cdc.gov/nchs/data/nhanes/nhanes_07_08/overviewbrochure_0708.pdf. Accessed February 2, 2012.
29. Parenteau MP, Sawada MC. The modifiable areal unit problem (MAUP) in the relationship between exposure to NO2 and respiratory health. Int J Health Geogr 2011;10:58.
30. Shields M, Connor Gorber S, Janssen I, Tremblay MS. Obesity estimates for children based on parent-reported versus direct measures. Health reports/Statistics Canada. Canadian Centre for Health Information 2011;22(3):47–58.

CHAPTER 2

UNEXPECTED PLATEAUING OF CHILDHOOD OBESITY RATES IN DEVELOPED COUNTRIES

MARTIN WABITSCH, ANJA MOSS, AND KATRIN KROMEYER-HAUSCHILD

2.1 INTRODUCTION

One of the most striking changes in human biology, starting from around 1980, has been the worldwide dramatic increase in prevalence rates of overweight and obesity in children [1]. This impressive development has recently been followed by stabilization or even decline in prevalence rates [2-10]. This commentary highlights the published data on the recent stabilization in childhood obesity rates. These data and their interpretation can serve as a basis for future prevention programs.

2.1.1 PAST AND RECENT TRENDS IN CHILDHOOD OBESITY

The body mass index (BMI), defined as weight/(height)^2 is a surrogate parameter for body fat mass in adults and in children [11]. There are only a

---

Unexpected Plateauing of Childhood Obesity Rates in Developed Countries. © *Wabitsch M, Moss A, and Kromeyer-Hauschild K.* BMC Medicine *12,17 (2014), doi:10.1186/1741-7015-12-17. Licensed under Creative Commons Attribution 2.0 Generic License, http://creativecommons.org/licenses/by/2.0.*

few datasets describing the cross-sectional development of BMI values in children over several decades before 1980. These data show a rather stable or slowly increasing prevalence of childhood obesity [12-15]. However, between 1980 and 2000, mean BMI values in children and the rates of childhood overweight and obesity increased dramatically in many countries [1]. This was paralleled by a steep increase in skinfold thickness, which is an anthropometric indicator of the amount of subcutaneous fat, and is widely used to assess body fat [16]. Skinfold thickness increased not only in overweight children, but also in normal and underweight children [17].

Along with the increase in obesity prevalence, the BMI distribution shifted in a skewed fashion, indicating that the heaviest children had become even heavier [18]. This matched the observation that the numbers of extremely obese children and adolescents (BMI >99th percentile) increased to a greater degree than those of individuals in other obesity categories (BMI 95th to 96.9th and BMI 97th to 98.9th percentile) [19,20].

Starting at around the year 2000, childhood obesity rates apparently reached a plateaue or even declined in developed countries [2-10]. This was an unexpected finding, because, for example, in the USA, it has been suggested that the prevalence rate of obesity in children will reach 30% by 2030 [21]. Recent data from the National Health and Nutrition Examination Survey (NHANES) now show that the rapid increase in obesity prevalence rates seen in the 1980s and 1990s has not continued [5]. When sex differences were analyzed, the flattening was more marked for girls than for boys. Furthermore, there were age-related differences, with prevalence declining more in preschool children (aged 2 to 5 or 6 years) compared with primary school aged children (6 to 11 or 12 years) or adolescents (12 to 19 years) [6]. However, it should be noted that extreme obesity is still increasing, despite the declining rates for lower obesity categories [19,20].

It is interesting that also in China, a developing country, stabilization of obesity rates has been observed. In the Jiangsu Province, no increase in the rate of overweight or obesity was seen in 12 to 14-year-old students in both urban and rural areas [6]. We have summarized all published data known to us that report a leveling off or a decline in prevalence rates of childhood overweight and obesity in Table 1. However, it should be noted that in all of the reported countries, the prevalence rates are still at a high level and still significantly higher than before 1980.

TABLE 1: Compilation of published data on stabilization or decline in prevalence rates of overweight and obesity in children in different countries

Author	Publication year	Country	Year	Age group, years
Olds et al.	2010	Australia	1985 to 2008	2 to 18
Shi et al.	2005	China-Jiangsu Province	2002 to 2007	12 to 14
Ministry of Health	2003; 2008	New Zealand	2002 to 2006/7	5 to 14
Lissner et al.	2010	Sweden	1999 to 2005	10 to 11
Murer et al.	2013	Switzerland	1999 to 2012	6 to 12
Aeberli et al.	2009	Switzerland	2002 to 2007	6 to 13
de Wilde et al.	2009	The Hague, Netherlands	1999 to 2007	3 to 16
NHS Information Centre (NCMP)	2010	England	1995 to 2007	2 to 15
Ministère de la Santé	2010	France	1999 to 2007	5 to 15
Salanave et al.	2009	France	2000 to 2007	7 to 9
Péneau et al.	2009	France	1996 to 2006	6 to 15
Lioret et al.	2009	France	1999 to 2007	3 to 14
Ogden et al. (NHANES)	2012	USA	1999 to 2010	2 to 19
Moss et al.	2012	Germany	1992 to 2009	5 to 7
Blüher et al.	2011	Germany	1999 to 2008	4 to 16
Schmidt Morgen et al.	2013	Denmark	1998 to 2011	3 mo to 16 yrs
Mitchell et al.	2007	Scotland	1997 to 2004	5,66
Tambalis et al.	2010	Greece	1997 to 2007	8 to 9
Schnohr et al.	2005	Greenland	1980 to 2004	6 to 7
CDC	2013	Anchorage, Alaska	2003/4 to 2010/11	5 to 12
Popkin et al.	2006	Russia	1995 to 2004	10 to 17,9

Abbreviations: CDC, Centers for Disease Control and Prevention; NHANES, National Health and Nutrition Examination Survey; NHS, National Health Service; NCMP, National Child Measurement Programme.

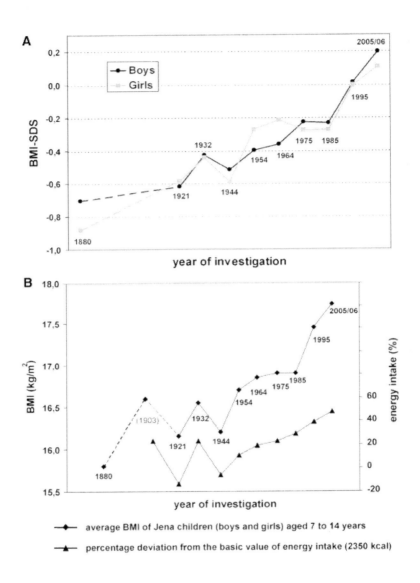

FIGURE 1: Changes in BMI parallel changes in living conditions and energy intake over time. (A) Development of body mass index standard deviation score (BMI SDS) of Jena schoolchildren (7 to 14 years of age) between 1880 and 2005. The children's average BMI SDS values increased slightly in the time period between 1880 and 2005/06, corresponding to a BMI increase of 1.8 kg/m^2 (0.14 kg/m2 per decade) in boys and of 2.1 kg/m^2 (0.17 kg/m^2 per decade) in girls. This increase did not occur continuously. The marked increase in

average BMI SDS between 1921 and 1932 indicates nutritional normalization following the famine due to World War I. This was followed by a downward shift in mean BMI between 1932 and 1944, reflecting a deterioration in living conditions during World War II. The marked increase in BMI SDS after 1985 was associated with a substantial increase in prevalence rate of obesity [22], and is a result of the dramatic changes in living conditions due to the German reunification. (B): Development and association of BMI and energy intake of Jena school children (7 to 14 years of age) between 1880 and 2005 (reproduced with permission from Zellner et al.[15]). The figure shows that BMI values as a surrogate of body fat mass paralleled the changes in energy intake over a time period of 100 years.

2.1.2 POSSIBLE CAUSES AND CONSEQUENCES OF THE OBSERVED TRENDS IN CHILDHOOD OBESITY

Changes in BMI as a surrogate of body fat mass parallel changes in living conditions and energy intake over time. This has been shown in a study of children in Jena over a period of more than 100 years (Figure 1) [15]. This study used measurements based on 10 anthropological investigations carried out between 1880 and 2005/2006. It belongs to the longest running longitudinal studies of schoolchildren in a single community worldwide, and provides a unique dataset to analyze secular changes in the physical development of schoolchildren.

The dramatic increases in obesity prevalence rates and body fat after 1980 are related to changes in individual behaviors of children. Children nowadays have decreased physical activity, and increased screen time and consumption of energy-dense foods and snacks [1]. These behavioral changes are probably related to social and environmental changes that affect the whole population [18].

In return, the recent decline in obesity prevalence rates in children in developed countries may be the result of a cumulative effect of programs designed to prevent childhood obesity [23-25]. After 1980, the recognition by healthcare professionals, schools, community organizations, industry, and governments of obesity as a health problem increased. Both at national level and at state and local level, programs focusing on reducing the consumption of energy-dense foods and television viewing, as well as increasing the daily physical activity have been developed to reduce environmental factors contributing to inappropriate weight gain [23-25]. Although it is possible that a biological plateau for obesity has been reached, there are several hints indicating that these initiated public health efforts have contributed to the leveling off of obesity rates.

A very recent study showed significant increases in daily physical activities and consumption of fruits and vegetables between 2001 and 2010 in a nationally representative cohort of students in grades 6 to 10. Television viewing and the consumption of sweets and sweetened beverages decreased during the same time period [26]. Another supporting example is the recently observed decline in the consumption of sugar-sweetened soft drinks by children, which parallels the decline in obesity prevalence rates [27,28]. These examples support the notion that in countries facing the childhood obesity epidemic over several years, the initiated public health programs have been able to stop the increasing obesity trends by influencing the lifestyle of children. If this can be confirmed in further analyses, such programs might even be improved in order to achieve a yet better success rate.

However, in contrast to these findings in developed countries, recent prevalence rates of overweight and obesity in children in developing low and middle income countries are still increasing at large [29]. This seems to be because the western lifestyle with easily available and low cost energy-dense food and increased motorization started to develop later in these countries, and had now become increasingly adopted [29]. These countries may be able to adapt public health programs from developed countries to their situation and launch them immediately in order to prevent further increases in childhood overweight and obesity rates, and possibly reach a plateau at a lower level than seen in developed countries.

2.2 CONCLUSIONS

The BMI of children is sensitive to living conditions and lifestyles, and the deep changes in children's living conditions and lifestyles in modern societies resulted in an extraordinary increase in childhood obesity rates from the 1980s. Unexpectedly, a plateau or even a decline in prevalence rates has been reported for several developed countries during the past 10 to 15 years. There are hints indicating that public health programs in these countries aiming at reducing obesity-promoting lifestyles might be responsible for the leveling off in obesity rates. However, it has to be recognized that despite the reported stabilization the prevalence rates of overweight and obesity in children, these rates remain at a high level and still represent a significant health issue.

REFERENCES

1. Lobstein T, Baur L, Uauy R: Obesity in children and young people: a crisis in public health. Obes Rev 2004, 5:4-104.
2. Matthiessen J, Velsing Groth M, Fagt S, Biltoft-Jensen A, Stockmarr A, Andersen JS, Trolle E: Prevalence and trends in overweight and obesity among children and adolescents in Denmark. Scand J Public Health 2008, 36:153-160.
3. Popkin BM, Conde W, Hou N, Monteiro C: Is there a lag globally in overweight trends for children compared with adults? Obesity (Silver Spring) 2006, 14:1846-1853.
4. Bluher S, Meigen C, Gausche R, Keller E, Pfaffle R, Sabin M, Werther G, Odeh R, Kiess W: Age-specific stabilization in obesity prevalence in German children: a cross-sectional study from 1999 to 2008. Int J Pediatr Obes 2011, 6:e199-206.
5. Ogden CL, Carroll MD, Kit BK, Flegal KM: Prevalence of obesity and trends in body mass index among US children and adolescents, 1999–2010. JAMA 2012, 307:483-490.
6. Olds T, Maher C, Zumin S, Peneau S, Lioret S, Castetbon K, Bellisle , de Wilde J, Hohepa M, Maddison R, et al.: Evidence that the prevalence of childhood overweight is plateauing: data from nine countries. Int J Pediatr Obes 2011, 6:342-360.
7. Moss A, Klenk J, Simon K, Thaiss H, Reinehr T, Wabitsch M: Declining prevalence rates for overweight and obesity in German children starting school. Eur J Pediatr 2012, 171:289-299.
8. Mitchell RT, McDougall CM, Crum JE: Decreasing prevalence of obesity in primary schoolchildren. Arch Dis Child 2007, 92:153-154.
9. Tambalis KD, Panagiotakos DB, Kavouras SA, Kallistratos AA, Moraiti IP, Douvis SJ, Toutouzas PK, Sidossis LS: Eleven-year prevalence trends of obesity in Greek children: first evidence that prevalence of obesity is leveling off. Obesity (Silver Spring) 2010, 18:161-166.
10. Schnohr C, Sorensen TI, Niclasen BV: Changes since 1980 in body mass index and the prevalence of overweight among inschooling children in Nuuk, Greenland. Int J Circumpolar Health 2005, 64:157-162.
11. Rolland-Cachera MF, Sempe M, Guilloud-Bataille M, Patois E, Pequignot-Guggenbuhl F, Fautrad V: Adiposity indices in children. Am J Clin Nutr 1982, 36:178-184.

12. Troiano RP, Flegal KM: Overweight children and adolescents: description, epidemiology, and demographics. Pediatrics 1998, 101:497-504.
13. Kuczmarski RJ, Flegal KM, Campbell SM, Johnson CL: Increasing prevalence of overweight among US adults. The National Health and Nutrition Examination Surveys, 1960 to 1991. JAMA 1994, 272:205-211.
14. Flegal KM, Carroll MD, Kuczmarski RJ, Johnson CL: Overweight and obesity in the United States: prevalence and trends, 1960-1994. Int J Obes Relat Metab Disord 1998, 22:39-47.
15. Zellner K, Ulbricht G, Kromeyer-Hauschild K: Long-term trends in body mass index of children in Jena, Eastern Germany. Econ Hum Biol 2007, 5:426-434.
16. Olds TS: One million skinfolds: secular trends in the fatness of young people 1951-2004. Eur J Clin Nutr 2009, 63:934-946.
17. Nagel G, Wabitsch M, Galm C, Berg S, Brandstetter S, Fritz M, Klenk J, Peter R, Prokopchuk D, Steiner R, et al.: Secular changes of anthropometric measures for the past 30 years in South-West Germany. Eur J Clin Nutr 2009, 63:1440-1443.
18. Flegal KM, Troiano RP: Changes in the distribution of body mass index of adults and children in the US population. Int J Obes Relat Metab Disord 2000, 24:807-818.
19. Wang YC, Gortmaker SL, Taveras EM: Trends and racial/ethnic disparities in severe obesity among US children and adolescents, 1976-2006. Int J Pediatr Obes 2011, 6:12-20.
20. Skelton JA, Cook SR, Auinger P, Klein JD, Barlow SE: Prevalence and trends of severe obesity among US children and adolescents. Acad Pediatr 2009, 9:322-329.
21. Wang Y, Beydoun MA, Liang L, Caballero B, Kumanyika SK: Will all Americans become overweight or obese? Estimating the progression and cost of the US obesity epidemic. Obesity (Silver Spring) 2008, 16:2323-2330.
22. Kromeyer-Hauschild K, Zellner K: Trends in overweight and obesity and changes in the distribution of body mass index in schoolchildren of Jena, East Germany. Eur J Clin Nutr 2007, 61:404-411.
23. Bae SG, Kim JY, Kim KY, Park SW, Bae J, Lee WK: Changes in dietary behavior among adolescents and their association with government nutrition policies in Korea, 2005-2009. J Prev Med Public Health 2012, 45:47-59.
24. Fernandes MM: A national evaluation of the impact of state policies on competitive foods in schools. J Sch Health 2013, 83:249-255.
25. Andreyeva T, Luedicke J, Tripp AS, Henderson KE: Effects of reduced juice allowances in food packages for the women, infants, and children program. Pediatrics 2013, 131:919-927.
26. Iannotti RJ, Wang J: Trends in physical activity, sedentary behavior, diet, and BMI among US adolescents, 2001-2009. Pediatrics 2013, 132:606-614.
27. Jensen BW, Nichols M, Allender S, de Silva-Sanigorski A, Millar L, Kremer P, Lacy K, Swinburn B: Consumption patterns of sweet drinks in a population of Australian children and adolescents (2003-2008). BMC Public Health 2012, 12:771.
28. Kit BK, Fakhouri TH, Park S, Nielsen SJ, Ogden CL: Trends in sugar-sweetened beverage consumption among youth and adults in the United States: 1999-2010. Am J Clin Nutr 2013, 98:180-188.
29. de Onis M, Blossner M, Borghi E: Global prevalence and trends of overweight and obesity among preschool children. Am J Clin Nutr 2010, 92:1257-1264.

CHAPTER 3

PREVALENCE, DISPARITIES, AND TRENDS IN OBESITY AND SEVERE OBESITY AMONG STUDENTS IN THE PHILADELPHIA, PENNSYLVANIA, SCHOOL DISTRICT, 2006–2010

JESSICA M. ROBBINS, GIRIDHAR MALLYA, MARCIA POLANSKY, AND DONALD F. SCHWARZ

3.1 INTRODUCTION

Childhood obesity increased dramatically in the latter part of the 20th century, making it a leading public health issue (1). In 2009–2010, 18.2% of US children aged 6 through 19 years were obese, although national data suggest that the prevalence of childhood obesity is plateauing (2). Arkansas data support this trend, while recent New York City data indicate that childhood obesity is decreasing (3-7); however, the long-term trends and applicability to other parts of the United States are uncertain.

Recent efforts have been made to assess the epidemic increases in childhood obesity in the United States through public health surveillance

---

Reprinted with permission from the Centers for Disease Control and Prevention. Robbins JM, Mallya G, Polansky M, Schwarz DF. Prevalence, Disparities, and Trends in Obesity and Severe Obesity Among Students in the Philadelphia, Pennsylvania, School District, 2006–2010. Preventing Chronic Disease *9 (2012), http://dx.doi.org/10.5888/pcd9.120118.*

methods. An important context in which such surveillance can take place is the school, because most children aged 5 through 18 years are enrolled in school and 90% of these students attend public schools (8). Many schools have nurses or other trained health personnel on site, and increasing numbers of school districts have mandated routine weight screening for students. The Centers for Disease Control and Prevention commissioned a report to provide guidance for school-based body mass index (BMI) measurement programs (9); Arkansas mandated school statewide BMI screening beginning in 2003, and as of 2009, a dozen other states had followed suit (9). Nonetheless, few communities have obtained and analyzed their data to track childhood obesity at the local level (10).

To identify the baseline prevalence and trends in childhood obesity locally, we analyzed height and weight data for students in kindergarten through grade 12 in the School District of Philadelphia. The school district includes approximately 300 public and charter schools, educating approximately 200,000 students. More than 80% of students are of racial/ethnic minorities, and more than 50% are eligible for free or reduced-price meals based on family income.

Our primary goals were to assess the prevalence of obesity and severe obesity among children in the School District of Philadelphia and to determine whether the prevalence of obesity and severe obesity changed between 2006–2007 and 2009–2010, the most recent school year for which data were available.

3.2 METHODS

School District of Philadelphia records cover all students enrolled in Philadelphia public schools at any point during the year, a number that varied from 189,913 in 2006–2007 to 177,499 in 2009–2010 (T. Williams, written communication, April 2012). Students who attended charter schools exclusively were not included. Analyses were limited to students aged 5 through 18 for whom valid height and weight measurements were recorded. These students represented an increasing percentage of the total school population over the 4 school years included, from 61.6% in 2006–2007 to

70.4% in 2009–2010. The demographics of the total school population are presented in the Appendix.

Students' heights and weights were measured by school nurses. Pennsylvania mandates that all children in kindergarten through grade 12 have their height and weight measured annually by a nurse or teacher. The Pennsylvania Department of Health's Division of Chronic Disease Intervention and Division of School Health have developed a manual to provide guidance to school districts and other educational entities on best practices in measuring and reporting these data (11). The measured heights and weights were entered into a secure school district database with the date of the examination. BMI measurements for girls whose records indicated a pregnancy were excluded from these analyses.

BMI was calculated as weight (kg)/height (m^2) and compared with sex and age-specific norms from CDC growth charts (12) to determine BMI percentile. Obesity was defined as a BMI at or above the 95th percentile. Severe obesity was defined as a BMI of 35 or higher or 120% or greater of the threshold for obesity, based on the recommendation of Flegal et al (13). The validity of the 99th percentile estimates that have been commonly used to characterize severe obesity among children is questionable; these estimates do not match well to the empirical data on which the CDC growth charts were based (13). We conducted a secondary analysis of BMI values above the 99th percentile criterion to assess the sensitivity of the results to the differences in definition of severe obesity.

The demographic variables examined were sex; race/ethnicity; socioeconomic status, using eligibility for free or reduced-price school meals as a proxy; and grade. Race/ethnicity patterns were different for boys and girls and are therefore presented separately by sex. Data were weighted for nonresponse so that the measured population would more accurately represent the entire school population. Weights were calculated by grade and racial/ethnic group.

Although no intentional sampling was conducted, we conducted significance tests using SAS version 9.2 (SAS Institute, Inc, Cary, North Carolina) to assess the likelihood that changes over time represented chance findings. We assessed the significance of changes across time by testing a linear variable for school year in multivariable models that included a race/ethnicity–sex term, age in years, grade, and eligibility for free or reduced-price meals, adjusted for clustering within schools. Separate models were also conducted for each demographic group to assess time trends within groups.

To assess the possibility of bias associated with missing data, we identified a subsample of schools in which missing data were minimized (defined as at least 75% of all enrolled students having been measured during the school year), calculated the prevalence of obesity in this high-response sample, and compared the results with those of the total study population.

3.3 RESULTS

Valid height and weight measurements were obtained for 61.6% of all students in 2006–2007, 66.4% in 2007–2008, 69.1% in 2008–2009, and 70.4% in 2009–2010. These figures exclude girls whose records indicated a pregnancy during the school year (n = 1,134 during all 4 school years, 0.48% of all measured female students).

The demographics of the study population were similar to those of the entire student population, except that a larger proportion of the total population was in grades 9 through 12 (31.5% in 2009–2010, compared with 26.4% of the measured population) and a smaller proportion was in kindergarten through grade 5 (46.7% compared with 51.0%) (Table 1). The demographic characteristics of the population were generally similar for all 4 years. Boys comprised approximately 51% of the student population throughout the study period. African Americans were the largest racial/ethnic group (60.1% of all students and 59.3% of those measured in 2009–2010), followed by Hispanics (17.6% of all students, 16.7% of those measured), non-Hispanic whites (13.6% of all students, 14.2% of those measured), and Asians (6.3% of all students, 7.2% of those measured). The most notable change over time was the increase in the proportion of students who were eligible for free or reduced-price meals (from 48.9% to 57.4% among all students and from 50.8% to 59.5% among those measured), a change that occurred primarily between the 2007–2008 school year and the 2008–2009 school year.

TABLE 1: Demographic Characteristics[a] of Students Aged 5 Through 18 Years Whose Weight Status Was Assessed, Philadelphia School District, 2006–2010

Characteristic	School Year, n (%)			
	2006–2007	2007–2008	2008–2009	2009–2010
Total	114,721 (100.0)	119,793 (100.0)	121,413 (100.0)	121,798 (100.0)
Grade				
K-5	57,222 (50.1)	59,568 (49.9)	60,342 (49.9)	61,940 (51.0)
6-8	28,724 (25.1)	28,331 (23.8)	26,825 (22.2)	27,436 (22.6)
9-12	28,322 (24.8)	31,404 (26.3)	33,856 (28.0)	31,984 (26.4)
Sex				
Male	58,679 (51.2)	61,152 (51.1)	61,940 (51.0)	62,223 (51.1)
Female	56,042 (48.8)	58,641 (49.0)	59,473 (49.0)	59,575 (48.9)
Race/ethnicity				
African American	68,310 (59.5)	71,629 (59.8)	72,911 (60.1)	72,182 (59.3)
Hispanic	19,485 (17.0)	20,305 (17.0)	20,514 (16.9)	20,375 (16.7)
Non-Hispanic white	18,111 (15.8)	18,084 (15.1)	17,554 (14.5)	17,330 (14.2)
Asian	7,263 (6.3)	7,849 (6.6)	8,105 (6.7)	8,774 (7.2)
Other	1,552 (1.4)	1,926 (1.6)	2,329 (1.9)	3,137 (2.6)
Eligiblility for free/reduced-price meals				
Eligible	58,296 (50.8)	59,542 (49.7)	71,184 (58.6)	72,484 (59.5)
Not eligible	56,425 (49.2)	60,251 (50.3)	50,229 (41.4)	49,314 (40.5)

Abbreviation: K, kindergarten. [a] Values may not sum to total due to missing data.

In 2009–2010, the prevalence of obesity among Philadelphia's public school students was 20.5% (Table 2). The prevalence was higher among students in grades 6 through 8 (23.0%), compared with both kindergarten through fifth grade (19.1%) and high school students (20.8%). Among boys in 2009-2010, Hispanics had the highest prevalence of obesity (25.6%), followed by whites (20.7%); among girls in 2009-2010, African Americans had the highest prevalence (22.7%), followed by Hispanics (20.6%). The lowest prevalence by far—less than half that of any other group—was among Asian females, at 8.9% in 2009-2010.

TABLE 2: Obesity[a] Prevalence, Students Aged 5 Through 18 Years, by Demographic Characteristics, Philadelphia School District, 2006–2010

Characteristic	School Year, %				P Value for Trend[b]	% Change 2006–2007 to 2009-2010
	2006–2007	2007–2008	2008–2009	2009–2010		
Total	21.5	21.3	20.6	20.5	<.001	−4.8
Grade						
K-5	20.3	20.2	19.1	19.1	<.001	−6.0
6-8	24.1	23.2	22.6	23.0	<.01	−4.7
9-12	21.4	21.4	21.2	20.8	.43	−2.4
Sex						
Male	21.7	21.3	20.3	20.4	<.001	−6.1
Female	21.3	21.3	20.8	20.6	.04	−3.3
Male race/ethnicity						
African American	20.7	20.1	19.1	19.1	<.001	−7.6
Hispanic	26.2	26.1	24.7	25.6	.13	−2.5
Non-Hispanic white	22.2	21.7	21.1	20.7	.01	−6.8
Asian	19.9	18.9	18.1	18.1	.01	−8.8
Other	20.4	20.7	19.5	19.3	.37	−5.7
Female race/ethnicity						
African American	23.0	22.9	22.8	22.7	.60	−1.2
Hispanic	22.3	22.4	21.1	20.6	<.01	−7.4
Non-Hispanic white	17.5	17.7	17.1	17.3	.45	−0.8
Asian	9.4	9.1	9.2	8.9	.57	−5.0
Other	18.6	18.8	17.4	17.1	.35	−8.2
Eligibility for free/reduced-price meals						
Eligible	21.4	21.3	20.5	20.7	.01	−3.3
Not eligible	21.6	21.2	20.7	20.2	<.001	−6.7

Abbreviations: K, kindergarten. [a] Obesity was defined as a body mass index ≥95th percentile, according to Centers for Disease Control and Prevention growth charts (12). Data were weighted for nonresponse so that the measured population would more accurately represent the entire school population. [b] Calculated using Wald χ^2 test. All tests were controlled for other variables shown in the table.

TABLE 3: Severe Obesity[a] Prevalence, by Demographic Characteristics, Students Aged 5 Through 18 Years, Philadelphia School District, 2006–2010

Characteristic	School Year, %				P Value for Trend[b]	% Change 2006–2007 to 2009-2010
	2006–2007	2007–2008	2008–2009	2009–2010		
Total	8.5	8.4	7.9	7.9	<.001	−7.7
Grade						
K-5	7.3	7.2	6.7	6.6	<.001	−8.7
6-8	10.0	9.7	9.0	9.1	<.001	−9.1
9-12	9.2	9.2	8.9	8.7	.29	−4.4
Sex						
Male	8.8	8.5	7.8	7.8	<.001	−11.9
Female	8.2	8.3	8.0	7.9	.10	−2.9
Male race/ethnicity						
African American	8.8	8.4	7.7	7.6	<.001	−13.8
Hispanic	10.7	10.4	9.4	9.8	<.01	−8.4
Non-Hispanic white	8.0	8.1	7.7	7.6	.12	−6.0
Asian	5.6	5.2	4.9	5.2	.26	−7.2
Other	8.8	7.4	6.8	6.3	.03	−28.0
Female race/ethnicity						
African American	9.2	9.5	9.2	9.2	.49	−0.1
Hispanic	8.3	8.1	7.7	7.5	.01	−10.2
Non-Hispanic white	6.1	5.8	6.2	6.2	.86	1.0
Asian	2.2	2.2	2.2	2.1	.61	−4.1
Other	6.1	6.7	5.4	5.3	.23	−11.7
Eligibility for free/reduced-price meals						
Eligible	8.6	8.6	8.0	8.1	<.01	−6.3
Not eligible	8.4	8.2	7.9	7.5	<.001	−10.2

Abbreviation: K, kindergarten. [a] Severe obesity was defined as a body mass index ≥35 kg/m² or being ≥120% of the threshold for obesity, based on the recommendation of Flegal et al (13). Data were weighted for nonresponse so that the measured population would more accurately represent the entire school population. [b] Calculated using Wald χ^2 test. All tests were controlled for other variables shown in the table.

Obesity declined slightly from 21.5% in 2006–2007 to 20.5% in 2009–2010, representing a 4.8% decrease (Table 2). Most of the decrease was between 2006–2007 and 2008–2009, followed by a leveling off in 2009–2010. This pattern varied by demographic group. At the beginning of the period, the prevalence of obesity was slightly higher among boys than girls (21.7% vs 21.3%); in the most recent school year this was reversed (20.4% among boys vs 20.6% among girls). Among high school students, the small decline in obesity was not significant. Trends within racial/ethnic–sex groups were significant for African American, non-Hispanic white, and Asian boys and for Hispanic girls. None of the subgroup changes between 2008–2009 and 2009–2010 was significant.

The prevalence of severe obesity in 2009–2010 was 7.9% (Table 3). Patterns of disparities in severe obesity were similar to those for obesity. Severe obesity was most prevalent among students in grades 6 through 8 (9.1% in 2009-2010), and the prevalence of severe obesity exceeded 9% among Hispanic boys and African American girls in 2009-2010. Trends over time in severe obesity were similar overall to those for obesity (Table 3). For the overall population, severe obesity prevalence decreased from 8.5% to 7.9% from 2006–2007 to 2009–2010, representing a 7.7% decrease. The largest significant changes were seen among African American boys and Hispanic girls. Results using the 99th percentile of BMI as a threshold (not shown) showed similar patterns, with slightly lower overall prevalence and somewhat larger declines over time (from 6.3% in 2006–2007 to 5.6% in 2009–2010).

Some groups that had shown declines in obesity, severe obesity, or both, including those with the highest prevalence of severe obesity, experienced small nonsignificant increases during the 2009–2010 school year. Most schools contributed at least 1 school year to the high-response subset with measurements for 75% or more of enrolled students. Analyses limited to this subset did not differ substantially from results for the complete data.

3.4 DISCUSSION

Analyses of annually collected height and weight data on more than 100,000 public school children in Philadelphia from 2006–2007 to 2009–

2010 demonstrated that the prevalence of obesity may be decreasing in small but potentially meaningful ways. However, trends were not consistent across subgroups, and obesity remains alarmingly high, particularly among some racial and ethnic minorities. Severe obesity, which confers the greatest short- and long-term risks to physical and emotional health, affects nearly 1 in 12 children in Philadelphia.

Some of these findings are consistent with national statistics on child overweight and obesity from the National Health and Nutrition Examination Surveys (NHANES) (2), although national rates of obesity in 2009–2010 were lower than those found among Philadelphia public school children. The differences were greatest for non-Hispanic whites, among whom 17.2% of boys and 13.0% of girls aged 6 to 19 years were obese nationally, compared with 20.7% of boys and 17.3% of girls aged 5 through 18 years in the School District of Philadelphia. This finding may reflect differences in socioeconomic status between whites in Philadelphia public schools and the US population overall. African Americans in the School District of Philadelphia had lower rates of obesity than those in the national data (19.1% for boys and 22.7% for girls in Philadelphia vs 25.4% for boys and 26.1% for girls nationally). In both the NHANES and School District of Philadelphia data, African American girls had higher rates of obesity than non-Hispanic white girls. In the NHANES data, African American boys also had higher rates of obesity than non-Hispanic white boys, although the opposite was true among Philadelphia public school children. This may again reflect the lower socioeconomic status of whites in the Philadelphia public schools compared with those in the national NHANES sample.

The NHANES study did not find evidence of any noticeable trends in obesity prevalence from 2007–2008 through 2009–2010. The differences seen between the School District of Philadelphia and NHANES data may reflect the different age ranges (5 through 18 in Philadelphia vs 6 through 19 in NHANES), different periods (2006–2010 vs 2007–2010), differences in measurement and methods, or genuine differences between Philadelphia public school children and national averages. The small size of the NHANES study population, which yielded 80% power to detect changes in obesity prevalence of 5% or more (14), may have precluded detecting declines in obesity over this period.

Routinely collected BMI data for public school children have been published only for a few jurisdictions, including New York City and Arkansas. The prevalence, disparities, and trends in obesity among public school children in New York City were similar to those seen here, with generally consistent small declines in obesity, including an apparent leveling off in both cities in 2009–2010. Among students in kindergarten through eighth grade, the prevalence of obesity in Philadelphia public school children was between 0.2% and 0.7% lower than among those in New York City in the same period. In 2009–2010, the prevalence of obesity in these grades was 20.3% in Philadelphia and 21.0% in New York City (7).

The prevalence of obesity found in Philadelphia public school children is also similar to statewide findings for public school children in Arkansas. The prevalence in the 2009–2010 school year was 21% in Arkansas and 20% in Philadelphia (3). Trends were generally declining or flat during the last several years. Many of the specific racial/ethnic differences noted, such as the marked sex disparity among Asian students, are consistent (3-6). Arkansas has not, however, reported the recent decline in obesity among African Americans noted in both Philadelphia and New York City.

Children affected by severe obesity face even greater health risks than obese children. Among children examined in the NHANES survey, those who were above the 99th percentile of BMI had higher mean blood pressures and insulin levels, lower mean high-density lipoprotein (HDL) cholesterol levels, and higher prevalence of metabolic syndrome than those who had BMI percentiles in the 95th to 97th range, putting them at greater risk of cardiovascular disease (15). In the HEALTHY study, a survey of primarily low-income and minority sixth-graders, students with BMI at or above the 99th percentile had higher blood pressure and insulin levels, lower HDL cholesterol levels, and larger waist circumferences than those who were moderately obese (16). Psychosocial comorbidities are also more severe among children and youth with severe obesity (17). Although the prevalence and consequences of severe obesity in children have prompted widespread interest in various interventions, including bariatric surgery for adolescents (18) and child welfare involvement (19), trends in severe obesity have been less widely studied or reported than those for overweight and obesity. Madsen et al, using different definitions of severe obesity (BMI ≥97th or ≥99th percentile), reported differing trends among subgroups of California students (20). Some of the patterns they found, such as continuing increases in severe obesity among African American girls, are not consistent with those found from analysis of School District of Philadelphia data. This inconsistency could reflect regional differences; our secondary analysis indicated that using BMI at or above the 99th percentile to define severe obesity would not affect these trends.

Many of the strengths and limitations of these data originate from the routine screening assessments of student populations conducted by school nurses. The data represent large, unselected populations and were collected by experienced clinical professionals; conversely, they were not collected under rigorous protocols or with consistent equipment, nor were they validated. Research on the accuracy of measurements taken in schools suggests that measurements taken by school nurses are of reasonably high quality (21). The substantial proportions of students that were not measured, especially in the higher grades, leave potential for selection bias, although our secondary analyses suggest that such bias is limited. Children who did not attend public schools during the school year, including those who attended private, parochial, and charter schools, were not included, and obesity prevalence and trends could differ in these groups. The similarities seen in both trends over time and disparities between racial/ethnic–sex groups when comparing the Philadelphia data with data from New York City and Arkansas strengthen our confidence in their accuracy.

Although these data do not allow us to say what is responsible for the apparent reversal of the trend toward increasing childhood obesity, greater attention has been paid to improving school health environments both nationally and in the School District of Philadelphia. Since 1999, the EAT. RIGHT.NOW. Pennsylvania Nutrition Education TRACKS program has provided nutrition education to all students and parents who are eligible for SNAP (the federal Supplemental Nutrition Assistance Program) and is now in more than 270 district schools (T.E. Wolford, written communication, March 2012). In 2004, the district beverage policy mandated the removal of all sodas and sugar-sweetened drinks from vending machines, and in 2006 snack standards were developed for á la carte and vending items. In 2006, the Philadelphia School Reform Commission passed a comprehensive School Wellness Policy with provisions for competitive foods, physical activity, and nutrition education. Finally, from 2009–2010,

School Food Services began offering "universal" or free breakfast to all students, discontinued the use of fryers, and switched from 2% to 1% low-fat milk. In 2010, the Philadelphia Department of Public Health (PDPH) launched the Get Healthy Philly (www.foodfitphilly.org) initiative to improve nutrition and physical activity through citywide policy and systems changes. PDPH has partnered with public and private sector organizations, including the School District of Philadelphia, to decrease the population-level burden of obesity and related diseases, particularly among children. Such comprehensive efforts may help accelerate the decreases in BMI found in the study reported here.

The inconsistency of findings between subgroups and the small increases in obesity, severe obesity or both in some groups in the most recent year of data indicate that it is not yet certain that the epidemic increases in child obesity are over. Continued surveillance is required to clarify whether we are seeing minor inconsistencies in a continuing crisis or a true change in the epidemic.

In either case, the prevalence of unhealthy weight remains unacceptably high among public school children in Philadelphia, and the evidence that some groups are facing exceptionally high health risks associated with obesity is sobering. When almost 9% of all teenage students are severely obese, identifying effective means of preventing obesity in our children, helping those already affected to attain a healthier weight, and preventing the serious chronic health problems associated with obesity remain urgent public health responsibilities.

REFERENCES

1. Ogden CL, Flegal KM, Carroll MD, Johnson CL. Prevalence and trends in overweight among US children and adolescents, 1999-2000. JAMA 2002;288(14):1728-32.
2. Ogden CL, Carroll MD, Kit BK, Flegal KM. Prevalence of obesity and trends in body mass index among US children and adolescents, 1999-2010. JAMA 2012;307(5):483-90.
3. Year eight assessment of childhood and adolescent obesity in Arkansas (fall 2010 - spring 2011). Little Rock (AK): Arkansas Center for Health Improvement; February 2012.

4. Year seven assessment of childhood and adolescent obesity in Arkansas (fall 2009-spring 2010). Little Rock (AK): Arkansas Center for Health Improvement; December 2010.
5. Year six assessment of childhood and adolescent obesity in Arkansas (fall 2008-spring 2009). Little Rock (AK): Arkansas Center for Health Improvement; December 2009.
6. Year five assessment of childhood and adolescent obesity in Arkansas (fall 2007–spring 2008). Little Rock (AK): Arkansas Center for Health Improvement; September 2008.
7. Centers for Disease Control and Prevention. Obesity in K-8 students — New York City, 2006-07 to 2010-11 school years. MMWR Morb Mortal Wkly Rep 2011;60(49):1673-8.
8. Strizek GA, Pittsonberger JL, Riordan KE, Lyter DM, Orlofsky GF. Characteristics of schools, districts, teachers, principals, and school libraries in the United States: 2003-04 Schools and Staffing Survey (NCES 2006-313). Washington (DC): US Government Printing Office, US Department of Education, National Center for Education Statistics; 2006.
9. Nihiser AJ, Lee SM, Wechsler H, McKenna M, Odom E, Reinold C, et al. BMI measurement in schools. Pediatrics 2009;124(Suppl 1):S89–S97.
10. Sheon A, Katta V, Costello B, Longjohn M, Mantinan K. Registry-Based BMI Surveillance: A Guide to System Preparation, Design, and Implementation. Altarum Institute, June 2011. http://www.altarum.org/files/imce/Chomp_BMI_FINAL_060811lr.pdf.
11. Johnson CB, Huff MK, Gray A. Procedures for the growth screening program for Pennsylvania's school-age population. Harrisburg (PA): Pennsylvania Department of Health; 2004.
12. Kuczmarski RJ, Ogden CL, Guo SS, Grummer-Strawn LM, Flegal KM, Mei Z, et al. CDC growth charts for the United States: methods and development. Vital Health Stat 11 2002;(246):1-190.
13. Flegal KM, Wei R, Ogden CL, Freedman DS, Johnson CL, Curtin LR. Characterizing extreme values of body mass index–for-age by using the 2000 Centers for Disease Control and Prevention growth charts. Am J Clin Nutr 2009;90(5):1314-20.
14. Ogden CL, Carroll MD, Curtin LR, Lamb MM, Flegal KM. Prevalence of high body mass index in US children and adolescents, 2007-2008. JAMA 2010;303(3):242-9.
15. Skelton JA, Cook SR, Auinger P, Klein JD, Barlow SE. Prevalence and trends of severe obesity among US children and adolescents. Acad Pediatr 2009;9(5):322-9.
16. Marcus MD, Baranowski T, DeBar LL, Edelstein S, Kaufman FR, Schneider M, et al. Severe obesity and selected risk factors in a sixth grade multiracial cohort: the HEALTHY study. J Adolesc Health 2010;47(6):604-7.
17. Zeller MH, Modi AC. Predictors of health-related quality of life in obese youth. Obesity (Silver Spring) 2006;14(1):122-30.
18. Brandt ML, Harmon CM, Helmrath MA, Inge TH, McKay SV, Michalsky MP. Morbid obesity in pediatric diabetes mellitus: surgical options and outcomes. Nat Rev Endocrinol 2010;6(11):637-45.
19. Murtagh L, Ludwig DL. State intervention in life-threatening childhood obesity. JAMA 2011;306(2):206-7.

20. Madsen KA, Weed AE, Crawford PB. Disparities in peaks, plateaus, and declines in prevalence of high BMI among adolescents. Pediatrics 2010;126(3):434-42.
21. Stoddard SA, Kubik MY, Skay C. Is school-based height and weight screening of elementary students private and reliable? J Sch Nurs 2008;24(1):43-8.

There are several supplemental files that are not available in this version of the article. To view this additional information, please use the citation on the first page of this chapter.

PART II

WHAT MAKES OUR CHILDREN OBESE AND OVERWEIGHT?

CHAPTER 4

PHYSICAL ACTIVITY, SCREEN TIME AND OBESITY STATUS IN A NATIONALLY REPRESENTATIVE SAMPLE OF MALTESE YOUTH WITH INTERNATIONAL COMPARISONS

ANDREW DECELIS, RUSSELL JAGO, AND KENNETH R. FOX

4.1 BACKGROUND

Physical activity is associated with improved physical and mental well-being among children and adolescents [1]. The percentage of children meeting the current PA guidelines of at least 60 minutes of moderate to vigorous physical activity (MVPA) a day [1] is low in many European countries, the United States and Canada [2,3]. A large percentage of children and adolescents spend considerable amounts of time being sedentary [3], and exceed the recommendation of not more than two hours of screen time per day [4].

There is inconclusive evidence of the association between physical activity and weight status among young people [5]. A recent review of

---

Physical Activity, Screen Time and Obesity Status in a Nationally Representative Sample of Maltese Youth with International Comparisons. © *Decelis A, Jago R, and Fox KR.* BMC Public Health, **14**,664 *(2014). doi:10.1186/1471-2458-14-664. Licensed under Creative Commons Attribution 2.0 Generic License, http://creativecommons.org/licenses/by/2.0/.*

cross-sectional studies conducted over the last ten years reported a negative relationship between PA and child weight status in some studies and no association in others. Sedentary behaviours were positively associated with higher weight status. However, results were inconsistent for total sedentary time and different types of screen time and effects varied for boys and girls [6,7]. A number of studies have reported that screen time is associated with body mass among children [8,9]. Thus, more information on the link between body mass and both physical activity and sedentary time is needed.

It is important to highlight that most of the studies that have assessed associations between physical activity, sedentary time and body mass have used self-reported measures of physical activity and screen time which are subject to response and recall bias [10]. Self-reported height and weight have been reported as underestimating overweight prevalence in comparison to measured height and weight [11]. This highlights the need for objective measurements of PA, sedentary time and weight status [6] as they provide a more precise estimate of these variables.

Current research is also limited by the location as most studies have been undertaken in North America, in Portugal and in the UK. As such, research is needed on physical activity and weight status using objective measures in other countries, particularly where there is a high prevalence of obesity.

Studies using self-report measures have suggested that Maltese children have the second highest prevalence of overweight and obesity at age 11 after USA [12]. Even though the problem of obesity in Maltese children and adults seems to be severe, data on lifestyle factors, including physical activity, sedentary behaviours and their association with obesity is limited. Furthermore, only one study has been published where activity and height and weight have been measured objectively and it has been limited to 11–12 year olds [13]. This was a pilot study by the authors and indicated very low physical activity levels, and high sedentary time, screen time and prevalence of obesity. However, the sample size was small and not nationally representative.

In the present study, we systematically selected a nationally representative sample of Maltese 10–11 year boys and girls and assessed through objective measures, PA, sedentary behaviour and screen time in different weight status categories. The resulting data were used to address the following research questions: 1) What are their physical activity levels? 2) What are their screen time (ST) patterns? 3) How do their physical activity and screen time levels compare to other EU and non EU countries? 4) How do their physical activity and screen time patterns differ by weight status (adjusting for socioeconomic status).

4.2 METHODS

Data are from the *Movement, Activity and Lifestyle—Tweens in Action* (MAL-TA) project, a cross-sectional study conducted between January and May 2012 with children in 54 schools in Malta [14]. A nationally representative sample of 1126 children was selected by the National Statistics Office (NSO) from a total population of 3890 (28.6%). This sample was stratified by regions of Malta and the neighbouring island of Gozo, type of school (495 from 35 state schools, 272 from 13 church schools, 107 from six independent schools) and gender (607 boys and 519 girls). One or two classes were chosen at random from each selected school and all children in each of these classes were invited to participate in the study. From the 1126 children invited, 901 children (80%) returned parental consent and the study was approved by the University of Malta research ethics committee.

4.2.1 CHILDREN'S QUESTIONNAIRE

Participants completed a questionnaire with pre-coded answer categories to assess the time spent watching television (TV), using a computer for chatting, internet, emails or homework, and playing games on a computer or games console. Separate questions were asked for use on weekdays and weekends and categories included none, 1 minute to 30 minutes, 31 minutes – 1 hour, 1–2 hours, 2–3 hours, 3–4 hours, and more than 4 hours. Questions were adapted from the Health Behaviour in School Children study (HBSC) [12]. A previous study [15] reported satisfactory test-retest reliability for these questions. Data for TV viewing were recoded into less than 2 hours, and 2 hours or more (i.e. exceeding American Academy of

Pediatrics guidelines [16]) while other ST was recoded into less than 1 hour and 1 hour or more. To facilitate comparison with data from the Health Behaviour of School Children study (HBSC) the data for 'playing games on a computer and games console' for over two hours was also analysed.

4.2.2 ANTHROPOMETRIC MEASUREMENTS

Body height and weight were measured with the child in light clothing and without shoes. Height was measured using a SECA 213 Leicester Stadiometer (SECA, Hamburg, Germany) and recorded to the nearest 0.1 cm. Weight was recorded using a SECA 813 Digital Scale to the nearest 0.1 kg. Body mass index was calculated (kg/m^2) and children were classified into normal weight, overweight and obese, using the age-related International Obesity Task Force criteria [17].

4.2.3 PHYSICAL ACTIVITY

Physical activity was assessed using Actigraph GT3X accelerometers (Actigraph, Pensacola, USA) set at 10 second epochs to capture children's intermittent physical activity [18]. Participants were instructed to wear the accelerometer on an elastic belt over the right hip for five consecutive days including three weekdays and two weekend days. The accelerometer data were then processed using Kinesoft version 3.3.62 with a valid day based on at least 600 minutes of monitor wear. Periods of at least 60 minutes of continuous zeros were considered to be non-wear time and were removed [19]. Participants who had at least three days of valid data were included in this study [20]. The following accelerometer variables were then derived: total physical activity per day (in counts per minute), mean minutes of sedentary time per day, and mean minutes of moderate to vigorous physical activity (MVPA) per valid day. Time spent in these thresholds was classified based on the Evenson criteria of <100 CPM for sedentary and >2296 for MVPA [21]. In a rigorous study by Trost these cutpoints were found to provide the best classification accuracy [22].

Data were filtered by different time periods to enable an analysis of activity patterns during weekdays and weekend days. The morning period before schools was from 5.30 am to 8.29 am; the period at school from 8.30 am to 1.59 pm; the afternoon period from 2.00 pm to 6.59 pm and the evening time from 7.00 pm to 11.59 pm.

A search of the Biosis Citation Index, Derwent Innovations Index, Medline and Scielo Citation Index online databases was conducted in July 2013 using Web of Science. This identified articles that had cited Evenson's 2008 [21] study. We manually screened the articles yielded from the search to identify articles which reported studies where a) accelerometry had been used to assess physical activity, b) comparable cutpoints for levels of intensity of activity had been used, and c) 10–11 year olds were the subjects of the study. While this was not a systematic review, it provided an opportunity to compare the results in the current study, with similar studies from other countries.

4.2.4 STATISTICAL ANALYSES

Group means and standard deviations (SDs) were calculated for physical activity and sedentary time, and percentages for screen time. Independent sample t-tests were used to explore gender differences in activity and Chi-square tests were used for gender differences in screen time. Distributions were checked and as all variables approximated normality with relatively small deviations, parametric tests were used. Differences in physical activity by weight categories were analysed using analyses of covariance (ANCOVA) with the model adjusted for socioeconomic status. Chi-square tests were used to compare ST by weight status groups. To facilitate the development of targeted intervention strategies, separate analyses were performed for boys and girls, for weekdays and weekends, and for different periods of the day. Follow-up Bonferroni pairwise comparisons for significant main effects were calculated. All analyses were carried out using the IBM Statistical Package for Social Sciences (SPSS) version 21 and a p value of 0.05 was used for statistical significance.

TABLE 1: Physical activity by gender for weekdays and weekends

Weekdays	Boys (n = 412)	sd	95% CI	Girls (n = 399)	sd	95% CI	Total (n = 769)	sd	95% CI	P value (t-test)
Total activity (counts/min)	475.2	138.1	461.8-488.5	383.7	101.3	373.7-393.6	430.2	129.7	421.2-439.1	<0.001
Sedentary (min/day)	569.0	110.1	558.3-579.6	601.1	98.0	591.4-610.7	584.8	105.5	577.5-592.1	<0.001
MVPA (min/day)	59.0	22.5	56.8-61.2	43.3	14.9	41.8-44.7	51.3	20.7	49.8-52.7	<0.001
MVPA (min/day)										
5.30 am-8.29 am	5.6	3.7	5.2-5.9	4.9	3.1	4.6-5.2	5.2	3.4	5.0-5.5	0.005
8.30 am-1.59 pm	20.8	8.8	20.0-21.7	15.2	6.3	14.6-15.8	18.1	8.1	17.5-18.6	<0.001
2.00 pm-6.59 pm	24.3	13.8	23.0-25.6	17.2	8.6	16.3-18.0	20.8	12.1	20.0-21.6	<0.001
7.00 pm-11.59 pm	7.8	6.9	7.1-8.5	5.7	5.0	5.2-6.2	6.8	6.1	6.4-7.2	<0.001
Weekends	Boys (n = 392)	sd	95% CI	Girls (n = 380)	sd	95% CI	Total (n = 774)	sd	95% CI	
Total activity (counts/min)	477.9	202.0	457.8-498.0	388.4	161.5	372.1-404.7	433.9	188.5	420.5-447.2	<0.001
Sedentary (min/day)	550.1	170.4	533.2-567.1	556.9	158.3	540.1-572.9	553.5	164.5	541.8-565.1	0.567
MVPA (min/day)	57.2	32.0	54.0-60.4	40.1	21.4	38.0-42.3	48.8	28.6	46.8-50.8	<0.001
MVPA (min/day)										
5.30 am-8.29 am	1.7	2.8	1.4-1.9	1.0	1.8	0.8-1.2	1.3	2.3	1.2-1.5	<0.001
8.30 am-1.59 pm	25.3	18.2	23.5-27.1	16.7	11.3	15.6-17.9	21.1	15.8	20.0-22.2	<0.001
2.00 pm-6.59 pm	23.1	16.7	21.5-24.8	16.4	11.7	15.2-17.6	19.8	14.8	18.7-20.8	<0.001
7.00 pm-11.59 pm	6.0	6.0	5.4-6.6	5.1	5.6	4.6-5.7	5.6	5.8	5.2-6.0	0.032

4.3 RESULTS

From the 901 children who provided consent to participate in this study, 874 (97%) were present during the data collection period, that is 78% of the total sample invited (1126). All these children provided data for screen time, and of these, 811 (93% of the recruited children and 72% of the sample who had been invited) (412 boys and 399 girls) provided at least three days of valid accelerometer data, while 772 (88% of the recruited participants and 69% of those invited) provided data for weekend activity, and were included in the analyses. Children who provided accelerometer data that met inclusion criteria (n=811) were not significantly different from those who failed to provide adequate data (n=57) in gender, region or BMI category but those providing data had significantly higher socio-economic status scores.

Using the International Obesity Task Force (IOTF) standards [17] 20.4% of the sample were overweight and 14.2% obese. A significantly greater percentage of boys than girls were overweight (24.2% v 16.4%) or obese (14.8% v 13.6%) (p=0.01).

4.3.1 PHYSICAL ACTIVITY

The means and standard deviations of boys and girls PA are presented separately for weekday and weekend days, in Table 1. The mean total PA for boys was 477.8 CPM (Confidence Interval [CI]–463.6-492.3) and for girls 385.0 CPM (CI–374.8-394.7) (p<0.001). Boys were engaged in 58.5 minutes of daily MVPA (CI–56.2-60.7), while girls' MVPA was 42.2 minutes (CI–40.7-43.5) (p<0.001). Only a quarter of the children in this study (24.7%) met the daily recommendation of over 60 minutes of MVPA, and the percentage was higher for boys (39%) than girls (10%).

Analysing the data by time-period, we found that boys were significantly more active than girls during all measured times. Weekday MVPA was highest during the period after school (2.00-6.59 pm), when boys were active for 24.3 minutes (CI–22.9-25.5), seven minutes more than girls (p<0.001). During the school day (8.30 am −1.59 pm), boys were engaged in 20.8 minutes of MVPA (CI–19.9-21.6), 5.6 minutes more than girls (p<0.001). On weekends, equal amounts of MVPA were obtained for the morning and afternoon periods for boys (25.3 and 23.1 minutes respectively), and for girls (16.7 and 16.4 minutes) (p<0.001).

4.3.2 SCREEN TIME

The number and proportion of boys and girls in each ST category are presented separately for weekday and weekend days in Table 2. A high prevalence of over one hour of playing games on a computer or games console was reported by boys on weekdays (44.8%) and on weekends (51.6%) and these values are considerably higher than those reported for girls (28.1% and 35.0%) (p<0.001). Almost a third of boys (29.3%) watched over two hours of TV on weekends, compared to 20.6% of girls (p<0.001) and this prevalence is double that on weekdays.

4.3.3 COMPARISON WITH OTHER COUNTRIES

Table 3 provides a comparison of the results of the current study and previously published studies. Using the same Evenson cut points [21], mean MVPA of Maltese boys and girls were marginally higher than those of children in Philadelphia, USA [23], while compared to data from Canberra, Australia [24], mean MVPA of Maltese boys and girls were considerably higher. In contrast, means were much lower than those in the PEACH study carried out in Bristol, England [25]. Comparing median MVPA values to those of children in a longitudinal study of the National Institute of Child Health and Human Development (NICHD) in ten geographical locations in the USA, Maltese children were again more active [26]. The percentage of Maltese children meeting recommendations for PA (60 minutes a day) was slightly lower than that of children in USA, while compared to Australian data, percentages were higher for Maltese boys and lower for Maltese girls.

TABLE 2: Screen time by gender for weekdays and weekends

Screen time	Boys n	%	Girls n	%	Total n	%	P value (chi-square)
Weekdays							
Watching TV	446		426		872		0.011
Less than 2 hours	375	84.1	383	89.9	758	86.9	
2 hours and more	71	15.9	43	10.1	114	13.1	
Using a computer for chatting, internet emails or homework	446		427		873		0.733
Less than 1 hour	316	70.9	307	71.9	623	71.4	
1 hour and more	130	29.1	120	28.1	250	28.6	
Playing games on a computer or games console	446		427		873		<0.001
Less than 1 hour	246	55.2	307	71.9	553	63.3	
1 hour and more	200	44.8	120	28.1	320	36.7	
Weekends							
Watching TV	444		422		866		0.003
Less than 2 hours	314	70.7	335	79.4	649	74.9	
2 hours and more	130	29.3	87	20.6	217	25.1	
Using a computer for chatting, internet emails or homework	447		427		874		0.873
Less than 1 hour	315	70.5	303	71.0	618	70.7	
1 hour and more	132	29.5	124	29.0	256	29.3	
Playing games on a computer or games console	446		426		872		<0.001
Less than 1 hour	216	48.4	277	65.0	493	56.5	
1 hour and more	230	51.6	149	35.0	379	43.5	

Comparing the percentages of children exceeding two hours of screen time on weekdays in this study to other countries in Europe, Canada and USA, using the Health Behaviour in School-aged children (HBSC) study [3] as a comparator, we found substantially lower rates in Maltese children. TV watching percentages for Maltese children were lower than children in all other countries, while for playing games on computers and games consoles, they were only higher than the lowest HBSC values observed in Switzerland (and boys in Luxembourg).

4.3.4 PHYSICAL ACTIVITY AND SCREEN TIME BY WEIGHT STATUS

Table 4 provides a presentation of PA by weight status. For weekdays the overall pattern is that MVPA and total PA differ by weight group. Follow-up tests indicated differences between the normal weight and obese and for boys on a weekday there were also differences between the overweight and obese groups. There were similar patterns when the analyses were repeated for the separate time periods. In all instances PA levels were lower in the obese group than the normal weight group. There were significant differences between the TV viewing times of boys in different weight categories on weekends only. Almost half of obese boys (45.5%) watched over two hours of TV compared to 30.8% of overweight and 24.7% of normal weight boys (p=0.004) (see Table 5). Obese boys (45.5%) were also more engaged in using a computer for chatting, emails or homework than overweight (28.0%) and normal weight boys (25.6%) (p=0.006), however this was significant only on weekdays. No significant differences were observed in the screen time of girls in different weight categories. In contrast, objectively measured overall sedentary time of overweight boys was significantly lower than that of normal weight boys both on weekdays and on weekends (see Table 4). Differences in girls were not statistically significant.

4.4 DISCUSSION

In this study we found that 39% of boys and 10% of girls met PA guidelines. Additionally, 29.3% of boys and 20.6% of girls exceeded the American Academy of Pediatrics (AAP) [27] guideline by watching more than 2 hours of TV per day on a weekend, and these percentages were double those observed for weekdays. Maltese children were found to be more active than children in the USA and Australia, were fewer active than English children, and spent fewer hours in front of a screen than children in other countries. As published elsewhere [14], a high percentage of children in this study were found to be overweight or obese, particularly boys, making them amongst the fattest in the world. The data from this study therefore indicate that although Maltese children are quite active compared to children in other countries, they are still more likely to be obese. Additionally, Maltese boys were more active than girls throughout the week and also less sedentary on weekdays, however boys are more overweight or obese. As concluded in a recent review by Wilks et al. [28] these international comparisons suggests that physical inactivity may not be the major contributor to the development of obesity in all children.

However, when categorised as BMI groups, the data reported here indicate that obese children engaged in a significantly lower total volume of activity and MVPA than overweight and normal weight children. Overweight and obese children also spent more hours in front of a screen compared to normal weight children. These results contribute to the debate on the relationship between PA and obesity, recently summarised in a review [6] which has reported mixed associations. The data therefore suggest that there are associations between PA/ST and obesity but the direction of causality of these associations cannot be delineated from this cross-sectional dataset. Although lower activity levels and greater time spent sedentary might contribute to weight gain in children, it is equally plausible that overweight and obese children become less active. Extra weight requires more exertion for physical tasks, and being overweight during activity may attract negative reactions from others, and cause discouragement. Moreover, one cannot determine fully that obesity is linked to increased screen time, or that it is due to behaviours such as increased snacking on energy dense food during screen time, particularly TV viewing.

This study found contrasting results for self-reported screen time and objectively measured sedentary behaviour. This confirms the recent findings of Verloigne et al. [7] that self-reported TV and computer time do not reflect total sedentary time in children. Accelerometry does not tell us what children are doing, therefore we need more studies that investigate other sedentary behaviours. Although screen time might be taking a good amount of children's time, children are also spending a considerable amount of time in other sedentary activities at school and in extra study at home.

TABLE 3: A comparison of objectively assessed MVPA using Evenson [21] cut-offs and screen viewing in other countries

Study	Age	Gender	n	Mean MVPA (min)	Median MVPA (min)	Meeting recommendation (%)
Present study 2012 - Malta	10.8	Boys	412	58.1	54.8	39
	10.7	Girls	399	41.7	39.7	10
Cooper et al.,2012 [25] - England	11.0	Boys	250	70.1		NR*
		Girls	315	56.0		
Trost et al.,2013 [23] - USA	10-11	Boys	201	57.5		41.5
		Girls	269	35.5		11.5
Mitchelle et al.,2013 - USA	11.0	Boys	369		46.7	NR
		Girls	382		32.4	NR
Telford et al.,2013 [24] – Australia	11.1	Boys	282	43.0		33
		Girls	266	31.0		18

*NR - Not reported

Percentage spending 2 hours or more of weekday screen viewing (all 11 years olds)

	Watching TV		Playing games on a computer and games console	
	Boys%	Girls%	Girls%	Boys%
Present study (Malta)	16	10	12	25
HBSC* Average	58	54	22	40
Highest HBSC				
Ukraine	69	71		

TABLE 3: *Cont.*

Study	Age	Gender	n	Mean MVPA (min)	Median MVPA (min)	Meeting recommendation (%)
Romania Lowest HBSC			43	57		
Switzerland	29	24	8	16		
Canada HBSC	64	56	25	45		
USA HBSC	56	50	17	31		

*HBSC - Health Behaviour in School-Aged Children study (Currie et al. [3]).

TABLE 4: MVPA during different times of the day by weight status (model adjusted for socioeconomic status)

	Normal weight	sd	95% CI	Over-weight	sd	95% CI	Obese	sd	95% CI	Total	sd	95% CI	P value (AN-COVA)	Post-hoc (Bon-ferroni)
Boys Weekdays	(n=254)			(n=99)			(n=59)			(n=412)				
MVPA (min/day)	61.2	22.2	58.6-64.0	59.2	23.8	54.4-64.0	49.1	18.8	44.6-54.3	59.0	22.5	56.9-61.2	0.001	B, C*
Sedentary (min/day)	582.2	112.9	568.5-596.0	544.5	106.9	524.5-565.0	552.7	94.3	529.6-577.8	569.0	110.1	558.2-579.1	0.009	A
Total activity (counts/min)	481.4	135.1	464.7-497.4	487.3	149.8	458.5-519.0	428.3	122.4	398.0-462.1	475.2	138.1	462.4-488.8	0.015	B, C
5.30 am-8.29 am (counts/min)	477.6	244.8	447.4-508.5	495.3	206.6	452.9-538.9	480.8	194.8	428.5-530.7	482.3	229.1	459.9-504.8	0.846	
8.30 am-1.59 pm (counts/min)	465.0	141.6	447.8-481.7	468.3	167.2	436.1-502.5	442.5	164.7	403.1-482.5	462.6	151.3	448.6-477.6	0.466	
2.00 pm-6.59 pm (counts/min)	581.2	250.8	550.7-610.8	581.8	235.3	534.4-631.3	470.4	173.7	425.5-518.4	565.5	240.2	540.5-588.6	0.004	B, C
7.00 pm-11.59 pm (counts/min)	391.9	244.4	362.1-422.0	382.7	211.6	342.8-426.1	341.6	151.2	305.5-377.4	382.4	225.7	360.5-404.9	0.301	

TABLE 4: Cont.

	Normal weight (n=241)	sd	95% CI	Over-weight (n=93)	sd	95% CI	Obese (n=57)	sd	95% CI	Total (n=391)	sd	95% CI	P value (AN-COVA)	Post-hoc (Bon-ferroni)
Weekends														
MVPA (min/day)	60.4	32.6	56.6-64.4	55.2	30.5	49.4-61.5	46.9	29.7	39.6-55.3	57.2	32.0	54.1-60.2	0.012	C
Sedentary (min/day)	572.3	185.8	549.9-597.2	512.6	133.1	487.0-538.4	518.0	140.8	484.9-554.1	550.1	170.4	534.0-567.9	0.005	A
Total activity (counts/min)	488.3	209.4	462.3-515.9	476.6	189.2	439.5-516.1	436.2	188.0	387.8-487.2	477.9	202.0	458.4-499.4	0.206	
5.30 am-8.29 am (counts/min)	382.6	522.0	310.6-468.4	465.7	464.0	365.4-581.3	344.2	281.5	266.8-427.9	396.4	479.5	341.8-455.4	0.316	
8.30 am-1.59 pm (counts/min)	567.7	289.1	533.0-605.4	617.9	341.8	549.5-684.4	484.4	231.4	430.3-541.5	567.5	297.1	538.5-598.5	0.028	B
2.00 pm-6.59 pm (counts/min)	578.9	324.9	542.2-625.2	495.8	224.2	449.3-542.9	486.5	269.0	422.0-562.5	545.6	298.1	517.8-575.8	0.017	A
7.00 pm-11.59 pm (counts/min)	329.0	193.7	301.6-356.6	306.5	151.9	273.7-337.6	373.2	255.0	312.1-448.8	330.0	195.4	309.3-350.3	0.168	

TABLE 4: *Cont.*

	Normal weight	sd	95% CI	Over-weight	sd	95% CI	Obese	sd	95% CI	Total	sd	95% CI	P value (AN-COVA)	Post-hoc (Bon-ferroni)
Girls														
Weekdays	(n=280)			(n=64)			(n=54)			(n=398)				
MVPA (min/day)	44.1	15.7	42.4-46.1	43.7	13.5	40.3-47.0	38.3	11.5	35.2-41.5	43.3	14.9	41.9-44.8	0.032	C
Sedentary (min/day)	603.4	96.6	592.2-614.7	583.6	75.7	565.3-602.3	610.3	125.0	580.7-644.8	601.2	98.1	591.3-610.2	0.21	
Total activity (counts/min)	387.8	103.4	375.5-400.0	393.2	95.5	369.5-418.5	351.3	93.1	327.3-376.8	383.7	101.4	374.4-393.4	0.034	C
5.30 am-8.29 am (counts/min)	430.7	187.6	409.6-454.0	423.9	177.1	383.0-473.3	436.6	164.3	391.8-481.2	430.4	182.5	412.3-448.9	0.956	
8.30 am-1.59 pm (counts/min)	365.5	122.3	352.3-379.8	354.8	105.4	331.6-381.6	345.3	114.9	316.2-377.5	361.0	118.7	350.1-372.3	0.466	
2.00 pm-6.59 pm (counts/min)	453.5	170.5	432.9-474.1	467.4	166.0	429.8-504.3	386.6	128.1	352.8-422.6	446.6	166.1	431.1-462.7	0.012	B, C
7.00 pm-11.59 pm (counts/min)	335.1	194.6	312.5-357.9	327.2	163.1	289.2-369.9	288.8	128.4	255.1-321.5	327.5	182.4	309.3-345.4	0.234	
Weekends	(n=267)			(n=61)			(n=50)			(n=378)				

TABLE 4: Cont.

	Normal weight	sd	95% CI	Over-weight	sd	95% CI	Obese	sd	95% CI	Total	sd	95% CI	P value (AN-COVA)	Post-hoc (Bon-ferroni)
MVPA (min/day)	41.8	22.8	39.0-44.5	38.2	17.1	34.3-42.4	33.7	17.4	29.1-38.6	40.1	21.4	38.0-42.4	0.049	C
Sedentary (min/day)	558.3	155.6	540.1-577.4	549.3	158.3	510.4-593.7	556.0	175.1	510.4-604.6	556.6	158.4	540.7-572.9	0.921	
Total activity (counts/min)	397.1	166.5	376.8-417.3	386.7	154.4	348.8-428.2	345.7	137.5	309.4-382.7	388.6	161.6	372.1-405.4	0.143	
5.30 am-8.29 am (counts/min)	385.2	549.9	312.6-467.1	279.2	257.1	194.2-369.6	474.2	601.0	322.4-720.1	381.8	527.4	321.2-450.6	0.299	
8.30 am-1.59 pm (counts/min)	444.0	209.6	418.6-469.1	418.5	191.5	372.9-466.7	373.9	162.7	331.7-419.2	430.7	202.1	410.2-450.9	0.084	
2.00 pm-6.59 pm (counts/min)	457.1	259.0	427.5-491.4	426.4	267.1	367.6-496.6	366.6	188.3	317.9-418.1	440.3	253.5	414.9-468.3	0.073	
7.00 pm-11.59 pm (counts/min)	306.9	212.2	281.0-332.7	318.8	178.1	273.6-366.7	279.8	147.1	236.4-324.2	305.2	199.1	284.7-328.2	0.563	

*A = Normal weight vs overweight p < .05. B = Overweight vs obese p < .05. C = Normal weight vs obese p < .05.

In this study we found that a low percentage of children, particularly girls meet daily PA guidelines. As found in other studies, girls were less active than boys throughout the week [29,30] stressing the need to provide them with more opportunities for physical activity, while aiming to raise the levels of activity of all the children. Verloigne et al. attributed these gender differences to the social context at particular time-periods [31]. Boys might be dominating playgrounds at school, and girls prefer to socialise during breaks [32], while after school, parents might be considering neighbourhoods to be safe for boys, but not for girls [33].

In contrast to previous research [29,30,34], the overall patterns of activity on weekends were not different from weekdays. Although children spend almost half their waking time at school, we found that they were only engaged in a quarter of the recommended hour of MVPA. Schools have been described as the providers of the best opportunity for a population-based approach to increasing physical activity [35]. Therefore adopting a whole school approach to increase physical activity through the development and implementation of physical activity policies is a priority. Girls should also be encouraged to be as active as boys and activities should be made appealing to them. Thirty minutes of daily MVPA at school is an achievable target for all children. This could be partly achieved through daily physical education lessons where at least 50% of the time is spent in MVPA, and this will result in long term benefits through the development of physical literacy which is key for lifelong physical activity. Introducing active breaks in class could also increase activity levels while having potential to stimulate improved academic performance [36]. As recommended by several researchers [37] more activity can be done during recess, when children can engage in up to twenty minutes of MVPA.

In the current dataset, the after school period provided only a few more minutes of activity than during school time. Half an hour of MVPA during this period [38,39], would result in children accumulating a total of one hour of daily MVPA. After-school sport programmes specifically targeting girls may provide one solution, together with more opportunities for unstructured play and access to open areas in the community. Furthermore, as suggested by Jago et al. [40], encouraging girls to support their friends' activity is important in order to help them sustain PA levels during periods of transition from primary to secondary schools. More opportunities for girls to be active on weekends, when they are about 15 minutes less active than boys, could be considered, although this would require strategies to engage parental support. Finally, another time-period when activity was very low is the period before school, when children can be encouraged to walk to school or be active while they wait outside or inside the school premises.

Weight category differences during periods after school hours might suggest the need for specific interventions to increase PA after school among overweight children. Although differences in total activity by weight status during school hours were not significant, the school still remains the place where activity for obese children can be increased, where they can gain the skills and confidence for being active outside school hours and throughout their life. Establishing a link between schools and clubs to encourage children of all abilities and sizes to become active would help. Holding such clubs on the school premises might provide a more reassuring environment for obese children, while providing more opportunities for unstructured play and physical activity in the community is also needed.

4.4.1 STRENGTHS AND LIMITATIONS

The strength of this study is its use of objective measurement of physical activity and weight status with a nationally representative sample of Maltese 10–11 year olds. A large percentage of the sample selected (80%) accepted to participate in this study, however a limitation might be that we do not know the weight status of those who did not provide consent. It is usually parents of obese children who refuse consent in studies on obesity [41]. Therefore if this is the case, the sample may be under representative of overweight and obese children. Although accelerometry has been used to provide measures of intensity and duration of physical activity, current data cannot describe what the participants are doing while they are sedentary or active and cannot assess some activities like swimming and cycling. This study has used Evenson's cutpoints and other higher accelerometer cutpoints would have produced lower prevalences of children meeting PA guidelines. A further limitation was that we were not able to calculate energy expenditure and the results provide simple estimates of movement. This underestimates the energy expenditure during activity of children who are heavier. Screen time was self-reported, and considering that children engage in many different types of screen time, the measure is likely to lack precision and accuracy. It is important to recognise that other factors including socio-economic position could also have affected the associations found in this study. We relied on evidence of the reliability and validity of sections of the questionnaire from other studies and cannot confirm how robust the measures were in our sample. Children were classified into different weight categories using the IOTF standards, and although these standards are used in many studies for international comparison, another study in Malta [14] has shown that these standards produce lower prevalence of overweight and obesity compared to WHO standards.

4.5 CONCLUSIONS

A low percentage of Maltese 10–11 year olds (39% of boys, 10% of girls), particularly girls, reached the recommended levels of daily MVPA and spent large amounts of time engaged in screen time. Obese children were less active than non-obese children, reaching significance at particular key periods during the week and also had higher levels of screen time. As children spend most of their waking time at school and that activity during this time is less than one third of the daily requirements, aiming to increase MVPA at school for all Maltese children is likely to be important and strategies to promote MVPA during this time periods may be helpful.

REFERENCES

1. Strong WB, Malina RM, Blimkie CJ, Daniels SR, Dishman RK, Gutin B, Hergenroeder AC, Must A, Nixon PA, Pivarnik JM, Rowland T, Trost S, Trudeau F: Evidence based physical activity for school-age youth. J Pediatr 2005, 146(6):732-737.
2. Van Lippevelde W, Te Velde SJ, Verloigne M, Van Stralen MM, De Bourdeaudhuij I, Manios Y, Bere E, Vik FN, Jan N, Fernandez Alvira JM, Chinapaw MJ, Bringof-Isler B, Kovacs E, Brug J, Maes L: Associations between family-related factors, breakfast consumption and BMI among 10- to 12-year-old European children: the cross-sectional ENERGY-study. PLoS One 2013, 8(11):e79550.

3. Currie C, Zanotti C, Morgan A, Currie D, de Looze M, Roberts C, Samdal O, Smith ORF, Barnekow V: Social determinants of health and well-being among young people. Health Behaviour in School-Aged children (HBSC) Study: International Report from the 2009/2010 survey. In Health Policy for Children and Adolescents. Copenhagen: WHO Regional Office for Europe; 2012.
4. Tremblay MS, Leblanc AG, Janssen I, Kho ME, Hicks A, Murumets K, Colley RC, Duggan M: Canadian sedentary behaviour guidelines for children and youth. Appl Physiol Nutr Metab 2011, 36(1):59-64.
5. Wareham NJ, Van Sluijs EM, Ekelund U: Physical activity and obesity prevention: a review of the current evidence. Proc Nutr Soc 2005, 64(2):229-247.
6. Prentice-Dunn H, Prentice-Dunn S: Physical activity, sedentary behavior, and childhood obesity: a review of cross-sectional studies. Psychol Health Med 2012, 17(3):255-273.
7. Verloigne M, Van Lippevelde W, Maes L, Yildirim M, Chinapaw M, Manios Y, Androutsos O, Kovacs E, Bringolf-Isler B, Brug J, De Bourdeaudhuij I: Self-reported TV and computer time do not represent accelerometer-derived total sedentary time in 10 to 12-year-olds. Eur J Public Health 2013, 23(1):30-32.
8. Jago R, Baranowski T, Baranowski JC, Thompson D, Greaves KA: BMI from 3–6 y of age is predicted by TV viewing and physical activity, not diet. Int J Obes (Lond) 2005, 29(6):557-564.
9. Tremblay MS, LeBlanc AG, Kho ME, Saunders TJ, Larouche R, Colley RC, Goldfield G, Connor Gorber S: Systematic review of sedentary behaviour and health indicators in school-aged children and youth. Int J Behav Nutr Phys Act 2011, 8:98.
10. Prince SA, Adamo KB, Hamel ME, Hardt J, Gorber SC, Tremblay M: A comparison of direct versus self-report measures for assessing physical activity in adults: a systematic review. Int J Behav Nutr Phys Act 2008, 5:56.
11. Sherry B, Jefferds ME, Grummer-Strawn LM: Accuracy of adolescent self-report of height and weight in assessing overweight status: a literature review. Arch Pediatr Adolesc Med 2007, 161(12):1154-1161.
12. Currie C, Gabhainn SN, Godeau E, Roberts C, Smith R, Currie D, Picket W, Richter M, Morgan A, Barnekow V: Inequalities in young people: HBSC International Report from the 2005–06 survey. In Health Policy for children and adolescents, No5. Edinburgh: World Health Organisation; 2008.
13. Decelis A, Jago R, Fox KR: Objectively assessed physical activity and weight status in Maltese 11–12 year-olds. Eur J Sport Sci 2014, 14(Suppl 1):S257-S266.
14. Decelis A, Fox K, Jago R: Prevalence of obesity among 10-11-year-old Maltese children using four established standards. Pediatr Obes 2013, 8(5):e54-e58.
15. Liu Y, Wang M, Tynjala J, Lv Y, Villberg J, Zhang Z, Kannas L: Test-retest reliability of selected items of Health Behaviour in School-aged Children (HBSC) survey questionnaire in Beijing, China. BMC Med Res Methodol 2010, 10:73.
16. American Academy of Pediatrics: Children, adolescents, and television. Pediatrics 2001, 107(2):423-426.
17. Cole TJ, Bellizzi MC, Flegal KM, Dietz WH: Establishing a standard definition for child overweight and obesity worldwide: international survey. BMJ 2000, 320(7244):1240-1243.

18. Reilly JJ, Penpraze V, Hislop J, Davies G, Grant S, Paton JY: Objective measurement of physical activity and sedentary behaviour: review with new data. Arch Dis Child 2008, 93(7):614-619.
19. Troiano RP, Berrigan D, Dodd KW, Masse LC, Tilert T, McDowell M: Physical activity in the United States measured by accelerometer. Med Sci Sports Exerc 2008, 40(1):181-188.
20. Van Sluijs EM, Skidmore PM, Mwanza K, Jones AP, Callaghan AM, Ekelund U, Harrison F, Harvey I, Panter J, Wareham NJ, Cassidy A, Griffin SJ: Physical activity and dietary behaviour in a population-based sample of British 10-year old children: the SPEEDY study (Sport, Physical activity and Eating behaviour: environmental Determinants in Young people). BMC Public Health 2008, 8:388.
21. Evenson KR, Catellier DJ, Gill K, Ondrak KS, McMurray RG: Calibration of two objective measures of physical activity for children. J Sports Sci 2008, 26(14):1557-1565.
22. Trost SG, Loprinzi PD, Moore R, Pfeiffer KA: Comparison of accelerometer cut points for predicting activity intensity in youth. Med Sci Sports Exerc 2011, 43(7):1360-1368.
23. Trost SG, McCoy TA, Vander Veur SS, Mallya G, Duffy ML, Foster GD: Physical activity patterns of inner-city elementary schoolchildren. Med Sci Sports Exerc 2013, 45(3):470-474.
24. Telford RM, Telford RD, Cunningham RB, Cochrane T, Davey R, Waddington G: Longitudinal patterns of physical activity in children aged 8 to 12 years: the LOOK study. Int J Behav Nutr Phys Act 2013, 10:91. doi:10.1186/1479-5868-10-81
25. Cooper AR, Jago R, Southward EF, Page AS: Active travel and physical activity across the school transition: the PEACH project. Med Sci Sports Exerc 2012, 44(10):1890-1897.
26. Mitchell JA, Pate RR, Beets MW, Nader PR: Time spent in sedentary behavior and changes in childhood BMI: a longitudinal study from ages 9 to 15 years. Int J Obes (Lond) 2013, 37(1):54-60.
27. American Academy of Pediatrics: American Academy of Pediatrics: Children, adolescents, and television. Pediatrics 2001, 107(2):423-426.
28. Wilks DC, Sharp SJ, Ekelund U, Thompson SG, Mander AP, Turner RM, Jebb SA, Lindroos AK: Objectively measured physical activity and fat mass in children: a bias-adjusted meta-analysis of prospective studies. PLoS One 2011, 6(2):e17205.
29. Rowlands AV, Pilgrim EL, Eston RG: Patterns of habitual activity across weekdays and weekend days in 9-11-year-old children. Prev Med 2008, 46(4):317-324.
30. Konharn K, Santos MP, Ribeiro JC: Differences between weekday and weekend levels of moderate-to-vigorous physical activity in Thai adolescents. Asia Pac J Public Health 2012. doi:10.1177/1010539512459946
31. Verloigne M, Van Lippevelde W, Maes L, Yildirim M, Chinapaw M, Manios Y, Androutsos O, Kovacs E, Bringolf-Isler B, Brug J, De Bourdeaudhuij I: Levels of physical activity and sedentary time among 10- to 12-year-old boys and girls across 5 European countries using accelerometers: an observational study within the ENERGY-project. Int J Behav Nutr Phys Act 2012, 9:34.
32. Boyle DE, Marshall NL, Robeson WW: Gender at play - Fourth-grade girls and boys on the playground. Am Behav Sci 2003, 46(10):1326-1345.

33. Carver A, Timperio A, Crawford D: Perceptions of neighborhood safety and physical activity among youth: the CLAN study. J Phys Act Health 2008, 5(3):430-444.
34. Treuth MS, Catellier DJ, Schmitz KH, Pate RR, Elder JP, McMurray RG, Blew RM, Yang S, Webber L: Weekend and weekday patterns of physical activity in overweight and normal-weight adolescent girls. Obesity (Silver Spring) 2007, 15(7):1782-1788.
35. Institute of Medicine: Preventing Childhood Obesity: Health in the Balance. Washington, D.C.: Institute of Medicine; 2004.
36. White PD, Goldsmith KA, Johnson AL, Potts L, Walwyn R, DeCesare JC, Baber HL, Burgess M, Clark LV, Cox DL, Bavinton J, Angus BJ, Murphy G, Murphy M, O'Dowd H, Wilks D, McCrone P, Chalder T, Sharpe M: Comparison of adaptive pacing therapy, cognitive behaviour therapy, graded exercise therapy, and specialist medical care for chronic fatigue syndrome (PACE): a randomised trial. Lancet 2011, 377(9768):823-836.
37. Ridgers ND, Stratton G, Fairclough SJ: Physical activity levels of children during school playtime. Sports Med 2006, 36(4):359-371.
38. Olds T, Wake M, Patton G, Ridley K, Waters E, Williams J, Hesketh K: How do school-day activity patterns differ with age and gender across adolescence? J Adolesc Health 2009, 44(1):64-72.
39. Tudor-Locke C, Lee SM, Morgan CF, Beighle A, Pangrazi RP: Children's pedometer-determined physical activity during the segmented school day. Med Sci Sports Exerc 2006, 38(10):1732-1738.
40. Jago R, Page AS, Cooper AR: Friends and physical activity during the transition from primary to secondary school. Med Sci Sports Exerc 2012, 44(1):111-117.
41. Mellor JM, Rapoport RB, Maliniak D: The impact of child obesity on active parental consent in school-based survey research on healthy eating and physical activity. Eval Rev 2008, 32(3):298-312.

Table 5 is not available in this version of the article. To view this additional information, please use the citation on the first page of this chapter.

CHAPTER 5

IMPULSIVITY, "ADVERGAMES," AND FOOD INTAKE

FRANS FOLKVORD, DOESCHKA J. ANSCHÜTZ, CHANTAL NEDERKOORN, HENK WESTERIK, AND MONIEK BUIJZEN

Rates of childhood obesity have increased greatly in the past 3 decades. [1] Although the causes of this trend are multifaceted, there is growing evidence that food commercials are a major contributor. [2] Food consumption can be activated by salient environmental cues in an automatic and difficult to control way. [3] Content analyses reveal that the majority of food products promoted are energy-dense and high in fat, sugar, and/or salt, which is in sharp contrast to (inter)national dietary guidelines. [2]

Cue reactivity theory states that food cues induce craving for food and actual eating behavior owing to the presence of sensory inputs associated with past consumption. [4,5] The sight, smell, or thought of tasty food induces appetite, and insuffcient inhibitory control causes failure in inhibition, leading to increased food intake. [6,7] Impaired behavioral inhibition (ie, impulsivity) might make it more difficult for children to resist the temptation of energy-dense food. [8,9] Impulsivity is generally defined as the tendency to control, think, and plan insufficiently. [10] Two aspects of

---

Reproduced with permission from Pediatrics, *Vol. 133, Page(s) 1007–1012, Copyright © 2014 by the AAP. Impulsivity, "Advergames," and Food Intake. Folkvord F, Anschütz DJ, Nederkoorn C, Westerik H, and Buijzen M. Pediatrics, **133**,6 (2014). doi: 10.1542/peds.2013-3384.*

impulsivity can be distinguished: insufficient inhibitory behavioral control and reward sensitivity or the inability to delay reward. [11] Being able to control impulsive behaviors can be an important explanation for the individual susceptibility to food advertisements, but this has not been examined before.

The objective of this study is to examine the role of impulsivity in the effect of advergames promoting energy-dense snacks on children's snack consumption. Advergames are online electronic games that are used to advertise a product or a brand. [12–14] Online games provide a highly involving, interactive, and entertaining brand experience. [12] We hypothesize that (H1) playing advergames promoting energy-dense snacks increases caloric intake, (H2a) stimulating response inhibition by rewarding refraining from eating decreases caloric intake, and (H2b) children who are rewarded for refraining from eating have a lower caloric intake when they play a nonfood advergame than when they play a food advergame. We also expect that (H3) impulsive children eat more. Specifically, we expect (H4) that rewarding refraining will have less influence on high impulsive children, especially when they are playing a food advergame.

5.1 METHODS

5.1.1 STUDY DESIGN

We used a factorial between-subject design: 2 (type of advergame: energy-dense snacks versus nonfood products) × 2 (inhibition task: reward to refrain from eating versus no reward) × 2 (impulsivity: high versus low). The dependent variable was caloric intake. While playing, 2 bowls of energy-dense snacks were presented: (1) jelly candy (cola bottles) and (2) milk chocolate candy shells. The jelly candy were identical to 1 of the food products shown in the advergame promoting energy-dense snacks.

We counterbalanced and randomly assigned children to 1 of 4 conditions, which involved playing [1] the energy-dense snacks advergame (ie, promoting a popular candy brand and 8 different sweets from this candy brand) without the inhibition task [2]; the energy-dense snacks advergame with the inhibition task [3]; the nonfood advergame (ie, promoting a popu-

Impulsivity, "Advergames," and Food Intake

lar Dutch toy brand and 8 individual toys from this brand) without the inhibition task [4]; and the nonfood advergame with the inhibition task. All games were identical, except for the advertised brands and products. The game involved an online memory game with 16 cards, whereby brand name and logos appeared on the back of the cards, and the individual products appeared on the front. These products clearly displayed the brand logos. For the candy products we used high-quality images of gummy cola bottles, bananas, cherries, frogs, licorice, and other gummy and jelly sweets. For the toys we used images of a trampoline, keyboard, basketball, teddy bear, drum kit, and other toys from this brand. Cards were laid out in a grid face down. On each turn, the child turned 1 card over, then a second. If the 2 cards matched, they remained open. If they did not match, the cards were turned back over and the child got another turn. The goal was to match the pairs of cards. When cards were turned over, it was important to remember where they were for when the matching card turned up later in the game. To enhance awareness of the brand, we showed it on the right side of the screen. To immerse the children into the game by exerting time pressure with a digital timer top-left of the screen and a time bar top-center of the screen. Furthermore, the game played an unpleasant sound when a child selected a false pair and a pleasant sound with a correct pair. The experimenter left the room every time the children played the advergame.

5.1.2 MEASURES

5.1.2.1 IMPULSIVITY

Impulsivity is a multifaceted construct, in which roughly 2 aspects can be distinguished: reward sensitivity and insufficient inhibitory behavioral control. [15] To measure impulsivity we used the door-opening task, which has been specially developed to measure reward sensitivity in young individuals, differentiating between normal children and children who have impulsive disorders like attention deficit hyperactivity disorder and conduct disorder. [16–19] The experimenter told the child that the aim of the task was to earn as many points as possible. When the child opened a door revealing a yellow smiley face the child received a point, but when the door revealed a blue sad smiley face, the child lost a point. In total, there were 90 doors to open. The tasks started with a 90% chance of winning, which decreased with 10% after every 10 doors. The chance was therefore 50% after 40 doors, being the most profitable moment to stop the game. Children who opened more than 40 doors were considered as highly impulsive. Because the child's aim was to earn as many points as possible, he or she should quit opening doors once the probability of a winning door dropped below 50%. When children continued the game, the chances of losing increased and winning decreased. If the child keeps opening doors in search for reward despite punishment, the reward system is considered dominant. [19]

5.1.2.2 BMI

We calculated BMI, measured as weight (kg)/height^2 (m). We measured weight to the nearest 0.1 kg and height to the nearest 0.5 cm while the children were wearing clothing but no shoes. We calculated whether the children were underweight, normal weight, overweight, or obese using international cut-off scores. [20]

5.1.2.3 CALORIC INTAKE

We weighed the amount of snack food that a child ate before each child entered the room and again after eating. We used a professional balance scale to estimate to the nearest 0.1 g. We calculated the number of grams that a child ate in kilocalories (kcal) for use as a dependent measure. The amount of energy-dense snack food that a child ate was the sum of the caloric intake of jelly candy and milk chocolate candy.

5.1.2.4 HUNGER

We controlled for individual differences in hunger by presenting the children with a visual analog scale (VAS; 14 cm) measuring the extent to which they felt hungry before the experiment began. The anchors were "not hungry at all" and "very hungry." VAS's have been used successfully and extensively to assess subjective appetite sensations, like hunger, prospective food consumption, and fullness in children. [14,21–23] Furthermore, VAS was compared with Likert scale measurements among children and found to be of comparable reliability. [24]

Attitude toward brand and foods shown in the advergames was assessed with 6 items (nice, stupid, tasteful, untasteful, cool, boring) on a VAS scale. This measurement has been established by Holbrook and Batra, [25] and tested extensively among (young) children [14,26] At the end of the experiment, we asked the children to indicate the goal of the research, but no child gave the correct answer.

5.1.3 SUBJECTS

Subjects were 266 children (grades 2–3) from 5 primary schools in the Netherlands. We obtained approval from the institute's ethical committee for social sciences and obtained informed consent from the schools and parents. More than 93% of the children were allowed to participate. Data collection occurred between January 2013 and March 2013. The experimenter brought 1 child to a separate classroom containing a computer where they started with an online questionnaire to assess gender, age, and pre-experimental hunger. Subsequently the child conducted the door-opening task and after this task played 1 version of the advergames. The child was instructed that (s)he would be playing a memory game for 5 minutes and should attempt to finish as many games as possible, which were unlimited. Then the experimenter placed the bowls with food and a glass of water at the same table as the computer. The experimenter told the children without the inhibition task that (s)he could eat as much as (s)he wanted, and the children with the inhibition task that (s)he could eat as much as (s)he wanted but that if (s)he would eat nothing (s)he would get a reward afterward. Further instructions stated that after each game, the time bar would stop, and the score would appear; then the time would continue when the new game started. The child signaled the experimenter when the game stopped after 5 minutes. To give the children an opportunity to snack, the children had a small break of 30 seconds after 2 finished games before they could start the next game. Subsequently, the second part of the questionnaire was filled out and length and height were measured. The experimenter asked all children to refrain from discussing the experiment with their classmates. After all children had finished participation, they were allowed to choose a pencil as reward. The children did not receive the reward immediately after the experiment and all children got the reward. After each session, the experimenter weighed the bowls to calculate caloric intake and refilled them before the next child entered.

TABLE 1: Variables Measured, By Condition

	Energy-Dense Snack Without Inhibition Task (n = 69)	Energy-Dense Snack With Inhibition Task (n = 65)	Nonfood Without Inhibition Task (n = 62)	Nonfood With Inhibition Task (n = 65)
Gender (boy = 1, girl = 0)	0.55 (0.5)	0.43 (0.5)	0.47 (0.5)	0.54 (0.5)
Hunger on VAS (cm)	2.8 (3.6)	3.7 (3.9)	3.6 (4.5)	3.2 (4.0)
Age (y)	7.8 (0.8)	7.8 (0.7)	7.7 (0.7)	7.6 (0.7)
BMI, corrected (kg/m^2)	1.25 (0.4)	1.29 (0.5)	1.16 (0.4)	1.29 (0.5)
Impulsivity	39.3 (28.9)	38.8 (26.2)	36.9 (28.5)	36.9 (25.5)
Total energy intake (kcal)	156.3 (135.2)	87.3 (114.3)	101.3 (74.1)	33.2 (74.4)

5.1.4 STATISTICAL ANALYSIS

Randomization checks using a 1-factor ANOVA were conducted for gender, hunger, age, BMI, impulsivity, and kcal energy intake (Table 1). Outlying scores on caloric intake were examined by computing residual scores and testing them for Mahal's distance, Cook's distance, and leverage scores, showing no indications for outlying scores. The main effects of type of advergame, impulsivity, and inhibition task were tested with analysis of covariance. An additional analysis of covariance tested the interaction effects between type of advergame, inhibition task, and impulsivity. Bonferroni-corrected post hoc test was used to examine the differences between the experimental conditions. We calculated effect sizes for Cohen's f and Cohen's d.

5.2 RESULTS

5.2.1 DESCRIPTIVES

The final sample consisted of 261 children, 50.2% boys. We excluded 5 children from the analyses because they had not finished the session (n = 3) or teachers had interrupted (n = 2). In our sample, 3.8% of children were underweight, 71.3% normal weight, 18.4% overweight, and 6.5% obese.

We found no differences between the experimental conditions for gender, hunger, BMI, age, and impulsivity. Brand recognition and attitudes toward the game, striving for the reward, and how much they wanted the reward did not differ between the type of advergame.

5.2.2 MAIN ANALYSES

Results confirmed our first hypothesis 1H showing a significant effect of type of advergame on caloric intake ($P < 0.01$) (Table 2). Children who played an advergame promoting energy-dense snacks ate significantly more ($P < 0.01$) than children who played an advergame promoting nonfood products. Children who were hungrier ate more ($P < 0.05$). Hypothesis H2a was also confirmed, showing a significant effect of the inhibition task on caloric intake ($P < .01$). Children who played 1 of the advergames without the inhibition task ate more than the children who played an advergame with the inhibition task. The post hoc results confirmed H2b, showing that children who played the advergame promoting energy-dense snacks with the inhibition task ate significantly more ($P < 0.01$) than the children who played the nonfood advergame with the inhibition task. Furthermore, we found that children who played the advergame promoting energy-dense snacks with the inhibition task had a lower caloric intake

(P < 0.01) compared with children who played the advergame promoting energy-dense snacks without the inhibition task. Children who played the advergame promoting nonfood products with the inhibition task ate less (P < 0.01) than children who played the nonfood advergame without the inhibition task. In contrast with H3, which stated that impulsive children would eat more, we found no effect for impulsivity (P > 0.05).

TABLE 2: Results From 2 Univariate Analyses of Covariance With Total Energy Intake as a Dependent Variable (n = 261)

	Total Energy Intake (kcal)	
Gender (boy = 1, girl = 0)	$F(1, 252) = 2.043$	$F(1, 248) = 1.369$
Hunger on VAS (cm)	$F(1, 252) = 5.046^a$	$F(1, 248) = 4.375^a$
Age (y)	$F(1, 252) = 1.310$	$F(1, 248) = 1.862$
BMI, corrected (kg/m²)	$F(1, 252) = 0.786$	$F(1, 248) = 0.510$
Advergames	$F(1, 252) = 18.541^b$	$F(1, 248) = 16.162^b$
Inhibition task	$F(1, 252) = 31.325^b$	$F(1, 248) = 26.439^b$
Impulsivity	$F(1, 252) = 2.704$	$F(1, 248) = 2.206$
Advergame*inhibition task		$F(1, 248) = 0.017$
Advergames*impulsivity		$F(1, 248) = 2.717$
Inhibition task*impulsivity		$F(1, 248) = 5.932^a$
Advergames*inhibition task*impulsivity		$F(1, 248) = 4.364^a$
Effect size[c]	0.18	0.22
Explained variance (%)	17.9	21.1

[a] $P < 0.05$. [b] $P < .01$. [c] Cohen's f.

Finally, we expected (H4) that rewarding refraining would have less influence on high impulsive children, particularly when they were playing an advergame promoting energy-dense snacks. Results showed that the 3-way interaction was significant (P < 0.05), shown in Table 2. Bonferroni corrected post hoc test (Table 3) showed that there was no difference for general caloric intake (P > .05) between the high impulsive children who played the advergame promoting energy-dense snacks with the inhibition task compared with the children without the inhibition task. In contrast, results showed that impulsive children who played the advergame promoting nonfood products with the inhibition task had a significantly lower caloric intake (P < 0.05) than those without the inhibition task. Low impulsive children who played the advergame promoting energy-dense snacks with the inhibition task had a significantly lower caloric intake (P < .01) than those without the inhibition task. Finally, low impulsive children who played the advergame promoting nonfood products with the inhibition task had a lower caloric intake (P < .01) than the children who did not have this inhibition task.

TABLE 3: Adjusted Means and SDs of Food Intake (in kcal) Controlled for Gender, Hunger, and Age, By Condition and Impulsivity (n = 261)

	Low Impulsivity[a]			High Impulsivity[b]		
	No Inhibition Task	With Inhibition Task		No Inhibition Task	With Inhibition Task	
Advergame promoting energy-dense snack	203.0* ± 16.4 (n = 37)	76.7† ± 16.0 (n = 39)	P < .001	104.6* ± 18.1 (n = 31)	94.6† ± 19.9 (n = 26)	P > .05
Advergame promoting nonfood products	101.9‡ ± 15.9 (n = 40)	32.4§ ± 15.5 (n = 42)	P < .001	99.4‡ ± 21.4 (n = 23)	39.2§ ± 21.0 (n = 23)	P < .05

[a] *ANOVA post hoc pairwise comparisons (Bonferroni) with food intake as the dependent variable showed significant differences between * and † (P < .001, Cohen's d = 0.97), and between ‡ and § (P < .001, Cohen's d = 0.91).* [b] *ANOVA post hoc pairwise comparisons (Bonferroni) with food intake as the dependent variable showed no significant differences between * and † (P > .05), and showed a significant difference between ‡ and § (P < .05, Cohen's d = 0.81).*

5.3 DISCUSSION

This is the first study examining the role of impulsivity in the effect of food advertisements on actual snack intake among young children. We found that food cues in advergames triggered eating behavior and that rewarding children to refrain from eating decreased caloric intake in both types of advergames, thereby supporting hypotheses 1 and 2a. From the children who were rewarded, children who played the food advergame ate more than the children who played the nonfood advergame, confirming hypothesis 2b. Impulsive children did not eat more than less impulsive children, which refutes hypothesis 3. Finally, we found that rewarding children to refrain from eating had less influence on high impulsive children than on low impulsive children, especially when they were playing an advergame promoting energy-dense snacks, supporting hypothesis 4. These findings imply that impulsive children have difficulties self-regulating their caloric intake during a food advertisement when they are rewarded to refrain from eating, but not when they are facing a nonfood advertisement. Furthermore, we found that less impulsive children had a lower caloric intake when they were rewarded to refrain from eating in both type of advergames. These latter findings mark the individual susceptibility to food advertising, which is a very interesting insight.

Cue reactivity theory states that food-related cues (eg, the sight or smell of food) act as conditioned stimuli that trigger conditioned responses, like craving and actual eating behavior. [4] This may mean that exposure to food-related cues results in cephalic phase responses and strong desires to eat, preparing children for food intake. Increased impulsivity might make it more difficult for children to resist the temptation of energy-dense food when craving for food is elicited by food commercials. This reasoning is in line with our hypotheses and earlier findings. [8,27,28] A remarkable finding was that low impulsive children playing the energy-dense advergame ate more than high impulsive children playing the same game when they were not asked to refrain from eating. A possible explanation is that conducting subsequent tasks may have led to a state of ego depletion. The high impulsive children did not inhibit their responses during the impulsivity task to the same extent as the low impulsive children. The latter were more successful in inhibiting their responses during the impulsivity task. Consequently, after successfully controlling reward sensitivity during the impulsivity task, a decrease in self-control could have occurred among the low impulsive children. [29]

Besides the large sample size, a strength of this study is its high external validity, as the advergames used are identical or comparable to advergames used by many (food) companies. Advergames are interactive entertainment, which makes it more difficult for children to recognize commercial message in the game. Because cognitive capacity is directed to playing the game, there is not enough capacity to think critically about the purpose of the game. [30] Moreover, we were able to test a large number of children and we successfully manipulated response inhibition so that we could conduct adequate analyses to examine the role of self-regulation when stimulated to inhibit responses during a food commercial.

5.4 CONCLUSIONS

This study showed that exposure to food cues in advergames influences caloric intake and that these food cues hamper self-regulation when young children are rewarded to refrain from eating. Children who played the advergame promoting energy-dense snacks did not report less motivation to self-regulate response inhibition, so an explanation could be that the food cues in the advergame signaled food intake, which led to failures in self-regulation of snack intake. Furthermore, impulsive children showed more difficulties in refraining from eating while playing an advergame promoting energy-dense snacks, supporting concerns from scholars that food commercials contribute to vulnerable children's snacking. [13] Future research should focus on whether children can be tutored by their parents to self-regulate their snack intake during or after advertising exposure. Active advertising-related parenting training children to cope with persuasive intentions of food advertisements can reduce undesired advertising effects. [31] Studies have shown that training self-regulation to control impulses for food is successful in learning adolescents and adults to control their food intake after temptations and tempting snacks, [32,33] so we might expect that children can also be trained to self-regulate their snack intake. A final recommendation to parents is reducing the availability of snack foods at home.

REFERENCES

1. Han JC, Lawlor DA, Kimm SYS. Childhood obesity. Lancet. 2010;375(9727):1737–1748
2. World Health Organization. WHO Report on Diet, Nutrition and the Prevention of Chronic Disease. Joint WHO/FAO Expert Consultation WHO Technical Report Series. Geneva, Switzerland: World Health Organization; 2003
3. Cohen DA. Neurophysiological pathways to obesity: below awareness and beyond individual control. Diabetes. 2008;57(7):1768–1773
4. Coelho JS, Jansen A, Roefs A, Nederkoorn C. Eating behavior in response to food-cue exposure: examining the cue-reactivity and counteractive-control models. Psychol Addict Behav. 2009;23(1):131–139
5. Jansen A. A learning model of binge eating: cue reactivity and cue exposure. Behav Res Ther. 1998;36(3):257–272
6. Jansen A, Nederkoorn C, van Baak L, Keirse C, Guerrieri R, Havermans R. High-restrained eaters only overeat when they are also impulsive. Behav Res Ther. 2009;47(2):105–110
7. Hofmann W, Malte F, Roefs A. Three ways to resist temptation: the independent contributions of executive attention, inhibitory control, and affect regulation to the impulse control of eating behavior. J Exp Soc Psychol. 2009;45:431–435
8. Nederkoorn C, Guerrieri R, Havermans RC, Roefs A, Jansen A. The interactive effect of hunger and impulsivity on food intake and purchase in a virtual supermarket. Int J Obes (Lond). 2009;33(8):905–912
9. Lawrence NS, Hinton EC, Parkinson JA, Lawrence AD. Nucleus accumbens response to food cues predicts subsequent snack consumption in women and increased body mass index in those with reduced self-control. Neuroimage. 2012;63(1):415–422
10. Solanto MV, Abikoff H, Sonuga-Barke E, et al. The ecological validity of delay aversion and response inhibition as measures of impulsivity in AD/HD: a supplement to the NIMH multimodal treatment study of AD/HD. J Abnorm Child Psychol. 2001;29(3):215–228
11. Dougherty DM, Mathias CW, Marsh DM, Jagar AA. Laboratory behavioral measures of impulsivity. Behav Res Methods. 2005;37(1):82–90
12. Culp J, Bell RA, Cassady D. Characteristics of food industry web sites and "advergames" targeting children. J Nutr Educ Behav. 2010;42(3):197–201
13. Nairn A, Hang H. Advergames: it's not child's play. A review of research. Family and parenting institute 2012. Available at: www.agnesnairn.co.uk/policy_reports/advergames-its-not-childs-play.pdf. Accessed June 28, 2013
14. Folkvord F, Anschütz DJ, Buijzen M, Valkenburg PM. The effect of playing advergames that promote energy-dense snacks or fruit on actual food intake among children. Am J Clin Nutr. 2013;97(2):239–245
15. Guerrieri R, Nederkoorn C, Jansen A. The interaction between impulsivity and a varied food environment: its influence on food intake and overweight. Int J Obes. 2008;32(4):708–714

16. Daugherty TK, Quay HC. Response perseveration and delayed responding in childhood behavior disorders. J Child Psychol Psychiatry. 1991;32(3):453–461
17. Matthys W, van Goozen SHM, de Vries H, Cohen-Kettenis PT, van Engeland H. The dominance of behavioural activation over behavioural inhibition in conduct disordered boys with or without attention deficit hyperactivity disorder. J Child Psychol Psychiatry. 1998;39(5):643–651
18. Shapiro SK, Quay HC, Hogan AE, Schwartz KP. Response perseveration and delayed responding in undersocialized aggressive conduct disorder. J Abnorm Psychol. 1988;97(3):371–373
19. Nederkoorn C, Braet C, Van Eijs Y, Tanghe A, Jansen A. Why obese children cannot resist food: the role of impulsivity. Eat Behav. 2006;7(4):315–322
20. Cole TJ, Bellizzi MC, Flegal KM, Dietz WH. Establishing a standard definition for child overweight and obesity worldwide: international survey. BMJ. 2000;320(7244):1240–1243
21. Dodd CJ, Welsman JR, Armstrong N. Energy intake and appetite following exercise in lean and overweight girls. Appetite. 2008;51(3):482–488
22. Moore MS, Dodd CJ, Welsman JR, Armstrong N. Short-term appetite and energy intake following imposed exercise in 9- to 10-year-old girls. Appetite. 2004;43(2):127–134
23. Rumbold PLS, Dodd-Reynolds CJ, Stevenson E. Agreement between paper and pen visual analogue scales and a wristwatch-based electronic appetite rating system (PRO-Diary©), for continuous monitoring of free-living subjective appetite sensations in 7-10 year old children. Appetite. 2013;69:180–185
24. van Laerhoven H, van der Zaag-Loonen HJ, Derkx BH. A comparison of Likert scale and visual analogue scales as response options in children's questionnaires. Acta Paediatr. 2004;93(6):830–835
25. Holbrook MB, Batra R. Assessing the role of emotions as mediators of consumer responses to advertising. J Consum Res. 1987;14(3):404–420
26. Panic K, Cauberghe V, de Pelsmacker P. Comparing TV ads and advergames targeting children: the impact of persuasion knowledge on behavioral responses. J Advert. 2013;42(2–3):264–273
27. Jasinska AJ, Yasuda M, Burant CF, et al. Impulsivity and inhibitory control deficits are associated with unhealthy eating in young adults. Appetite. 2012;59(3):738–747
28. Francis LA, Susman EJ. Self-regulation and rapid weight gain in children from age 3 to 12 years. Arch Pediatr Adolesc Med. 2009;163(4):297–302
29. Baumeister RF. Yielding to temptation: self-control failure, impulsive purchasing, and consumer behavior. J Consum Res. 2002;28(4):670–676
30. Rozendaal E, Lapierre MA, van Reijmersdal EA, Buijzen M. Reconsidering advertising literacy as a defense against advertising effects. Media Psychol. 2011;14(4):333–354
31. Buijzen M. The effectiveness of parental communication in modifying the relation between food advertising and children's consumption behaviour. Br J Dev Psychol. 2009;27(Pt 1):105–121
32. Kroese FM, Adriaanse MA, Evers C, De Ridder DTD. "Instant success": turning temptations into cues for goal-directed behavior. Pers Soc Psychol Bull

CHAPTER 6

ASSESSING CAUSALITY IN THE ASSOCIATION BETWEEN CHILD ADIPOSITY AND PHYSICAL ACTIVITY LEVELS: A MENDELIAN RANDOMIZATION ANALYSIS

REBECCA C. RICHMOND, GEORGE DAVEY SMITH, ANDY R. NESS, MARCEL DEN HOED, GEORGE MCMAHON, AND NICHOLAS J. TIMPSON

6.1 INTRODUCTION

Cross-sectional studies have shown that objectively measured physical activity is associated with childhood adiposity [1]–[6], and a strong inverse dose–response association with body mass index (BMI) has been found [1]. However, confounding or reverse causation (where adiposity influences inactivity, rather than vice versa) may explain part of the association [7],[8]. Indeed, there may be a bidirectional relationship between adiposity and physical activity, and this would imply that only a small change in

---

Assessing Causality in the Association between Child Adiposity and Physical Activity Levels: A Mendelian Randomization Analysis. © Richmond RC, Smith GD, Ness AR, den Hoed M, McMahon G, and Timpson NJ. PLoS Medicine **11**,3 *(2014),* doi:10.1371/journal.pmed.1001618. Licensed under a Creative Commons Attribution 4.0 International License, http://creativecommons.org/licenses/by/4.0/.

adiposity or physical activity may be required to initiate a cycle of weight gain and increased inactivity [9].

There are few randomized trials examining the effectiveness of physical activity interventions for weight loss [10]. Those that exist report smaller, if any, effects on BMI [11]–[14] than predicted by observational associations. However, the efficacy of BMI as a measure of adiposity is subject to debate, and some improvements in other measures of fatness such as skinfold thickness have been demonstrated in school-based physical activity interventions, without an accompanying reduction in BMI [14]. Nevertheless, the small effect seen in these trials suggests that reverse causation may in part have generated the association between physical activity and adiposity observed in cross-sectional studies. These findings, together with the quality of the trials—which has been limited by short trial duration, lack of assessment of trial adherence, or a limited difference in activity achieved between intervention and control groups [12]—call for further investigation and the use of genetic instruments as a better surrogate for adiposity.

To address the issue of reverse causation, prospective studies have measured activity and adiposity at multiple time points in children [7],[15]–[22], although few studies have investigated bidirectional associations between activity and fatness in childhood and adolescence. Of those that have, one showed a lack of longitudinal association between physical activity and body composition [21], while three showed that whereas physical activity could not predict fatness, fatness was predictive of future physical inactivity [7],[20],[22]. Sample size and poorly assessed activity have limited the ability to infer the causal direction of effects, even where longitudinal data are available.

Mendelian randomization (MR) can be used to assess whether adiposity causally affects activity levels [23]. MR is an approach that applies instrumental variable methods, using genetic variants as a proxy for environmentally modifiable exposures. This technique, which is analogous to a randomized trial where randomization to genotype takes place at conception, is not susceptible to reverse causation or confounding and so may be used to reassess observational associations and strengthen causal inference [23]–[26].

The Association Between Child Adiposity and Physical Activity

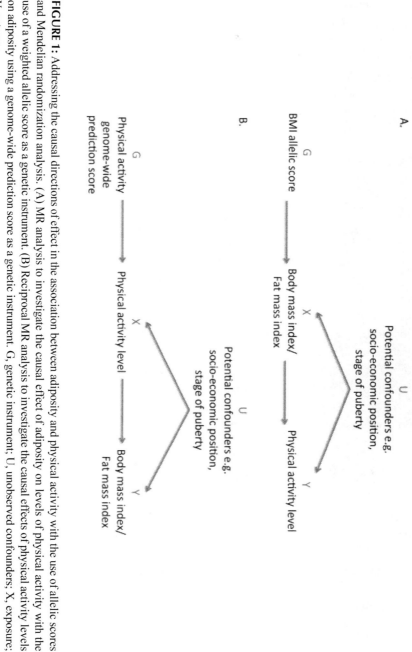

FIGURE 1: Addressing the causal directions of effect in the association between adiposity and physical activity with the use of allelic scores and Mendelian randomization analysis. (A) MR analysis to investigate the causal effect of adiposity on levels of physical activity with the use of a weighted allelic score as a genetic instrument. (B) Reciprocal MR analysis to investigate the causal effects of physical activity levels on adiposity using a genome-wide prediction score as a genetic instrument. G, genetic instrument; U, unobserved confounders; X, exposure; Y, outcome.

Previous MR studies investigating the effect of adiposity on various outcomes have used one or a few of the common genetic locus variants with the largest effect sizes to serve as instruments [27]–[32]. In this study, we aimed to use 32 independent genetic correlates of BMI, confirmed in a large-scale meta-analysis of genome-wide association studies (GWASs) [33], to elucidate the causality and magnitude of the effect of adiposity on activity levels in children (Figure 1A).

6.2 METHODS

6.2.1 STUDY SAMPLE

The Avon Longitudinal Study of Parents and Children (ALSPAC) is a prospective birth cohort that enrolled over 13,000 pregnant women in the former County of Avon, UK, with an expected delivery date between April 1991 and December 1992 [34],[35]. Detailed information has been collected on these women and their offspring using self-administered questionnaires, research clinic examinations, data extraction from medical notes, and linkage to routine information systems. The study website contains details of all available data through a fully searchable data dictionary (http://www.bristol.ac.uk/alspac/researchers/data-access/data-dictionary/). Ethical approval was obtained from the ALSPAC Law and Ethics Committee and local research ethics committees.

6.2.2 EXPOSURE VARIABLES

Body composition was measured at a clinic where the children's average age was 11.7 y [1]. BMI, the primary exposure variable, was calculated as weight (in kilograms) divided by height (in meters) squared. BMI as a measure of adiposity has well-recognised limitations [36],[37], and of particular concern for this analysis is that BMI does not distinguish between fat and lean mass, since lean mass correlates positively with levels of activity [2]. Therefore, phenotypic refinement was employed through the use of total body fat, assessed using a Lunar Prodigy dual energy X-ray absorptiometry scanner [1]. The fat mass index (FMI) was subsequently calculated as fat mass (in kilograms) divided by height (in meters) squared.

6.2.3 OUTCOME VARIABLES

All children who attended the age 11-y clinic were asked to wear an MTI Actigraph AM7164 2.2 accelerometer for 7 d [38]. Only data from children who wore the Actigraph for at least 10 h/d for 3 d were included in this analysis. Movement counts were detected as a combined function of the frequency and intensity of movements. Activity was expressed as the total daily volume of physical activity averaged over the period of valid recording (counts/minute), and as time spent on moderate-to-vigorous-intensity physical activity (>3,600 counts/min) [39] and sedentary time (<199 counts/min) in minutes/day [40].

6.2.4 GENOTYPING

9,912 ALSPAC children were genotyped using the Illumina HumanHap550 quad genome-wide single nucleotide polymorphism (SNP) genotyping platform by the Wellcome Trust Sanger Institute (Cambridge, UK) and the Laboratory Corporation of America (Burlington, North Carolina, US). Individuals with incorrect sex assignments, extreme heterozygosity (<0.320 and >0.345 for Wellcome Trust Sanger Institute data and <0.310 and >0.330 for Laboratory Corporation of America data), disproportionate levels of individual missingness (>3%), evidence of cryptic relatedness (>10% identity by descent), or non-European ancestry were excluded. The resulting dataset consisted of 8,365 individuals. Of 609,203 SNPs, those with a minor allele frequency of <1%, with a call rate of <95%, or not in Hardy–Weinberg equilibrium ($p<5\times10^{-7}$) were removed, leaving 500,527 SNPs that passed quality control. Established BMI variants that had not been genotyped directly were imputed with MACH 1.0.16 Markov Chain Haplotyping software [41],[42] using CEPH individuals from HapMap phase 2 (release 22) as a reference set.

From these genome-wide data, a weighted allelic score was created using 32 independent variants shown to be robustly associated with BMI in a large-scale GWAS meta-analysis [33] (Table S1). The dose of the effect allele at each locus was weighted by the effect size of the variant in this independent meta-analysis [33], and these doses were summed to reflect the average number of BMI-increasing alleles carried by an individual. This weighted allelic score was created to act as an instrumental variable in MR analysis, and explained a greater proportion of variance in BMI than single SNPs [43]. The allelic score was also used as an instrument for FMI.

6.2.5 STATISTICAL METHODS

Means and standard deviations (SD) were calculated for continuous variables to describe baseline characteristics. The distribution of moderate-to-vigorous activity was skewed and was therefore log-transformed to achieve normality. All adiposity and activity values were converted to sex-specific SD (z) scores.

Observational associations between adiposity and activity measures were assessed using linear regression adjusted for age. Additional analyses were adjusted for potentially confounding factors that have been found to be independently associated with obesity [44], including maternal pre-pregnancy BMI, estimated gestational age at birth, infant birth weight, maternal education level, parental social class, maternal smoking during pregnancy, child's stage of puberty at age 11 y, total daily dietary intake, and intake of main food groups.

For investigating associations between the allelic score and standardised phenotypes, continuous effects were estimated using linear regression with adjustment for age. An additive genetic model was assumed since there was no evidence for interaction effects among the SNPs combined in the allelic score [33]. MR analysis may generally forego the need for inclusion of other covariates, which are anticipated to be randomly distributed with respect to genotype [23]. Despite this, we examined associations between the confounding factors and genotypes to check the core instrumental variable assumption that the instrument (genotype) is independent of factors that potentially confound the observational association [25],[26].

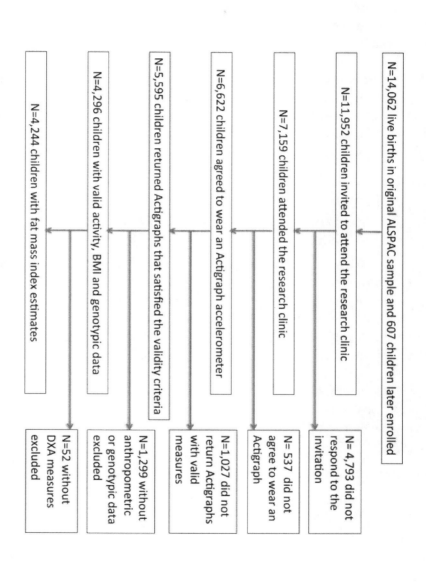

FIGURE 2: Participants in ALSPAC and in the analyses presented in this paper. DXA, dual energy X-ray absorptiometry.

For MR analyses, we performed two-stage least squares using the weighted allelic score as an instrument for adiposity and implementing the "ivreg2" function in Stata. F-statistics from the first-stage regression between genotype and adiposity were examined to check the instrumental variable assumption that the instrument is sufficiently associated with the exposure, in order to reduce the possibility of weak instrument bias [45]. The Durbin-Wu-Hausman (DWH) test for endogeneity [46] was used to compare effect estimates from the second stage of the instrumental variable analysis and observational analysis. Stata 12 (StataCorp) was used for all analyses.

6.2.6 SENSITIVITY ANALYSES

6.2.6.1 MULTIPLE INDEPENDENT INSTRUMENTS.

The existence of pleiotropy, where a genetic instrument has an effect on an outcome (activity) independent of its effect on the exposure (adiposity), would have implications for assumptions made in MR analyses [47]. Similar instrumental variable estimates acquired using independent instruments would provide suggestive evidence against an influence of pleiotropic effects, as it is unlikely that they have shared pleiotropy [43],[48]. The two independent genetic instruments generated were rs1558902 in *FTO*, the individual SNP with the largest effect size in the meta-analysis of GWASs for BMI [33], and a weighted allelic score constructed from the remaining 31 BMI-associated SNPs.

6.2.6.2 GENOME-WIDE PREDICTION FOR PHYSICAL ACTIVITY.

An exploratory MR analysis investigating the association between adiposity and activity levels may provide evidence for causality in this direction. However, it does not exclude the possibility that physical activity has a causal effect on adiposity levels. A genetic instrument for activity is required to test the relationship in a bidirectional manner (Figure 1B) [31],[32]. No meta-analysis of GWASs has so far been reported for physical activity, and no genetic variants have been robustly associated with activity to date [49],[50]. Genome-wide prediction scores, which examine the aggregated contribution of genome-wide variation in a trait, have the potential to recover some of the information lost by dismissing false-negative results in GWASs [51]–[55] and may be used as instruments in MR analysis.

Before the generation of a genetic instrument for physical activity, the heritability of activity in ALSPAC was assessed to consider the plausibility of a genetic contribution to activity. GCTA (Genome-wide Complex Trait Analysis) (version 1.04) [56] was used to estimate the total amount of variance captured by all 500,527 SNPs in the genotypic data for the activity measures. The approach first involves the estimation of a genetic relationship matrix for individuals based on autosomal genotype information, with a further cryptic relatedness cutoff of 2.5% applied to reduce the potential for biased estimates. The variance of each activity trait attributable to all SNPs was estimated using restricted maximum likelihood. Given evidence of a heritable contribution to observed variance in activity measures (Table S2), genome-wide prediction scores were generated for total physical activity, moderate-to-vigorous activity, and sedentary time. Individuals in the complete sample were randomized into two subgroups. Using activity and genotypic data from the first subgroup (n = 2,148), genetic variants yielding a p-value$\leq$0.1 in a GWAS for each activity variable were extracted, and prediction scores were constructed using profile scoring and the "–score" command within PLINK (version 1.07) [57]. The prediction score is a sum across SNPs of the number of reference alleles multiplied by the weight for that SNP, which is its effect size in the GWAS with activity.

We used split sample analysis, where the physical activity prediction scores from the first subgroup (composed of one half of the sample) were applied to individuals in the second independent subgroup (composed of the other half of the sample) and used in two-stage least squares instrumental variable analysis to assess a causal effect of activity on adiposity. This method was repeated with prediction scores generated from data in the second subgroup and applied to instrumental variable analysis in the first [58]. The results of these two instrumental variable analyses were meta-analysed using the inverse variance-weighted method with a fixed-effects model. A test for heterogeneity [59] was performed to investigate similarity between instrumented effects in the two independent subgroups.

We performed all of the above analyses stratified by sex because a sex interaction for the associations between adiposity and activity levels has been shown previously [1] (Tables S11, S12, S13).

6.3 RESULTS

Of the 11,952 children who were invited to attend the research clinic, 7,159 (59.9%) came to the clinic. 6,622 of the 7,159 (92.5%) agreed to wear an Actigraph accelerometer, and 5,595 of the 6,622 (84.5%) returned Actigraph accelerometer data that satisfied the validity criteria. Of the 5,595, BMI and genotypic data were available for 4,296 children (76.8%). FMI estimates were available for 4,244 children (75.8%) (Figure 2).

Of the individuals included in this analysis, 22.1% (950/4,296) were defined as being overweight and 4.2% (181/4,296) as obese, according to age- and sex-specific cutoffs proposed by the International Obesity Task Force [60]. A comparison of the baseline characteristics of individuals who did and did not attend the age 11-y clinic has been described in detail elsewhere [1]. Differences in baseline characteristics between the subset of children included in this analysis and those who did not attend the age 11-y clinic are shown in Table S3. The children included in this analysis were more likely to be girls and had a higher birth weight, higher gestational age at birth, higher social class, higher dietary intake at age 10 y and mothers who were less likely to be smokers and were more highly educated.

6.3.1 OBSERVATIONAL ANALYSIS

From observational analysis of baseline characteristics, objectively assessed activity levels were higher for boys than girls for total physical activity (664.6 versus 555.1 mean movement counts/min, $p<0.001$) and for moderate-to-vigorous activity (25.8 versus 16.0 median min/d, $p<0.001$).

Sedentary time was higher for girls than for boys (435.6 versus 418.2 mean min/d, p<0.001), as were mean values of BMI (19.1 versus 18.7 kg/m^2, p<0.001) and fat mass (12.7 versus 10.2 kg, p<0.001) (Table 1). BMI and FMI were strongly correlated (Pearson's correlation coefficient = 0.94).

A 3.3 kg/m^2 (1 SD) higher BMI was associated with 22.3 (95% CI, 17.0, 27.6) counts/min less total physical activity (p = 1.6×10^{-16}), 2.6 (2.1, 3.1) min/d less moderate-to-vigorous activity (p = 3.7×10^{-29}), and 3.5 (1.5, 5.5) min/d more sedentary time (p = 5.0×10^{-4}). These associations were stronger when using FMI instead of BMI and were largely unaltered by adjusting for additional confounders (Table 2). In observational analyses stratified by sex, effect estimates were larger in boys for all activity phenotypes (Table S11).

6.3.2 DIRECT GENOTYPIC ASSOCIATIONS

The BMI allelic score was normally distributed, with a mean of 29.6, SD of 3.9, and range of 16.3–42.3 (Figure S1). A per (average BMI-increasing) allele change in the allelic score was associated with a 0.14 (95% CI, 0.12, 0.17) kg/m^2 increase in BMI (p = 5.5×10^{-29}), and a 0.11 (0.09, 0.13) kg/m^2 increase in FMI (p = 2.3×10^{-25}) (Table 3). The BMI allelic score explained 2.8% of the variance in standardised BMI in this cohort, and 2.5% of the variance in FMI.

In contrast to BMI and FMI, confounding factors were not associated with the genotypes in this cohort (Table S4). Although the allelic score showed some weak associations with reported dietary intake and certain food groups and macronutrients (Table S5), these associations are largely driven by the inclusion of FTO in the score. As dietary intake is a known mediator in the association between FTO and adiposity [61], adjustment in instrumental variable analysis would not be appropriate.

A per allele change in the BMI allelic score was associated with a decrease of 1.4 (95% CI, 0.0, 2.8) counts/min of total physical activity (p = 0.05), an approximate decrease of 0.1 (0.0, 0.2) min/d of moderate-to-vigorous activity (p = 0.05), and an increase of 0.6 (0.1, 1.1) min/d of sedentary time (p = 0.03) (Table 3).

TABLE 1: Baseline characteristics of children.

Variable	All (n = 4,296)		Boys (n = 2,044)		Girls (n = 2,252)	
	Mean or Percent	SD	Mean or Percent	SD	Mean or Percent	SD
Age (mo)	140.8	2.8	140.8	2.8	140.8	2.7
Height (cm)	150.7	7.2	150.0	7.1	151.3	7.2
Weight (kg)	43.3	9.7	42.4	9.5	44.2	9.8
BMI (kg/m^2)	18.9	3.3	18.7	3.2	19.1	3.4
Fat mass (kg) measured by DXA	11.5	6.5	10.2	6.4	12.7	6.4
FMI (kg/m^2)	5.0	2.7	4.5	2.6	5.5	2.6
Body fat percentage (fat mass [kg]/weight [kg])	25.4	9.1	22.5	9.2	27.3	8.4
Total physical activity (counts/min)	607.2	178.4	664.6	187.9	555.1	151.7
Moderate-to-vigorous-intensity physical activity (min/d)[a]	20.0	12.0–31.4	25.8	15.9–38.5	16.0	9.9–24.9
Sedentary time (min/d)	427.3	66.6	418.2	68.5	435.6	63.7
Birth weight (g)	3,433.8	526.7	3,483.5	568.3	3,388.3	481.2
Gestational age at birth (wk)	39.5	1.8	39.4	1.9	39.6	1.6
Maternal BMI (kg/m^2)	22.9	3.7	23.0	3.7	22.9	3.7
Total daily dietary intake (kcal/d)	1,862.0	377.3	1,953.5	389.8	1,778.3	344.9
Maternal smoking during pregnancy						
No	80.1%		80.1%		80.1%	
Yes	19.9%		19.9%		19.9%	
Maternal education						
Education up to age 16 y with certificate of secondary education or vocational training	20.0%		21.0%		19.1%	
Education up to age 16 y with general certificate of education (Ordinary level)	35.1%		34.4%		35.8%	
Education up to age 18 y with general certificate of education (Advance level)	27.2%		26.8%		27.5%	
University degree	17.7%		17.8%		17.6%	
Parental social class[b]						
I Professional occupations	16.3%		16.5%		16.2%	
II Managerial and technical occupations	45.9%		45.5%		46.3%	

TABLE 1: *Cont.*

Variable	All (n = 4,296)		Boys (n = 2,044)		Girls (n = 2,252)	
	Mean or Percent	SD	Mean or Percent	SD	Mean or Percent	SD
III(NM) Skilled non-manual occupations	24.4%		24.8%		24.0%	
III(M) Skilled manual occupations	9.6%		9.9%		9.4%	
IV Partly skilled occupations	3.3%		2.9%		3.6%	
V Unskilled occupations	0.5%		0.5%		0.5%	
Stage of puberty[c]						
Stage 1	47.7%		66.7%		33.2%	
Stage 2	35.0%		28.8%		39.8%	
Stage 3	13.7%		4.2%		21.0%	
Stage 4	3.1%		0.4%		5.2%	
Stage 5	0.5%		0%		0.8%	

Total sample sizes rnage from 3,121 to 4,098 depending on the availability of the data. [a]*Median and interquartile ranges are displayed for this variable because it is skewed.* [b]*Based on parent with highest social class, as defined by the 1991 British Office of Population Censuses and Surveys classification.* [c]*Based on highest Tanner scale developmental stage of breasts and pubic hair for females and pubic hair for males. DXA = dual energy X-ray absorptiometry.*

6.3.3 MENDELIAN RANDOMIZATION

Instrumental variable analysis using the BMI allelic score showed that a 3.3 kg/m^2 higher BMI was associated with 32.4 (95% CI, 0.9, 63.9) counts/min less total physical activity (p = 0.04) (equivalent to 5.3% of the mean counts/min), 2.8 (0.1, 5.5) min/d less moderate-to-vigorous activity (p = 0.04), and 13.2 (1.3, 25.2) min/d more sedentary time (p = 0.03) (F-statistic = 124.9; partial R^2 = 0.03).

TABLE 2: Associations between measures of adiposity and physical activity levels.

Adiposity	Activity		Model A[a]				Model B[b]		
		N	Z-Score Value Coefficient (95% CI)[c]	Difference in Activity, Raw Units (95% CI)[c]	p-value	N	Z-Score Value Coefficient (95% CI)[c]	Differences in Activity, Raw Units (95% CI)[c]	p-value
BMI (kg/m^2)	Total physical activity (counts/min)	4,296	−0.12 (−0.15, −0.10)	−22.3 (−27.6, −17.0)	1.6×10^{-16}	1,338	−0.13 (−0.20, −0.05)	−22.8 (−36.6, −8.7)	0.002
	Moderate-to-vigorous activity (min/d)[d]		−0.17 (−0.20, −0.14)	−2.6 (−3.1, −2.1)	3.7×10^{-29}		−0.17 (−0.24, −0.09)	−2.6 (−3.7, −1.4)	1.8×10^{-5}
	Sedentary time (min/d)		0.05 (0.02, 0.08)	3.5 (1.5, 5.5)	5.0×10^{-4}		0.07 (−0.01, 0.15)	4.6 (−0.5, 9.7)	0.06
FMI (kg/m^2)	Total physical activity (counts/min)	4,244	−0.18 (−0.21, −0.15)	−32.3 (−37.6, −27.1)	1.5×10^{-33}	1,320	−0.22 (−0.29, −0.14)	−39.1 (−52.4, −25.8)	7.9×10^{-9}
	Moderate-to-vigorous activity (min/d)[d]		−0.22 (−0.25, −0.19)	−3.4 (−3.8, −2.9)	2.4×10^{-48}		−0.24 (−0.31, −0.17)	−3.7 (−4.8, −2.6)	4.0×10^{-11}
	Sedentary time (min/d)		0.09 (0.06, 0.12)	5.8 (3.8, 7.7)	5.4×10^{-6}		0.14 (0.07, 0.21)	9.5 (4.8, 14.2)	1.1×10^{-4}

[a]Model A: adjusted for age. [b]Model B: adjusted for age, birth weight, gestational age at birth, maternal smoking during pregnancy, maternal education, parental social class, maternal BMI, stage of puberty, total daily dietary intake, and intake of main food groups. [c]Coefficients are displayed as sex-specific z-scores for both measures of adiposity and activity levels and have also been rescaled to give more meaningful outcomes relating to the raw units of these variables. The raw-unit difference was computer by multiplying the z-score value by the SD of the variable, taken from Table 1. [d]Moderate-to-vigorous activity was log transformed for analysis.

TABLE 3: Associations between the weighted allelic score for 32 SNPs and body mass index/fat mass index and activity measures.

Outcome	N	Per Allele Effects					
		Z-Score Value Coefficient (95% CI)[b]	Difference in Adiposity or Activity Raw Units (95% CI)[b]	p-value	Z-Score Value Coefficient (95% CI)[b]	Difference in Adiposity or Activity, Raw Units (95% CI)[b]	p-value
BMI (kg/m^2)	4,296	0.04 (0.04, 0.05)	0.14 (0.12, 0.17)	5.5×10^{-29}	0.04 (0.03, 0.05)	0.14 (0.11, 0.16)	4.2×10^{-28}
FMI (kg/m^2)	4,244	0.04 (0.03, 0.05)	0.11 (0.09, 0.13)	2.3×10^{-25}	0.04 (0.03, 0.05)	0.10 (0.08, 0.12)	2.3×10^{-24}
Total physical activity (counts/min)	4,296	−0.01 (0.00, −0.02)	−1.4 (−2.8, −0.03)	0.05			
Moderate-to-vigorous activity (min/d)[c]	4,296	−0.01 (−0.02, 0.00)	−0.12, (−0.24, −0.00)	0.05			
Sedentary time (min/d)	4,296	0.01 (0.00, 0.02)	0.57 (0.06, 1.1)	0.03			

Regression results were adjusted for age. Per (average BMI-increasing) allele effects were obtained by linear regression for all of these continuous outcome variables. [a]*Activity variables were total physical activity, moderate-to-vigorous and minutes of sedentary time.* [b]*Coefficients are displayed as sex-specific z-scores for both measures of adiposity and activity levels and have also been rescaled to give more meaningful outcomes relating to the raw units of these variables. The raw-unit difference was computer by multiplying the z-score value by the SD of the variable, taken from Table 1.* [c]*Moderate-to-vigorous activity was log transformed for analysis.*

There was no evidence of a departure of instrumental-variable-derived estimates from observational results, as demonstrated by DWH tests (p≥0.10), indicating similarity between observational and MR estimates in the effect of BMI on physical activity levels. Furthermore, point estimates for effect sizes from the instrumental variable analysis were equal to or greater than those derived from basic observational analyses for all traits, though wider confidence intervals for the instrumental variable estimates resulted in larger pvalues.

Similar results were found when FMI was instrumented (Table 4). In addition, similar results were found when using physical activity and adiposity data for individuals at age 13 y, though the number of individuals at this time point was smaller (Table S6). In sensitivity analyses stratified by sex, wide confidence intervals for instrumental variable estimates did not allow the resolution of differences between boys and girls (Table S11).

6.3.4 MULTIPLE INDEPENDENT INSTRUMENTS

An analysis of the alleles included in the BMI allelic score showed that rs1558902 (FTO) was the variant contributing most to its association with BMI (Figure 3). Results of instrumental variable analysis using this genetic variant were compared with those of a weighted allelic score consisting of the 31 genetic variants excluding FTO (Tables 5 and 6). The instrumented effect for FTO showed some difference to observational estimates, especially for sedentary time, where the instrumental variable analysis produced larger effect estimates than the observational analysis (p = 0.01 for DWH test). However, there was no strong statistical evidence that the instrumented effects of BMI on activity levels were different from one another (p for heterogeneity ≥0.06). An additional analysis was run that showed that independent pairs of variants from the 32 SNPs have normally distributed instrumental variable effects. Although pairs of variants including FTO lie at the lower end of this distribution, indicating that variation in FTO produces a larger-than-average effect in the instrumental variable analysis, this effect is not an outlier (Figure S2). Similar results were found when FMI was instrumented.

The Association Between Child Adiposity and Physical Activity

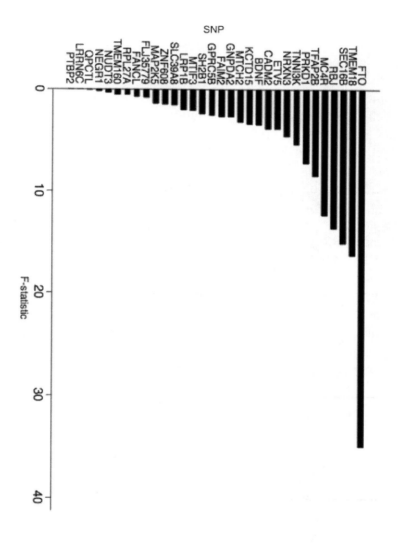

FIGURE 3: Strength of individual genetic variants for BMI as genetic instruments in instrumental variable analysis. F-statistic derived from first-stage regression in two-stage least squares analysis

6.3.5 GENOME-WIDE PREDICTION FOR PHYSICAL ACTIVITY

The additive heritability of activity measures was estimated to be 17%–25% (Table S2), indicating a non-negligible contribution of genetic variation to variance in physical activity levels. Genome-wide prediction scores were generated for each of the activity measures and applied in instrumental variable analysis to independent subgroups. Physical activity scores were normally distributed and showed some association with their respective activity measures in the other subgroups (Table S7). The physical activity scores had no substantive correlation with the BMI allelic score (Table S8), providing evidence that the instruments for adiposity and physical activity were independent of each other.

There was no strong statistical evidence that the instrumented effects of activity on adiposity in the subgroups were different from each other (p for heterogeneity ≥ 0.11). A meta-analysis of both instrumental variable analyses, unlike observational analysis, found no strong evidence for a causal effect of physical activity on BMI at age 11 y (regression coefficient 0.27 [95% CI, −0.41, 0.94], p = 0.44, for total physical activity; −0.03 [−0.72, 0.66], p = 0.93, for moderate-to-vigorous activity; −0.51 [−1.24, 0.22], p = 0.17, for sedentary time, with z-standardised units of BMI and activity measures) (Table S9). Results were similar when FMI was the outcome (Table S10). However, confidence intervals were wide, and small F-statistics indicated that caution should be applied when using these instruments for physical activity ($F \leq 6.80$).

6.4 DISCUSSION

This study used a MR approach to investigate a causal role for elevated BMI and FMI in lower physical activity levels in children. In agreement with previous findings that adiposity loci identified by GWASs in adults are associated with childhood anthropometric traits [62],[63], the allelic score derived from established genetic variants for BMI was strongly associated with both exposures of interest (BMI and FMI). The allelic score explained a larger proportion of the variation in BMI compared with FMI. Nonetheless, the F-statistic for the association between the allelic score and FMI was large (>100), supporting previous findings for consistent associations between the 32 BMI-associated loci and other measures of adiposity [64].

The similarity between observational and instrumental variable estimates for the association between BMI and physical activity provides evidence suggesting that increasing adiposity leads to a causal reduction in total and moderate-to-vigorous physical activity, and a causal increase in the length of sedentary time. Associations from instrumental variable analysis were marginally stronger between FMI and activity levels, as expected given that BMI does not differentiate between fat and lean mass, and lean mass correlates positively with levels of activity. These results are in line with findings from recent prospective studies that show that fatness is predictive of reduced physical activity at later time points [7],[20],[22].

The finding that the calculated effect sizes in this MR analysis account for a substantial proportion of the association between adiposity and activity identified in observational studies [1]–[6] has important public health implications. Whilst the mechanisms of this pathway are unclear and may constitute both physiological and psychological factors [65],[66], evidence that adiposity is a causal risk factor for low physical activity is important, since it has been recommended that children spend at least 60 min in moderate-to-vigorous-intensity physical activity each day in order to maintain their physical health [67]–[73]. In particular, this evidence highlights the importance of developing programmes targeting body weight in order to increase physical activity levels in overweight children [74].

A limitation of the study was that we were not able to collect physical activity, body composition, or genetic data on a substantial number of children originally enrolled in the study. These missing data can lead to a bias if the causal effect of adiposity on physical activity (and vice versa) is different in the children who did not take part. Whilst we cannot fully exclude such a bias, associations were not altered by adjustment for factors associated with missing data [1]. Possible limitations to the MR analysis in general include the possibility of population stratification, canalization, power deficiency, pleiotropy, and linkage disequilibrium [23],[47]. Major population stratification is unlikely since this analysis was completed in unrelated individuals of European ancestry. A pleiotropic association of a genetic variant included in the allelic score with the outcome, or linkage disequilibrium with a functional variant associated with the outcome, would violate the assumptions of MR analysis. Multiple independent instruments were used to provide evidence against the existence of shared pleiotropy and against the influence of linkage-disequilibrium-induced confounding [48]. Whereas instrumental variable estimates for the association between adiposity and physical activity obtained using the 31-SNP allelic score (excluding FTO) were consistently similar to observational effect sizes, the estimates produced using the FTO variant as an instrument were generally larger than observational findings. However, there was no strong statistical evidence for a difference between the instrumented estimates, arguing against a pleiotropic effect. It should be emphasised that this investigation does not provide definitive evidence against the existence or impact of pleiotropy, and more functional knowledge of the variants is required to assess this more comprehensively.

With evidence for causality in the direction from adiposity to activity levels, further analyses were undertaken to address the reciprocal association between physical activity and levels of adiposity in children at age 11 y. The absence of a causal effect of physical activity on adiposity goes some way towards explaining the lack of impact of short-term physical activity intervention trials on adiposity levels in children [11]–[13]. It is also in line with the fact that there is little evidence that there has been a major decline in physical activity during the course of the obesity epidemic [75], compared with stronger evidence that there has been an increase in energy intake in the same time period [76]. Although no causal effect was shown in our preliminary analysis, this analysis is likely to suffer from limitations of small sample sizes and inadequacy of the prediction scores for physical activity in terms of the association between genotype and physical activity [77]–[79], genetic confounding, or pleiotropy. In addition, split sample instrumental variable methods have been shown to generate estimates that are biased towards the null [58]. Before we can confirm or refute a complete lack of effect of activity levels on adiposity using MR analysis, a well-powered study with strong genetic instruments for physical activity variables is required. Therefore, findings from this secondary analysis do not exclude lower physical activity also leading to increases in adiposity and a "vicious cycle" being initiated [9].

Results of our main analysis suggest that increased adiposity leads to a reduction in physical activity. Although further work is required to determine a more accurate estimate of the causal effect in the reverse direction, this study provides insight into the causal contributions of adiposity to activity levels in children and supports research into the targeting of BMI in efforts to increase childhood activity levels.

REFERENCES

1. Ness AR, Leary SD, Mattocks C, Blair SN, Reilly JJ, et al. (2007) Objectively measured physical activity and fat mass in a large cohort of children. PLoS Med 4: e97. doi: 10.1371/journal.pmed.0040097
2. Ekelund U, Sardinha LB, Anderssen SA, Harro M, Franks PW, et al. (2004) Associations between objectively assessed physical activity and indicators of body fatness in 9- to 10-y-old European children: a population-based study from 4 distinct regions in Europe (the European Youth Heart Study). Am J Clin Nutr 80: 584–590.
3. Dencker M, Thorsson O, Karlsson MK, Linden C, Eiberg S, et al. (2006) Daily physical activity related to body fat in children aged 8–11 years. J Pediatr 149: 38–42. doi: 10.1016/j.jpeds.2006.02.002
4. Trost SG, Kerr LM, Ward DS, Pate RR (2001) Physical activity and determinants of physical activity in obese and non-obese children. Int J Obes Relat Metab Disord 25: 822–829. doi: 10.1038/sj.ijo.0801621
5. Ortega FB, Ruiz JR, Sjostrom M (2007) Physical activity, overweight and central adiposity in Swedish children and adolescents: the European Youth Heart Study. Int J Behav Nutr Phys Act 4: 61. doi: 10.1186/1479-5868-4-61
6. Jimenez-Pavon D, Kelly J, Reilly JJ (2010) Associations between objectively measured habitual physical activity and adiposity in children and adolescents: systematic review. Int J Pediatr Obes 5: 3–18. doi: 10.3109/17477160903067601
7. Metcalf BS, Hosking J, Jeffery AN, Voss LD, Henley W, et al. (2011) Fatness leads to inactivity, but inactivity does not lead to fatness: a longitudinal study in children (EarlyBird 45). Arch Dis Child 96: 942–947. doi: 10.1136/adc.2009.175927
8. Luke A, Cooper RS (2013) Physical activity does not influence obesity risk: time to clarify the public health message. Int J Epidemiol 42: 1831–1836. doi: 10.1093/ije/dyt159
9. Christiansen E, Swann A, Sorensen TI (2008) Feedback models allowing estimation of thresholds for self-promoting body weight gain. J Theor Biol 254: 731–736. doi: 10.1016/j.jtbi.2008.07.004
10. Cook CM, Schoeller DA (2011) Physical activity and weight control: conflicting findings. Curr Opin Clin Nutr Metab Care 14: 419–424. doi: 10.1097/mco.0b013e328349b9ff
11. Kamath CC, Vickers KS, Ehrlich A, McGovern L, Johnson J, et al. (2008) Behavioral interventions to prevent childhood obesity: a systematic review and metaanaly-

ses of randomized trials. J Clin Endocrinol Metab 93: 4606–4615. doi: 10.1210/jc.2006-2411
12. Harris KC, Kuramoto LK, Schulzer M, Retallack JE (2009) Effect of school-based physical activity interventions on body mass index in children: a meta-analysis. CMAJ 180: 719–726. doi: 10.1503/cmaj.080966
13. McGovern L, Johnson JN, Paulo R, Hettinger A, Singhal V, et al. (2008) Clinical review: treatment of pediatric obesity: a systematic review and meta-analysis of randomized trials. J Clin Endocrinol Metab 93: 4600–4605. doi: 10.1210/jc.2006-2409
14. Sun C, Pezic A, Tikellis G, Ponsonby AL, Wake M, et al. (2013) Effects of school-based interventions for direct delivery of physical activity on fitness and cardiometabolic markers in children and adolescents: a systematic review of randomized controlled trials. Obes Rev 14: 818–838. doi: 10.1111/obr.12047
15. Riddoch CJ, Leary SD, Ness AR, Blair SN, Deere K, et al. (2009) Prospective associations between objective measures of physical activity and fat mass in 12–14 year old children: the Avon Longitudinal Study of Parents and Children (ALSPAC). BMJ 339: b4544. doi: 10.1136/bmj.b4544
16. Moore LL, Gao D, Bradlee ML, Cupples LA, Sundarajan-Ramamurti A, et al. (2003) Does early physical activity predict body fat change throughout childhood? Prev Med 37: 10–17. doi: 10.1016/s0091-7435(03)00048-3
17. Remmers T, Sleddens EF, Gubbels JS, de Vries SI, Mommers M, et al. (2014) Relationship between physical activity and the development of body mass index in children. Med Sci Sports Exerc 46: 177–184. doi: 10.1249/mss.0b013e3182a36709
18. Reichert FF, Baptista Menezes AM, Wells JC, Carvalho Dumith S, Hallal PC (2009) Physical activity as a predictor of adolescent body fatness: a systematic review. Sports Med 39: 279–294. doi: 10.2165/00007256-200939040-00002
19. Wilks DC, Sharp SJ, Ekelund U, Thompson SG, Mander AP, et al. (2011) Objectively measured physical activity and fat mass in children: a bias-adjusted meta-analysis of prospective studies. PLoS ONE 6: e17205. doi: 10.1371/journal.pone.0017205
20. Ekelund U, Luan J, Sherar LB, Esliger DW, Griew P, et al. (2012) Moderate to vigorous physical activity and sedentary time and cardiometabolic risk factors in children and adolescents. JAMA 307: 704–712. doi: 10.1001/jama.2012.156
21. Hallal PC, Reichert FF, Ekelund U, Dumith SC, Menezes AM, et al. (2012) Bidirectional cross-sectional and prospective associations between physical activity and body composition in adolescence: birth cohort study. J Sports Sci 30: 183–190. doi: 10.1080/02640414.2011.631570
22. Hjorth MF, Chaput JP, Ritz C, Dalskov SM, Andersen R, et al. (2013) Fatness predicts decreased physical activity and increased sedentary time, but not vice versa: support from a longitudinal study in 8- to 11-year-old children. Int J Obes (Lond) E-pub ahead of print. doi: 10.1038/ijo.2013.229
23. Davey Smith G, Ebrahim S (2003) 'Mendelian randomization': can genetic epidemiology contribute to understanding environmental determinants of disease? Int J Epidemiol 32: 1–22. doi: 10.1093/ije/dyg070
24. Davey Smith G, Lawlor DA, Harbord R, Timpson N, Day I, et al. (2007) Clustered environments and randomized genes: a fundamental distinction between conventional and genetic epidemiology. PLoS Med 4: e352. doi: 10.1371/journal.pmed.0040352

25. Lawlor DA, Harbord RM, Sterne JA, Timpson N, Davey Smith G (2008) Mendelian randomization: using genes as instruments for making causal inferences in epidemiology. Stat Med 27: 1133–1163. doi: 10.1002/sim.3034
26. Didelez V, Sheehan N (2007) Mendelian randomization as an instrumental variable approach to causal inference. Stat Methods Med Res 16: 309–330. doi: 10.1177/0962280206077743
27. Timpson NJ, Harbord R, Davey Smith G, Zacho J, Tybjaerg-Hansen A, et al. (2009) Does greater adiposity increase blood pressure and hypertension risk?: Mendelian randomization using the FTO/MC4R genotype. Hypertension 54: 84–90. doi: 10.1161/hypertensionaha.109.130005
28. Lawlor DA, Harbord RM, Tybjaerg-Hansen A, Palmer TM, Zacho J, et al. (2011) Using genetic loci to understand the relationship between adiposity and psychological distress: a Mendelian randomization study in the Copenhagen General Population Study of 53,221 adults. J Intern Med 269: 525–537. doi: 10.1111/j.1365-2796.2011.02343.x
29. Lawlor DA, Timpson NJ, Harbord RM, Leary S, Ness A, et al. (2008) Exploring the developmental overnutrition hypothesis using parental-offspring associations and FTO as an instrumental variable. PLoS Med 5: e33. doi: 10.1371/journal.pmed.0050033
30. Nordestgaard BG, Palmer TM, Benn M, Zacho J, Tybjaerg-Hansen A, et al. (2012) The effect of elevated body mass index on ischemic heart disease risk: causal estimates from a Mendelian randomisation approach. PLoS Med 9: e1001212. doi: 10.1371/journal.pmed.1001212
31. Timpson NJ, Nordestgaard BG, Harbord RM, Zacho J, Frayling TM, et al. (2011) C-reactive protein levels and body mass index: elucidating direction of causation through reciprocal Mendelian randomization. Int J Obes (Lond) 35: 300–308. doi: 10.1038/ijo.2010.137
32. Welsh P, Polisecki E, Robertson M, Jahn S, Buckley BM, et al. (2010) Unraveling the directional link between adiposity and inflammation: a bidirectional Mendelian randomization approach. J Clin Endocrinol Metab 95: 93–99. doi: 10.1210/jc.2009-1064
33. Speliotes EK, Willer CJ, Berndt SI, Monda KL, Thorleifsson G, et al. (2010) Association analyses of 249,796 individuals reveal 18 new loci associated with body mass index. Nat Genet 42: 937–948.
34. Boyd A, Golding J, Macleod J, Lawlor DA, Fraser A, et al. (2013) Cohort profile: the 'children of the 90s'—the index offspring of the Avon Longitudinal Study of Parents and Children. Int J Epidemiol 42: 111–127. doi: 10.1093/ije/dys064
35. Fraser A, Macdonald-Wallis C, Tilling K, Boyd A, Golding J, et al. (2013) Cohort profile: the Avon Longitudinal Study of Parents and Children: ALSPAC mothers
36. Garn SM, Leonard WR, Hawthorne VM (1986) Three limitations of the body mass index. Am J Clin Nutr 44: 996–997.
37. Prentice AM, Jebb SA (2001) Beyond body mass index. Obes Rev 2: 141–147. doi: 10.1046/j.1467-789x.2001.00031.x
38. Riddoch CJ, Mattocks C, Deere K, Saunders J, Kirkby J, et al. (2007) Objective measurement of levels and patterns of physical activity. Arch Dis Child 92: 963–969. doi: 10.1136/adc.2006.112136

39. Mattocks C, Leary S, Ness A, Deere K, Saunders J, et al. (2007) Calibration of an accelerometer during free-living activities in children. Int J Pediatr Obes 2: 218–226. doi: 10.1080/17477160701408809
40. Mattocks C, Ness A, Leary S, Tilling K, Blair SN, et al. (2008) Use of accelerometers in a large field-based study of children: protocols, design issues, and effects on precision. J Phys Act Health 5 (Suppl 1) S98–S111.
41. Li Y, Willer C, Sanna S, Abecasis G (2009) Genotype imputation. Annu Rev Genomics Hum Genet 10: 387–406. doi: 10.1146/annurev.genom.9.081307.164242
42. Li Y, Willer CJ, Ding J, Scheet P, Abecasis GR (2010) MaCH: using sequence and genotype data to estimate haplotypes and unobserved genotypes. Genet Epidemiol 34: 816–834. doi: 10.1002/gepi.20533
43. Palmer TM, Lawlor DA, Harbord RM, Sheehan NA, Tobias JH, et al. (2012) Using multiple genetic variants as instrumental variables for modifiable risk factors. Stat Methods Med Res 21: 223–242. doi: 10.1177/0962280210394459
44. Reilly JJ, Armstrong J, Dorosty AR, Emmett PM, Ness A, et al. (2005) Early life risk factors for obesity in childhood: cohort study. BMJ 330: 1357–1359. doi: 10.1136/bmj.38470.670903.e0
45. Staiger D, Stock JH (1997) Instrumental variables regression with weak instruments. Econometrica 65: 557–586. doi: 10.2307/2171753
46. Baum C, Schaffer M, Stillman S (2007) IVENDOG: Stata module to calculate Durbin-Wu-Hausman endogeneity test after ivreg. Statistical Software Components S494401. Boston: Boston College Department of Economics.
47. Davey Smith G, Ebrahim S (2004) Mendelian randomization: prospects, potentials, and limitations. Int J Epidemiol 33: 30–42. doi: 10.1093/ije/dyh132
48. Davey Smith G (2011) Use of genetic markers and gene-diet interactions for interrogating population-level causal influences of diet on health. Genes Nutr 6: 27–43. doi: 10.1007/s12263-010-0181-y
49. De Moor MH, Liu YJ, Boomsma DI, Li J, Hamilton JJ, et al. (2009) Genome-wide association study of exercise behavior in Dutch and American adults. Med Sci Sports Exerc 41: 1887–1895. doi: 10.1249/mss.0b013e3181a2f646
50. Kim J, Oh S, Min H, Kim Y, Park T (2011) Practical issues in genome-wide association studies for physical activity. Ann N Y Acad Sci 1229: 38–44. doi: 10.1111/j.1749-6632.2011.06102.x
51. Evans DM, Visscher PM, Wray NR (2009) Harnessing the information contained within genome-wide association studies to improve individual prediction of complex disease risk. Hum Mol Genet 18: 3525–3531. doi: 10.1093/hmg/ddp295
52. Purcell SM, Wray NR, Stone JL, Visscher PM, O'Donovan MC, et al. (2009) Common polygenic variation contributes to risk of schizophrenia and bipolar disorder. Nature 460: 748–752. doi: 10.1038/nature08185
53. de los Campos G, Gianola D, Allison DB (2010) Predicting genetic predisposition in humans: the promise of whole-genome markers. Nat Rev Genet 11: 880–886. doi: 10.1038/nrg2898
54. Yang J, Benyamin B, McEvoy BP, Gordon S, Henders AK, et al. (2010) Common SNPs explain a large proportion of the heritability for human height. Nat Genet 42: 565–569. doi: 10.1038/ng.608

55. Wray NR, Yang J, Hayes BJ, Price AL, Goddard ME, et al. (2013) Pitfalls of predicting complex traits from SNPs. Nat Rev Genet 14: 507–515. doi: 10.1038/nrg3457
56. Yang J, Lee SH, Goddard ME, Visscher PM (2011) GCTA: a tool for genome-wide complex trait analysis. Am J Hum Genet 88: 76–82. doi: 10.1016/j.ajhg.2010.11.011
57. Purcell S, Neale B, Todd-Brown K, Thomas L, Ferreira MAR, et al. (2007) PLINK: a tool set for whole-genome association and population-based linkage analyses. Am J Hum Genet 81: 559–575. doi: 10.1086/519795
58. Angrist JD, Krueger AB (1995) Split-sample instrumental variables estimates of the return to schooling. J Bus Econ Stat 13: 225–235. doi: 10.1080/07350015.1995.10524597
59. DerSimonian R, Laird N (1986) Meta-analysis in clinical trials. Control Clin Trials 7: 177–188. doi: 10.1016/0197-2456(86)90046-2
60. Cole TJ, Bellizzi MC, Flegal KM, Dietz WH (2000) Establishing a standard definition for child overweight and obesity worldwide: international survey. BMJ 320: 1240–1243. doi: 10.1136/bmj.320.7244.1240
61. Timpson NJ, Emmett PM, Frayling TM, Rogers I, Hattersley AT, et al. (2008) The fat mass- and obesity-associated locus and dietary intake in children. Am J Clin Nutr 88: 971–978.
62. den Hoed M, Ekelund U, Brage S, Grontved A, Zhao JH, et al. (2010) Genetic susceptibility to obesity and related traits in childhood and adolescence: influence of loci identified by genome-wide association studies. Diabetes 59: 2980–2988. doi: 10.2337/db10-0370
63. Bradfield JP, Taal HR, Timpson NJ, Scherag A, Lecoeur C, et al. (2012) A genome-wide association meta-analysis identifies new childhood obesity loci. Nat Genet 44: 526–531. doi: 10.1038/ng.2247
64. Kilpelainen TO, Zillikens MC, Stancakova A, Finucane FM, Ried JS, et al. (2011) Genetic variation near IRS1 associates with reduced adiposity and an impaired metabolic profile. Nat Genet 43: 753–760. doi: 10.1038/ng.866
65. Sallis JF, Prochaska JJ, Taylor WC (2000) A review of correlates of physical activity of children and adolescents. Med Sci Sports Exerc 32: 963–975. doi: 10.1097/00005768-200005000-00014
66. Szendroedi J, Roden M (2008) Mitochondrial fitness and insulin sensitivity in humans. Diabetologia 51: 2155–2167. doi: 10.1007/s00125-008-1153-2
67. Janssen I, LeBlanc AG (2010) Systematic review of the health benefits of physical activity and fitness in school-aged children and youth. Int J Behav Nutr Phys Act 7: 40. doi: 10.1186/1479-5868-7-40
68. Strong WB, Malina RM, Blimkie CJ, Daniels SR, Dishman RK, et al. (2005) Evidence based physical activity for school-age youth. J Pediatr 146: 732–737. doi: 10.1016/j.jpeds.2005.01.055
69. Leary SD, Ness AR, Davey Smith G, Mattocks C, Deere K, et al. (2008) Physical activity and blood pressure in childhood—findings from a population-based study. Hypertension 51: 92–98. doi: 10.1161/hypertensionaha.107.099051
70. Ekelund U, Brage S, Froberg K, Harro M, Anderssen SA, et al. (2006) TV viewing and physical activity are independently associated with metabolic risk in children: the European Youth Heart Study. PLoS Med 3: 2449–2457. doi: 10.1371/journal.pmed.0030488

71. Brage S, Wedderkopp N, Ekelund U, Franks PW, Wareham NJ, et al. (2004) Objectively measured physical activity correlates with indices of insulin resistance in Danish children. the European Youth Heart Study (EYHS). Int J Obes 28: 1503–1508. doi: 10.1038/sj.ijo.0802772
72. Andersen LB, Riddoch C, Kriemler S, Hills A (2011) Physical activity and cardiovascular risk factors in children. Br J Sports Med 45: 871–876. doi: 10.1136/bjsports-2011-090333
73. Luke A, Dugas LR, Durazo-Arvizu RA, Cao GC, Cooper RS (2011) Assessing physical activity and its relationship to cardiovascular risk factors: NHANES 2003–2006. BMC Public Health 11: 387. doi: 10.1186/1471-2458-11-387
74. Deforche B, Haerens L, de Bourdeaudhuij I (2011) How to make overweight children exercise and follow the recommendations. Int J Pediatr Obes 6: 35–41. doi: 10.3109/17477166.2011.583660
75. Westerterp KR, Speakman JR (2008) Physical activity energy expenditure has not declined since the 1980s and matches energy expenditures of wild mammals. Int J Obes (Lond) 32: 1256–1263. doi: 10.1038/ijo.2008.74
76. Swinburn B, Sacks G, Ravussin E (2009) Increased food energy supply is more than sufficient to explain the US epidemic of obesity. Am J Clin Nutr 90: 1453–1456. doi: 10.3945/ajcn.2009.28595
77. Stubbe JH, Boomsma DI, De Geus EJ (2005) Sports participation during adolescence: a shift from environmental to genetic factors. Med Sci Sports Exerc 37: 563–570. doi: 10.1249/01.mss.0000158181.75442.8b
78. Franks PW, Ravussin E, Hanson RL, Harper IT, Allison DB, et al. (2005) Habitual physical activity in children: the role of genes and the environment. Am J Clin Nutr 82: 901–908.
79. Fisher A, van Jaarsveld CH, Llewellyn CH, Wardle J (2010) Environmental influences on children's physical activity: quantitative estimates using a twin design. PLoS ONE 5: e10110. doi: 10.1371/journal.pone.0010110

There are several tables and supplemental files that are not available in this version of the article. To view this additional information, please use the citation on the first page of this chapter.

CHAPTER 7

ASSOCIATIONS BETWEEN EATING FREQUENCY, ADIPOSITY, DIET, AND ACTIVITY IN 9–10-YEAR-1OLD HEALTHY-WEIGHT AND CENTRALLY OBESE CHILDREN

AMY JENNINGS, AEDÍN CASSIDY, ESTHER M. F. VAN SLUIJS, SIMON J. GRIFFIN, AND AILSA A. WELCH

7.1 INTRODUCTION

Worldwide childhood obesity rates are reaching epidemic proportions with established health consequences that include both the presence of cardiovascular risk factors and strong links to adult morbidity and mortality (1). The distribution of body fat is also thought to predict cardiovascular disease risk with central (abdominal) obesity being more strongly related than total adiposity (2). Evidence also suggests that measures of central obesity, in particular waist-to-height ratio, predict adverse health outcomes including cardiovascular disease independently of BMI. Waist-to-height ratio is also associated with percentage body fat in children (3).

Reprinted with permission from Jennings A, Cassidy A, van Sluijs EMF, Griffin SJ, and Welch AA. Associations Between Eating Frequency, Adiposity, Diet, and Activity in 9–10 year old Healthy-Weight and Centrally Obese Children. Obesity **20**,7 *(2012), DOI: 10.1038/oby.2012.72.*

Poor diet, next to lack of physical activity, has been implicated as a key determinant of obesity (1); however, it is not clear which specific aspects of dietary behavior, such as eating frequency (EF), should be targeted to reduce obesity (4,5). In order to develop effective strategies for obesity prevention, it is critical to determine how different aspects of children's diet relate to body composition and body fat distribution to enable more specific guidance and intervention strategies in the future.

EF (number of eating occasions/meals per day) is one aspect of the diet that is thought to be associated with both weight status and with risk factors associated with chronic diseases (6). Studies in adults have shown that increased EF is associated with improved weight status, although the evidence is equivocal (7,8,9,10,11) perhaps due to the use of different methodologies (12), different definitions of intake occasions (12), underreporting (13), or limited data on energy expenditure (7). The evidence in children is more consistent with four previous studies showing that EF is associated with reduced obesity status (14,15,16,17). These studies, however, have only used questionnaires to examine EF and physical activity meaning they have been unable to concurrently examine distribution and content of meals and snacks and objectively measured physical activity throughout the course of the day. These data would allow us to examine whether the mechanisms proposed to explain the association between increased EF and improved weight status in adults, including elevated physical activity levels (7), and better adjustment of energy intake (EI) in response to preceding eating occasions (7,14,18) also act in children. To date, it has been suggested that the specific distribution of meals and snacks may be important in the maintenance of body weight in children with data showing that increased snacking and breakfast consumption are associated with reduced risk of overweight and obesity (19,20). However, studies have not investigated the composition of foods within eating occasions.

The aims of the current cross-sectional study were as follows: first, to assess whether, in a well-characterized population-based sample of children aged 9–10 years, EF was associated with objectively measured parameters of adiposity when children were stratified by central obesity status. Second, to examine whether any observed associations might be attributable to differences in the composition of the diet or physical activity levels in an attempt to elucidate the potential mediating mechanisms whereby EF might influence bodyweight. Because breakfast consumption and snacking have been highlighted as key meals in terms of weight control and energy regulation, we chose to focus specifically on dietary intake at these meals (19,20,21). It was hypothesized that the children who ate more frequently would have more favorable adiposity status, dietary behaviors, and physical activity levels as compared with children who ate less frequently.

7.2 METHODS AND PROCEDURE

7.2.1 PARTICIPANTS

A total of 92 schools in the county of Norfolk, UK, agreed to take part in the SPEEDY study (Sport, Physical activity and Eating behaviour: Environmental Determinants in Young people), which was designed to quantify dietary habits, physical activity, and their correlates in a population-based sample of 9- to 10-year-old children. A total of 2,064 children participated and detailed descriptions of the sampling strategy, participation rates, and measurement procedures have been previously reported (22). Briefly, children aged 9–10 years were recruited from schools during the 12-week summer term of 2007 (April to July). Trained researchers took anthropometric measurements, and instructed children on how to complete questionnaires and diaries, and how to use an accelerometer. The University of East Anglia local research ethics committee approved the study protocol and the written consent of all participating children and their parents was obtained.

7.2.2 PROCEDURE

Assessment of dietary intake. Dietary intake was recorded using a 4-day food and drink diary where children, with assistance from their parents, were asked to record everything they ate and drank over a 4-day period (including two weekend days). This method has previously been used and validated with children aged 9–10 years (23). Estimated weights of portions were then calculated using published values, including those specific to children (24,25), and mean nutrient intakes estimated using the WISP nutritional analysis software, version 3.0 (Tinuviel Software, Warrington, UK) using nutrient values from McCance and Widdowson's the Composition of Foods (26).

Children were asked to record their food and drink consumption in predefined time periods (6–9 am, 9 am–12 pm, 12–2 pm, 2–5 pm, 5–8 pm, 8–10 pm, 10 pm–6 am). Daily EF was defined as the number of time periods in which children reported consuming any food or drink. Breakfast was defined as consuming any food or drink during the first eating period (between 6 am and 9 am), a mid-day meal as any food or drink consumed in the third eating period (between 12 pm and 2 pm) and an evening meal as food and drink consumed in the fifth eating period (between 5 pm and 8 pm). A snack was defined as food or drink consumed at any other time.

Underreporting of EI was assessed by calculating the ratio of reported EI to estimated energy requirements (EERs), which were estimated using equations from the Food and Agriculture Organization/World Health Organization/United Nations University Expert Consultation Report on Human Energy Requirements (27). A 95% confidence interval for the accuracy of EI:EER was calculated by taking into account the amount of variation inherent in the methods used to estimate EI and EER (28). For the SPEEDY data, the 95% confidence interval for EI:EER was 0.71–1.30 and, therefore, reports of EI within 71–130% of EER were considered to be in the range of normal measurement. As excluding children who underreport can distort dietary intake data, energy reporting quality (ratio of EI:EER) was examined as a continuous variable in all statistical models (29).

Assessment of anthropometry variables. Portable Leicester height measures (Seca, Hamburg, Germany) were used to assess height to the nearest millimeter. A nonsegmental bioimpedance scale (type TBF-300A; Tanita, Tokyo, Japan) was used to measure weight (to the nearest 0.1 kg) and impedance. Previously validated and published equations were used to calculate percentage body fat (30). BMI was calculated as weight in kilograms divided by height in meters squared and transformed to standardized z-scores using the least mean square method and the 1990 British Growth Reference data (31). Waist circumference was measured twice to the nearest millimeter (or three times if a discrepancy of more than 3 cm was observed) at the midpoint between the lower costal margin and the level of the anterior superior iliac crests, using a calibrated measuring tape (Seca, Birmingham, UK), a 0.5-cm correction was applied to account for clothing. Waist-to-height ratio was calculated as waist (cm) divided by height (cm) and used to classify children as centrally obese (>0.46 boys and >0.45 girls) or healthy weight ($\leq$0.46 boys and $\leq$0.45 girls) using recently developed age-appropriate cutoffs to define central obesity (3). We chose to use waist-to-height ratio as the measurement to define obesity in this study for a number of reasons. First, there is substantial evidence that abdominal obesity is a better predictor of cardiovascular risk than BMI in children (2,32,33). Second, waist-to-height ratio has benefits over waist circumference when defining central obesity as it is known that height influences the observations of fat accumulation and distribution. Third, the use of waist-to-height ratio has also been highlighted as a useful public health tool in that very similar cutoff values can be used in different age, gender, and ethnic groups (34). A greater interest in and advocacy for the use of waist-to-height ratio to define obesity has, therefore, been observed in recent years (34).

Assessment of confounding variables. Information on highest parental education (in categories) was obtained from parental self-report. Free-living physical activity was assessed over 1 week with the ActiGraph activity monitor (GTIM; ActiGraph, Pensacola, FL) using a recording epoch of 5 s. Children were fitted with the monitor on the measurement day at school and received both verbal and written instructions regarding its use. They were instructed to wear the monitor during all waking hours, except while engaged in water-based activities. A special written program (MAHUffe; www.mrc epid.cam.ac.uk) was used for data cleaning, reduction, and further analyzes. Zero activity periods of 10 min or longer were interpreted as "not worn time" and these periods were removed from the summation of activity in line with previous research (35). Participants who did not manage to record valid data for at least 500 min per day for at least 3 days were excluded from further analyses. Physical activity was defined as mean daily activity counts per minute, an indicator of overall energy expenditure, and minutes in activity of moderate (2,000–3,999 counts/min) and vigorous activity (>4,000 counts/min).

TABLE 1: Characteristics of 1,700 healthy-weight and centrally obese children aged 9–10 years from the SPEEDY study

	All children (n = 1,700)	Healthy-weight children (n = 1,034)	Centrally obese children (n = 666)
Gender (% girls)	56	53	62[a]
Age (years)	10.3 (0.3)	10.3 (0.3)	10.2 (0.3)
Parental education (%)			
None or school leaving certificate	7	5	9
GCSE (exams usually taken at age 16 years)	51	49	55
A-level (exams usually taken at age 18 years)	25	28	21
University	17	18	15a
Height (cm)	141 (6.6)	140 (6.3)	142 (6.9)[a]
Weight (kg)	36.6 (8.3)	32.7 (4.9)	42.7 (8.9)[a]
BMI (kg/m^2)	18.2 (3.1)	16.5 (1.4)	21.0 (3.1)[a]
BMI (z-score)	0.4 (1.1)	−0.3 (0.8)	1.4 (0.8)[a]
Waist (cm)	64.1 (8.1)	59.4 (3.6)	71.5 (7.7)[a]
Waist: height (cm)	0.454 (0.051)	0.422 (0.109)	0.504 (0.044)[a]
Body fat (%)	30.6 (7.9)	26.1 (4.9)	37.7 (6.1)[a]
Eating occasions			
Eating frequency (occasions/day)	4.3 (0.8)	4.4 (0.7)	4.3 (0.7)
Snacking frequency (occasions/day)	1.57 (0.68)	1.58 (0.68)	1.56 (0.69)
Breakfast frequency (% days)	89.2 (18.0)	89.8 (17.6)	88.3 (18.7)
Composition of the diet			
Energy density (kcal/g)	1.97 (0.31)	1.98 (0.31)	1.97 (0.32)
Total fat (% energy/day)	37.0 (4.6)	36.9 (4.4)	37.2 (4.7)
Carbohydrate (% energy/day)	48.6 (5.1)	48.9 (5.0)	48.3 (5.1)[a]
Protein (% energy/day)	14.3 (2.3)	14.2 (2.3)	14.5 (2.3)[a]
Fiber (g/day)	9.7 (3.4)	9.7 (3.4)	9.7 (3.4)
Fruit and vegetable (g/day)	196 (115)	198 (115)	192 (115)
Physical activity			
Moderate activity (min/day)	48.3 (14.3)	49.2 (14.5)	47.0 (13.9)[a]
Vigorous activity (min/day)	25.0 (13.2)	26.9 (13.9)	22.0 (11.5)[a]
Total activity (counts/min)	668 (218)	691 (227)	631 (197)[a]

Values are mean (SD) or %, n = 1,700. GCSE, General Certificate of Secondary Education; SPEEDY, Sport, Physical activity, and Eating behavior: Environmental Determinants in Young people. [a]Significant difference between healthy-weight and overweight children (P<0.05; independent sample t-test or χ^2 test for categorical data).

7.2.3 STATISTICAL ANALYSIS

As overweight children have been shown to have different dietary and physical activity patterns to healthy-weight children (36), and differences in meal frequencies have been shown between obese and healthy-weight adults (37), we examined the relationships between EF and adiposity separately in healthy-weight and centrally obese children using stratified analyses. Independent sample t-tests and χ^2 test for categorical data were used to examine the differences between characteristics of the healthy-weight and centrally obese children. Associations between EF and children's adiposity status were evaluated using multiple regression analysis after adjustment for relevant confounders. The distribution and nutritional composition of breakfast and snacks, and physical activity levels, were determined in quartile categories of EF. Mean percentage differences, adjusted for relevant confounders, are presented between the highest and lowest quartile (Q4–Q1), with statistical comparisons made using analysis of covariance. Potential confounders included gender, parental educational attainment, underreporting (EI:EER), EI (kcal), and physical activity (counts/min). Statistical analyses were performed using SPSS, version 16.0 for windows (SPSS, Chicago, IL).

7.3 RESULTS

Descriptive statistics for demographic and physical characteristics of the children are shown in Table 1. Of the 2,064 children recruited for the SPEEDY study 1,700 (82%) had adiposity measurements taken, completed diet diaries, provided valid physical activity data, and data on relevant confounders. All the children were aged between 9 and 10 years (10.3 ± 0.3 years) and 56% were girls. The included children did not differ in age to those who were excluded, although there were differences by gender (56% girls included sample v 50% girls excluded sample; $\chi^2 = 4.71$; P = 0.030). Centrally obese children were more likely to be girls ($\chi^2 = 12.6$; P < 0.001) and have parents with lower levels of education ($\chi^2 = 22.1$; P = 0.001). As expected, the healthy-weight children had significantly lower anthropometric measures (all P < 0.05) and higher physical activity levels (t = 6.05; P < 0.001) than the centrally obese children. There were no clear differences in the nutrient intake of the two groups although the healthy-weight children consumed more energy from carbohydrate (t = 2.42; P = 0.015) and less energy from protein (t = −2.31; P = 0.021), as compared with the centrally obese children.

Mean EF was 4.3 eating occasions/day (SD 0.8, range 2.3–6.0). There was no significant difference in reported frequency of meals and snacks between the healthy-weight and centrally obese children (4.4 eating occasions/day, SD 0.7, range 2.3–6.0 vs. 4.3 eating occasions/day SD 0.7, range 2.5–6.0; t = −0.31; P = 0.308), and the distribution of EF in each subgroup was similar (Figure 1). The mean number of snacks reported was 1.6/day in this sample (SD 0.68, range 0.0–3.0). The observed relationship between EF and adiposity differed between the healthy-weight children and the centrally obese children (Table 2). In healthy-weight children, increased EF was associated favorably with adiposity; each unit increase in EF was inversely associated with weight (β = −0.78 kg; P = 0.001), BMI (β = −0.17 kg/m^2; P = 0.020), BMI z-score (β = −0.10; P = 0.014), and waist circumference (β = −0.38 cm; P = 0.031). In centrally obese children, each increase in eating occasion was positively associated with BMI z-score (β = 0.09; P = 0.047) and waist-to-height ratio (β = 0.005 cm; P = 0.036).

EF was significantly associated with both the number of snacks consumed and the nutritional composition of the snacks. As compared with the least-frequent eaters, the most-frequent eaters consumed more snacks (healthy-weight children 188% Q4–Q1, P < 0.001; centrally obese children 200% Q4–Q1, P < 0.001). Moreover, their snacks were lower in energy density (healthy-weight children −35% Q4–Q1, P < 0.001; centrally obese children −33% Q4–Q1, P < 0.001) and higher in carbohydrate (healthy-weight children 10% Q4–Q1, P < 0.001; centrally obese children 15% Q4–Q1, P < 0.001), fiber (healthy-weight children 57% Q4–Q1, P < 0.001; centrally obese 62% Q4–Q1, P < 0.001), and fruit and vegetables (healthy-weight children 201% Q4–Q1, P < 0.001; centrally obese children 209% Q4–Q1, P < 0.001; Figure 2).

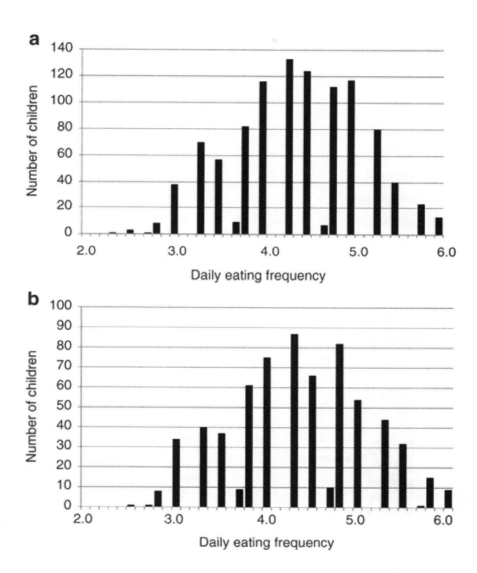

FIGURE 1: Distribution of eating frequency in 1,700 children aged 9–10 years. (a) Healthy-weight children (n = 1,034). (b) Centrally obese children (n = 666).

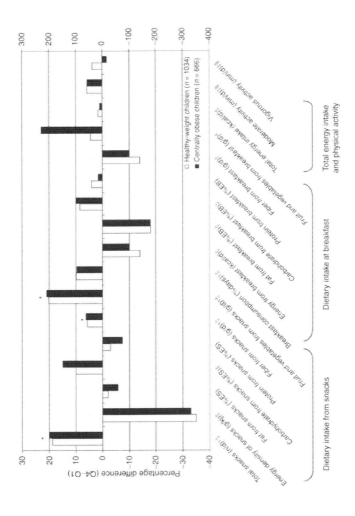

FIGURE 2: Mean percentage differences in dietary intake at specified meals and physical activity by eating frequency. Comparisons were made between the 4th and 1st quartile (healthy-weight children: n = 269 for Q1 and 273 for Q4; centrally obese children: n = 191 for Q1 and 155 for Q4). Values were adjusted for gender, parental education, underreporting, physical activity, and energy intake. %EB, percentage of total energy from breakfast; %ES, percentage of total energy from snacks. *Categories were plotted on the secondary axis. †Values adjusted for energy intake. ‡The difference between the 4th and 1st quartile was significantly different P <0.05 (analysis of covariance) in healthy weight and centrally obese children, or in §healthy-weight children only.

TABLE 2: Association between daily eating frequency and adiposity in 1,700 healthy-weight and centrally obese children aged 9–10 years

	All children (n = 1,700)			Healthy-weight children (n = 1,034)			Centrally obese children (n = 666)		
	β	SE	P value	β	SE	P value	β	SE	P value
Weight (kg)	−0.02	0.31	0.479	−0.78	0.24	0.001	0.64	0.52	0.220
BMI (kg/m^2)	0.02	0.12	0.867	−0.17	0.07	0.020	0.30	0.18	0.088
BMI (z-score)	−0.03	0.04	0.556	−0.10	0.04	0.014	0.09	0.05	0.047
Waist circumference (cm)	0.41	0.31	0.893	−0.38	0.17	0.031	0.71	0.45	0.118
Waist: height (cm)	0.002	0.002	0.313	0.000	0.001	0.849	0.005	0.003	0.036
Body fat (%)	−0.03	0.27	0.992	−0.20	0.21	0.347	0.40	0.33	0.226

Values are β coefficients and SE for a one unit increase in eating frequency, multivariate linear regression adjusted for gender, parental education, underreporting, energy intake, and physical activity.

Breakfast consumption was reported on an average of 89.2% of days (SD 18.0, range 0–100%). EF was associated with the number of days that breakfast consumption was reported with children in the highest quartile of EF reporting breakfast consumption most frequently (healthy-weight children 10% Q4–Q1, P < 0.001; centrally obese children 9% Q4–Q1, P < 0.001). The nutritional composition of food and drinks reported at breakfast time also differed by EF. As compared with the least-frequent eaters (quartile 1) the most-frequent eaters (quartile 5) reported lower EI (healthy-weight children −14% Q4–Q1, P < 0.001; centrally obese children −10% Q4–Q1, P = 0.044), lower total fat intake (healthy-weight children −18% Q4–Q1, P < 0.001; centrally obese children −18% Q4–Q1, P < 0.001), and higher carbohydrate intake at breakfast (healthy-weight children 9% Q4–Q1, P < 0.001; centrally obese children 10% Q4–Q1, P = 0.001; Figure 2).

The percentage differences in EI between extreme EF quartiles were similar for both healthy-weight (1.5% Q4–Q1, P < 0.001) and centrally obese children (1.1% Q4–Q1, P = 0.035), as were differences in activity of moderate intensity (healthy-weight children 6% Q4–Q1, P = 0.040 and overweight children 6% Q4–Q1, P = 0.104). The direction of differences in high-intensity activity differed between the two groups, however, with the healthy-weight children who ate most frequently reporting significantly higher levels of vigorous activity than the children who ate least frequently (4% Q4–Q1, P = 0.033), with the converse observed for overweight children, although this did not reach statistical significance (−2% Q4–Q1, P = 0.801; Figure 2).

7.4 DISCUSSION

Using a large population-based sample of 9- to 10-year-old children, we observed that increased EF was associated with improved body weight, BMI, and waist circumference in healthy-weight children with relative mean differences of −2.4% for body weight, −1.0% for BMI, −33% for BMI z-score, and −0.6% for waist circumference detected. Conversely, increased EF was associated with a higher BMI z-score and waist-to-height ratio in centrally obese children, with relative mean differences of 6% and 1%, respectively. Increased EF was also associated with the more favorable nutritional composition of breakfast and snacks in both groups, with children in the highest quartiles of EF reporting improved fruit and vegetable, fat, fiber, and carbohydrate intakes at these meals, as compared with the children in the lowest quartiles. Finally, an inverse association between high-intensity physical activity and EF was seen for the healthy-weight, but not the centrally obese children. These findings were all independent of covariates known to be associated with obesity including gender, EI, physical activity, parental education, and underreporting.

Despite the large amount of work examining the associations between dietary intake and weight status in children, it is not entirely clear how different eating behaviors relate to measures of adiposity in children, or the mechanisms behind these associations. To our knowledge, this is the first time a study has examined the behaviors that may be associated with EF in a large cohort of children using food diaries and objectively measured physical activity. Previous studies in children have shown daily meal frequency to be associated with a lower prevalence of obesity in German children aged 5–6 years (14), lower BMI z-score in German children aged

7–14 years (15), and with lower BMI in Portuguese girls aged 13–17 years (16). Furthermore snacking frequency has shown to be associated with overweight status in the National Health and Nutrition Examination Survey (NHANES) study (19). The current study builds on the results of this previous work by showing EF to be differentially associated with adiposity in healthy-weight and centrally obese children. The magnitude of our findings may have potential clinical relevance as reductions in BMI z-score similar to those observed in the current study have previously been associated with reductions in cardiometabolic risk factors in children of a similar age. Specifically, a decrease in BMI z-score of 0.1 has been associated with significantly lower insulin (−19 pmol/l), and total (−0.1 mmol/l) and low-density lipoprotein cholesterol levels (−0.12 mmol/l; ref. 38).

Our data also suggest that there may be a favorable impact of increased EF on fruit and vegetable, fat, fiber, and carbohydrate intake at the specific meal times examined in this study. These food groups and nutrients are known to be important in terms of weight control in children and are the dietary components forming the basis of public health policy relating to the prevention and treatment of childhood obesity (39). We have also shown that intake of these foods and nutrients are improved at specific meals that have been highlighted as important in terms of reducing obesity in children (19,20).

The positive relationship observed between EF and adiposity in centrally obese children does not appear to have been reported previously in the literature. It is possible that the differences observed in the associations between EF and adiposity between healthy-weight and obese children were linked to disparities in how the children were compensating EI and energy expenditure as our data show no association between physical activity and EF in centrally obese children. This could indicate that centrally obese children who were eating more frequently were, unlike the healthy-weight children, not compensating for their increased EI by being physically active. Previous studies have shown that children are generally good energy compensators, although this ability declines with age, and there is some evidence that overweight children compensate less well than healthy-weight children (40). A further possibility is that some of the centrally obese children were eating fewer meals as a strategy for weight loss, which could make it appear that there were positive associations between frequency of eating and adiposity in this group.

Strengths of this study are robust methodologies that allowed us to collect data on EF, the composition of the diet, and objectively measured physical activity concurrently. Unlike previous studies that have investigated EF, we were able to examine the composition of foods and nutrients within eating occasions. There was also a large sample recruited using a population-based sampling strategy. Underreporting is common in nutritional studies, especially among those who are overweight or obese (29), by using underreporting as a covariate we were able to control for the effect misreporting may have had on any reported associations.

The limitations include the cross-sectional design that means we cannot determine whether reverse causality was a factor. Furthermore, although our sample included children from a diverse range of urban and rural environments and areas of varying deprivation, Norfolk does not have large cities, and is culturally less varied than some parts of the country, as there are a low proportion of families from different ethnic backgrounds. Lower rates of overweight and obesity were also found in the current sample as compared with national averages (22). We acknowledge that our findings would not be generalizable to more ethnically diverse populations and further work is needed to see whether these findings are replicated in other samples. Finally, although food diaries have been shown to provide a valid measure of food intake in this age group (23), underreporting was accounted for in the present analysis and substantial assistance from parents was requested, we cannot entirely eliminate measurement error or the possibility of reporting bias by the children or parents. Furthermore, our definition of EF was restrictive (to a maximum of six eating occasions), although more detailed than previous studies, and it is possible that some children consumed more than one meal or snack in the time periods we considered. This misclassification may have underestimated the magnitude of associations between EF, measures of adiposity, diet, and physical activity in this sample. If EF was more precisely defined, the associations observed may have been of an even greater magnitude.

In conclusion, we found that increased EF was favorably associated with body weight and adiposity measures in healthy-weight children but not centrally obese children. The healthy-weight children who ate most frequently reported significantly higher physical activity levels and improved composition of snacks and breakfast in terms of fruit and vegetables, fat, fiber, and carbohydrates, as compared with the children who ate least frequently. In contrast, our data show no association between objectively measured physical activity and EF in centrally obese children. It is, therefore, important that public health messages supporting increased EF in children, such as those that promote breakfast or snacking consumption, should focus on promoting dietary quality and the importance of physical activity in balancing EI. The findings of this study suggest that future obesity interventions should consider the mediating role of physical activity and diet quality in the relationship between EF and in children, however, further evidence from prospective studies is needed to confirm the findings of this study.

REFERENCES

1. World Health Organization. Obesity: Preventing and Managing the Global Epidemic. Report of a WHO Consultation. World Health Organization: Geneva, 2000.
2. Mokha JS, Srinivasan SR, Dasmahapatra P et al. Utility of waist-to-height ratio in assessing the status of central obesity and related cardiometabolic risk profile among normal weight and overweight/obese children: the Bogalusa Heart Study. BMC Pediatr 2010;10:73.
3. Nambiar S, Hughes I, Davies PS. Developing waist-to-height ratio cut-offs to define overweight and obesity in children and adolescents. Public Health Nutr 2010;13:1566–1574.
4. National Institute for Health and Clinical Excellence. Obesity: Guidance on the Prevention, Identification, Assessment and Management of Overweight and Obesity in Adults and Children. London, 2006.
5. Scottish Intercollegiate Guidelines Network. Management of Obesity. A National Clinical Guideline. Scottish Intercollegiate Guidelines Network: Edinburgh, UK, 2010.
6. Titan SM, Bingham S, Welch A et al. Frequency of eating and concentrations of serum cholesterol in the Norfolk population of the European prospective investigation into cancer (EPIC-Norfolk): cross sectional study. BMJ 2001;323:1286–1288.
7. Duval K, Strychar I, Cyr MJ et al. Physical activity is a confounding factor of the relation between eating frequency and body composition. Am J Clin Nutr 2008;88:1200–1205.
8. Drummond SE, Crombie NE, Cursiter MC, Kirk TR. Evidence that eating frequency is inversely related to body weight status in male, but not female, non-obese adults reporting valid dietary intakes. Int J Obes Relat Metab Disord 1998;22:105–112.
9. Yannakoulia M, Melistas L, Solomou E, Yiannakouris N. Association of eating frequency with body fatness in pre- and postmenopausal women. Obesity (Silver Spring) 2007;15:100–106.

10. Ma Y, Bertone ER, Stanek EJ 3rd et al. Association between eating patterns and obesity in a free-living US adult population. Am J Epidemiol 2003;158:85–92.
11. Ruidavets JB, Bongard V, Bataille V, Gourdy P, Ferrières J. Eating frequency and body fatness in middle-aged men. Int J Obes Relat Metab Disord 2002;26:1476–1483.
12. Bertéus Forslund H, Lindroos AK, Sjöström L, Lissner L. Meal patterns and obesity in Swedish women-a simple instrument describing usual meal types, frequency and temporal distribution. Eur J Clin Nutr 2002;56:740–747.
13. Summerbell CD, Moody RC, Shanks J, Stock MJ, Geissler C. Relationship between feeding pattern and body mass index in 220 free-living people in four age groups. Eur J Clin Nutr 1996;50:513–519.
14. Toschke AM, Küchenhoff H, Koletzko B, von Kries R. Meal frequency and childhood obesity. Obes Res 2005;13:1932–1938.
15. Würbach A, Zellner K, Kromeyer-Hauschild K. Meal patterns among children and adolescents and their associations with weight status and parental characteristics. Public Health Nutr 2009;12:1115–1121.
16. Mota J, Fidalgo F, Silva R et al. Relationships between physical activity, obesity and meal frequency in adolescents. Ann Hum Biol 2008;35:1–10.
17. Nicklas TA, Morales M, Linares A et al. Children's meal patterns have changed over a 21-year period: the Bogalusa Heart Study. J Am Diet Assoc 2004;104:753–761.
18. Bellisle F. Impact of the daily meal pattern on energy balance. Scand J Nutr 2004;48:114–118.
19. Keast DR, Nicklas TA, O'Neil CE. Snacking is associated with reduced risk of overweight and reduced abdominal obesity in adolescents: National Health and Nutrition Examination Survey (NHANES) 1999–2004. Am J Clin Nutr 2010;92:428–435.
20. Rampersaud GC, Pereira MA, Girard BL, Adams J, Metzl JD. Breakfast habits, nutritional status, body weight, and academic performance in children and adolescents. J Am Diet Assoc 2005;105:743–60; quiz 761.
21. McCrory MA, Campbell WW. Effects of eating frequency, snacking, and breakfast skipping on energy regulation: symposium overview. J Nutr 2011;141:144–147.
22. van Sluijs EM, Skidmore PM, Mwanza K et al. Physical activity and dietary behaviour in a population-based sample of British 10-year old children: the SPEEDY study (Sport, Physical activity and Eating behaviour: environmental Determinants in Young people). BMC Public Health 2008;8:388.
23. Crawford PB, Obarzanek E, Morrison J, Sabry ZI. Comparative advantage of 3-day food records over 24-hour recall and 5-day food frequency validated by observation of 9- and 10-year-old girls. J Am Diet Assoc 1994;94:626–630.
24. Crawley H. Food Portion Sizes. H.M. Stationary Office: London, 2002.
25. Wrieden WL, Longbottom PJ, Adamson AJ et al. Estimation of typical food portion sizes for children of different ages in Great Britain. Br J Nutr 2008;99:1344–1353.
26. Food Standards Agency. McCance and Widdowsons's the Composition of Foods, 6th edn. Royal Society of Chemistry: Cambridge, 2002.
27. Torun B. Energy requirements of children and adolescents. Public Health Nutr 2005;8:968–993.

28. Black AE, Cole TJ. Within- and between-subject variation in energy expenditure measured by the doubly-labelled water technique: implications for validating reported dietary energy intake. Eur J Clin Nutr 2000;54:386–394.
29. Rennie KL, Coward A, Jebb SA. Estimating under-reporting of energy intake in dietary surveys using an individualised method. Br J Nutr 2007;97:1169–1176.
30. Tyrrell VJ, Richards G, Hofman P et al. Foot-to-foot bioelectrical impedance analysis: a valuable tool for the measurement of body composition in children. Int J Obes Relat Metab Disord 2001;25:273–278.
31. Cole TJ, Freeman JV, Preece MA. British 1990 growth reference centiles for weight, height, body mass index and head circumference fitted by maximum penalized likelihood. Stat Med 1998;17:407–429.
32. Kahn HS, Imperatore G, Cheng YJ. A population-based comparison of BMI percentiles and waist-to-height ratio for identifying cardiovascular risk in youth. J Pediatr 2005;146:482–488.
33. Savva SC, Tornaritis M, Savva ME et al. Waist circumference and waist-to-height ratio are better predictors of cardiovascular disease risk factors in children than body mass index. Int J Obes Relat Metab Disord 2000;24:1453–1458.
34. Browning LM, Hsieh SD, Ashwell M. A systematic review of waist-to-height ratio as a screening tool for the prediction of cardiovascular disease and diabetes: 0·5 could be a suitable global boundary value. Nutr Res Rev 2010;23:247–269.
35. Riddoch CJ, Bo-Andersen L, Wedderkopp N et al. Physical activity levels and patterns of 9- and 15-yr-old European children. Med Sci Sports Exerc 2004;36:86–92.
36. Oellingrath IM, Svendsen MV, Brantsaeter AL. Eating patterns and overweight in 9- to 10-year-old children in Telemark County, Norway: a cross-sectional study. Eur J Clin Nutr 2010;64:1272–1279.
37. Bertéus Forslund H, Torgerson JS, Sjöström L, Lindroos AK. Snacking frequency in relation to energy intake and food choices in obese men and women compared to a reference population. Int J Obes (Lond) 2005;29:711–719.
38. Kolsgaard ML, Joner G, Brunborg C et al. Reduction in BMI z-score and improvement in cardiometabolic risk factors in obese children and adolescents. The Oslo Adiposity Intervention Study — a hospital/public health nurse combined treatment. BMC Pediatr 2011;11:47.
39. Parliamentary Office of Science and Technology. Childhood obesity. Postnote 2003;205. <http:www.parliament.ukdocumentspostpn205.pdf>.
40. Cecil JE, Palmer CN, Wrieden W et al. Energy intakes of children after preloads: adjustment, not compensation. Am J Clin Nutr 2005;82:302–308.

CHAPTER 8

ROLE OF DEVELOPMENTAL OVERNUTRITION IN PEDIATRIC OBESITY AND TYPE 2 DIABETES

DANA DABELEA AND CURTIS S. HARROD

8.1 INTRODUCTION

Childhood obesity continues to be a significant public health burden, with almost one-third of children in the United States classified as overweight or obese (≥85th percentile of weight for height).[1] The original "Barker hypothesis"[2] (also known as the fetal origins of adult disease hypothesis) postulated, based on epidemiological evidence available in the early 1990s, that fetal life was a critical period for the development of later, adult chronic diseases. Later on, empirical evidence began to accumulate identifying developmental pathways and mechanisms that increase the likelihood of excess adiposity and increased risk of type 2 diabetes (T2D) among offspring. Epidemiologic studies have demonstrated that both low- and high-birth weight offspring have increased obesity in later life, though this is likely through different mechanisms. Thus, intrauterine exposures resulting in both restricted and exacerbated fetal growth also lead to in-

---

Reprinted with permission from Dabelea D and Harrod CS. Role of Developmental Overnutrition in Pediatric Obesity and Type 2 Diabetes. Nutrition Reviews *71,S1 (2013), DOI: 10.1111/nure.12061.*

creased adiposity later in the life course.[3, 4] Fetal growth restriction occurs as a result of inadequate fuel substrates and oxygenation, resulting in a phenotypically undernourished infant. Excessive fetal growth occurs when the fetus is overnourished by excess maternal fuels, which can deregulate the fetus' adipoinsular axis, resulting in altered energy and appetite regulation, and disordered adipocyte metabolism.[5] The adipoinsular axis, which involves the hormones insulin and leptin, may play a significant role in the development of adiposity and diabetes. The pathway related to excess maternal fuels results in increased fetal and neonatal fat mass and subsequent childhood obesity, which increases the likelihood of cardiovascular disease (CVD), T2D, metabolic syndrome, and other morbidities later in life. Studies have shown that developmental overnutrition can occur as a result of the fetus being exposed to an excess of maternal fuels from maternal diabetes,[6-8] maternal prepregnancy overweight and obesity,[9, 10] and excess gestational weight gain (GWG).[11-13] Based on this and other evidence reviewed herein, it appears that a transgenerational vicious cycle is set in motion, which perpetuates and likely contributes to the rise in the prevalence and risk for early-onset obesity and T2D.[14, 15]

The present review examines the evidence that an altered intrauterine environment results in long-term consequences for the offspring. It also explores the history and concept of developmental overnutrition along with the evidence of the effect it has on childhood adiposity and T2D, public health consequences, potential preventive approaches, and future directions for research.

8.2 OBESITY AND TYPE 2 DIABETES AMONG CHILDREN AND ADOLESCENTS IN THE UNITED STATES

The potential roles of developmental overnutrition and the transgenerational vicious cycle must be seen in the context of current trends in obesity and T2D among children and adolescents in the United States. In recent decades, the prevalence of obesity (≥95th percentile of weight for height) has increased dramatically among US children and adolescents.[16] Currently, the prevalence of obesity is close to 20% in youth older than 6 years of age, which results in an enormous burden on health resources and overall population health. Furthermore, obese individuals often have comorbidities such as T2D, which is also on the rise.[17] The most recent data come from the multicenter, population-based, prospective registry study SEARCH for Diabetes in Youth, where investigators explored the incidence of T2D by age and race-ethnicity among US youth.[18] Native Americans had the highest incidence of T2D among both 10–14 and 15–19 year olds, followed by other minority youth; the lowest rates were seen among non-Hispanic white youth. Additionally, 15–19 year olds had a higher incidence of T2D than 10–14 year olds[18] in all race/ethnic groups. Few data exist on trends for T2D in youth, though recent data from the SEARCH study suggest it is increasing among Hispanics and non-Hispanic whites.[19]

8.3 CONCEPT OF DEVELOPMENTAL OVERNUTRITION

The fuel-mediated teratogenesis hypothesis,[20] first proposed in the 1950s by Pederson, postulates that intrauterine fetal exposure to hyperglycemia in women with diabetes in pregnancy causes permanent fetal changes, leading to malformations, greater birth weight, and an increased risk of developing T2D and obesity in later life. A likely mechanism occurs through intrauterine exposure to a hyperglycemic environment, which induces hyperinsulinemia. Insulin is an adipogenic hormone; thus, this type of environment would catalyze excessive fetal growth, increasing the risk of macrosomia. In the 1980s, this hypothesis was broadened to include the possibility that other fuels, in addition to glucose, such as free fatty acids, ketone bodies, and amino acids also increase fetal growth.[20] More recently, it has been suggested that fetal overnutrition may also occur in nondiabetic but obese pregnancies, and that it has consequences on offspring that extend beyond those apparent at birth.[21] Most recently, scientists have started to refer to this theory as "developmental overnutrition,"[22] in recognition of the likelihood that overnutrition occurring during other developmentally sensitive periods, such as early postnatal life, may also have long-term consequences on offspring.

8.4 EFFECTS ON CHILDHOOD ADIPOSITY

It is well known that infants born to mothers with diabetes have increased birth length and weight. However, it is less clear whether developmental overnutrition leads to increased adiposity later in life. Pettitt et al.[23] analyzed the weight of 5–19-year-old offspring of Pima Indian women, a population with one of the highest T2D risks in the world. A unique aspect of this study was that the investigators knew whether the offspring were the product of nondiabetic, prediabetic, or diabetic pregnancies from serial testing over many years. After adjusting for maternal and offspring characteristics, 5–9-, 10–14-, and 15–19-year-old offspring of mothers who were diabetic during pregnancy all had significantly greater relative weight compared to the offspring of women who were either prediabetic ($P<0.001$) or nondiabetic during pregnancy ($P<0.002$).[23] Because it was possible to determine a prediabetic pregnancy (i.e., a mother that did not have diabetes during pregnancy, but developed it after the birth of the child), it was possible to examine the in utero role of overnutrition independent of a genetic predisposition to later diabetes. At all ages from birth to 19 years, there was no difference in relative weight for offspring of prediabetic compared to nondiabetic mothers ($P<0.20$).[23] Interestingly, no effect was seen among offspring aged 20 years and older; this is likely because obesity is extremely prevalent in this population during adulthood. [24] There is now substantial evidence that these effects are present in other populations with lower obesity and T2D risks than the Pima Indians.

The retrospective cohort study, Exploring Perinatal Outcomes among Children (EPOCH), consisted of 461 multiethnic offspring, 82 of whom were exposed to GDM and 379 youth who were unexposed.[25] The results showed that offspring exposed to GDM had significantly increased BMI, waist circumference, visceral and subcutaneous adipose tissue (by magnetic resonance imaging), and a more central subscapular-to-triceps skinfold thickness ratio, after adjusting for maternal and offspring characteristics.[25] Not only did the study confirm the relationships of exposure to diabetes in utero with increased adiposity during childhood and early adolescence, it also showed that adipose tissue is more centrally distributed in exposed offspring. Not surprisingly, the relationships were attenuated when adjustments were made for maternal prepregnancy BMI. Evidence described below shows that maternal obesity and maternal fuels, in addition to glucose, are also related to developmental overnutrition. Thus, it is likely that maternal obesity is part of a common causal pathway linking maternal obesity and diabetes, through elevated maternal fuels, to offspring outcomes. Therefore, adjustment for prepregnancy BMI is likely an overadjustment.

Childhood overweight and obesity are not the only morbidities associated with developmental overnutrition. Boney et al.[26] explored whether developmental overnutrition was associated with development of metabolic syndrome in a longitudinal cohort study of 179 children followed from birth to early adolescence. Of the participants, 84 were born large for gestational age (LGA) and 95 were average for gestational age (AGA). Compared with AGA offspring, those born LGA had a twofold increased hazard for metabolic syndrome by the age of 11 years. Additionally, independent of maternal diabetes, maternal obesity increased the risk of metabolic syndrome by 1.8-fold.[26] These findings provide evidence of metabolic factors that contribute to excess adiposity in childhood and early adolescence among offspring of obese pregnant women, independent of GDM presence.

8.5 EFFECTS ON CHILDHOOD TYPE 2 DIABETES

The first study of the long-term consequences of maternal diabetes in utero on risk of T2D in offspring again came from the Pima Indian study.[27] The results showed that the odds of being exposed to maternal diabetes in utero was 10.4 times greater (95% confidence interval [CI] 4.3–25.1) among offspring with T2D compared to offspring without such exposure. Furthermore, the researchers estimated that maternal diabetes was responsible for 35.4% of all T2D cases among exposed offspring.[27] More recently, the SEARCH case-control study tested if these associations existed in an ethnically diverse population of youth aged 10–22 years in Colorado and South Carolina. After adjusting for offspring age, sex, and race/ethnicity, the odds of exposure to diabetes in utero was 7.3 times greater (95%

CI 3.2–16.8) among offspring with T2D than controls, with similar results in non-Hispanic whites, Hispanics, and African Americans.[28] Thus, the effects of developmental overnutrition on pediatric T2D are detectable in both high- and low-risk populations.

8.6 ASSOCIATIONS REFLECT SPECIFIC INTRAUTERINE EFFECTS

Clearly, fetal development takes place in an environment shaped both by parental genetics and environmental influences. What evidence is there that the associations described above reflect specific intrauterine effects and that the outcomes are not primarily due to parental genetics or shared familial behaviors? In an attempt to test this hypothesis of specificity of the intrauterine effects, Dabelea et al.[6] selected nuclear Pima Indian families with at least one offspring born before and one after the mother was diagnosed with T2D. Siblings born after a maternal diagnosis of diabetes (exposed) had a BMI that was 2.6 kg/m^2 higher (P=0.003) than that of siblings born before diabetes was diagnosed (unexposed). However, there were no significant differences in offspring BMI among those who were born before or after paternal diagnosis of diabetes (P=0.50).[6]

Next, the researchers explored the presence of T2D among siblings who were born before and after maternal and paternal diagnosis of diabetes. Siblings exposed to maternal diabetes in utero were 3.0 times more likely to have T2D than those born before the mother developed diabetes (P=0.02).[6] No significant differences in T2D risk in the offspring were found between siblings born before or after the diagnosis of paternal T2D (odds ratio 1.3, P=0.80).[6] These results clearly indicate that exposure to an in utero diabetic environment (developmental overnutrition) increases the likelihood that the offspring will develop obesity and T2D, independent of genetic or familial factors.

8.7 POTENTIAL MECHANISMS

While it is clear that developmental overnutrition increases the likelihood of excess adiposity and early-onset T2D among exposed offspring, and that these associations exist over and above genetic and familial factors, what are some of the potential mechanisms that may explain these intrauterine effects?

8.7.1 ROLE OF MATERNAL FUELS

Pregnancy is a state of relative insulin resistance, which spares glucose, amino acids, and fatty acids for placental-fetal transport.[29] Therefore, obese or diabetic pregnant women, who have severe insulin resistance, transport an excess of nutrients, such as glucose, to the fetus.[20] Increased transfer of glucose across the placental barrier in obese or diabetic pregnancies results in the fetal pancreas secreting excess insulin, which acts as a growth hormone and may result in excessive growth or macrosomia in the offspring. This process is presumed to increase the risk of obesity later in life.

Several studies have explored specific maternal fuels, such as glucose and free fatty acids (FFA). In 2007, Hillier et al.[30] analyzed 9,439 multiethnic mother-offspring pairs. All mothers received a 50 g, 1-h glucose challenge test as screening for GDM, followed by a diagnostic test using a 3-h, 100 g oral glucose tolerance test. Offspring weight was measured at 5–7 years of age. Sex-specific weight-for-age percentiles were calculated and shown to be linearly associated with maternal glucose levels, even among mothers with a normal glucose challenge test during screening.[30] These results showed that maternal glucose may represent one of the important fuels involved in developmental overnutrition.

However, maternal glucose is not the only fuel believed to be involved. Schaffer-Graf et al.[31] studied 150 pregnant women and their offspring to examine whether several maternal fuels, including FFA and triglyceride levels, were associated with neonatal outcomes. The authors found positive correlations between maternal FFA levels and fetal abdominal circumference ($r=0.22$, $P=0.02$), FFA in cord blood ($r=0.28$, $P=0.004$), and neonatal fat mass ($r=0.27$, $P=0.01$).[31] Thus, maternal FFAs appear to be associated with neonatal adiposity. However, it is important to note that no studies have thus far explored whether maternal FFAs are associated with obesity or T2D later in life.

8.7.2 ROLE OF THE ADIPOINSULAR AXIS

The adipoinsular axis is a dual-hormone feedback loop based on the adipocytokine, leptin, and the adipogenic hormone insulin. The endocrine feedback loop links the brain (i.e., autonomic nervous system [ANS] and hypothalamus) and endocrine pancreas with other peripheral leptin- and insulin-sensitive tissues in the regulation of feeding behavior, metabolic regulation, and energy expenditure.[32, 33] Leptin, which is produced and secreted by adipocytes, occurs at levels proportionate to the amount of fat stored. As adiposity and leptin levels concurrently increase, insulin secretion decreases due to central and direct actions on pancreatic β-cells.[33] When the adipoinsular axis is regulated appropriately, nutrient balance may be maintained; however, if dysregulation of the axis occurs, then obesity and hyperinsulinemia resulting in the development of diabetes may occur.[33] In animal[32, 34] and human studies,[35-37] increasing circulating leptin levels, which is a biologic indicator of leptin resistance, has been shown to be associated with CVD, hyperphagia, insulin resistance, and obesity.

8.8 PUBLIC HEALTH CONSEQUENCES

Historically, T2D was uncommonly diagnosed among children; however, an increase in T2D among children and adolescents has occurred in the past few decades.[17, 38] In the first population-based study to explore the changes in T2D prevalence in youth, Dabelea et al.[27] analyzed 5,274 Pima Indian children from 1967 to 1996 to determine potential trends in the prevalence of early-onset T2D. The authors found that the prevalence of T2D increased almost threefold over the past three decades, especially among 15–19 year olds. They next explored the potential role of developmental overnutrition (exposure to maternal diabetes) in explaining these trends.[27] From 1967–1976 to 1987–1996, the prevalence of exposure to maternal diabetes in utero increased from 2% of all pregnancies to 7.5%. This was associated with a doubling of the population-attributable fraction (PAF), which represents the proportion of T2D in the population that may be due to exposure. This translated into a PAF of 35.4%, which means that over one-third of Pima Indian youth with T2D in 1987–1996 may have developed T2D because they were exposed to maternal diabetes in utero. Together, increasing weight and increasing frequency of exposure to diabetes in utero accounted for most of the increase in T2D prevalence in Pima Indian children over the past 30 years.[27]

Dabelea et al.[28] later replicated these findings in a tri-ethnic population in the SEARCH case-control study. Here, they separately estimated the proportion of T2D in youth attributable to exposure to maternal diabetes, to maternal obesity, and to both. The results showed that 4.7% of T2D among youth aged 10–22 years was attributable to maternal diabetes (in the absence of obesity), 19.7% was attributable to maternal obesity (in the absence of diabetes), and 22.8% was attributable to exposure to both maternal morbidities. Overall, an estimated 47.2% of T2D in youth was attributable to intrauterine exposure to maternal diabetes and obesity,[28] which is similar to that seen among the Pimas. Clearly, developmental overnutrition has a significant public health impact. These results also support the idea of a vicious cycle of obesity and diabetes leading to obesity and its comorbidities in the next generation.

8.9 POSTNATAL MODIFICATION OF EFFECTS

The role of postnatal life in mediating or modifying the effects of developmental overnutrition has not been studied extensively. Recently, the EPOCH study explored growth trajectories after birth among offspring exposed and not exposed to maternal diabetes in utero.[39] During an in-person research visit, current height and weight of children aged 6–13 years were measured. Historical recumbent length (up to 2 years of age) and height and weight measures were abstracted from medical records. These data were used to estimate BMI and BMI growth trajectory.[39] On average, BMI growth trajectories during early stages of life (birth to 26 months of age) were not significantly different between exposed and unexposed offspring (P=0.48). Although there were no immediate and consistently observed differences in mean BMI or growth trajectory up to the age of 26 months, both were significantly greater among exposed offspring from the age of 27 months to 13 years (P=0.01; P=0.008, respectively).[39] Furthermore, the difference in BMI based on maternal diabetes exposure status became much more evident around puberty. The largest difference in BMI growth trajectories between exposed and unexposed offspring was around 10–13 years of age ($\beta=1.05$; $P=0.005$). This highlights the fact that other developmentally sensitive periods, such as the pubertal period, may modify the long-term consequences of intrauterine exposures, supporting the concept of developmental overnutrition.

Other postnatal periods and factors must also be considered. One such period is early life and one such factor is breastfeeding, both of which are known to affect offspring obesity and T2D status.[40] The role of breastfeeding status as a potential moderator of the association between exposure to maternal diabetes in utero and childhood BMI, skinfold measures (subscapular and triceps), waist circumference, and visceral and subcutaneous fat was also explored in the EPOCH study.[41] Breastfeeding status was calculated as breast milk-months (similar to pack-years with regard to smoking), which accounts for both the duration and exclusivity of breastfeeding. Analyses were stratified based on breastfeeding status categorized as low (<6 breast milk-months) or adequate (≥6 breast milk-months). Among offspring with low breastfeeding status, exposure to diabetes in utero was associated with significantly higher adiposity parameters in childhood. However, among offspring with adequate breastfeeding history, all of the statistically significant excesses of adiposity among offspring exposed to diabetes in utero were substantially attenuated and no longer statistically significant.[41] Thus, breastfeeding appears to reduce the harmful influence of in utero exposure to maternal diabetes on offspring adiposity measures.

8.10 HOW CAN THESE EFFECTS BE PREVENTED?

Although no studies have directly addressed preventing the vicious cycle, studies have suggested possible approaches. In a study by Hillier et al.[30] results suggested that maternal glucose levels above 122 mg/dL were associated with childhood overweight and obesity; however, levels below that were not significantly associated with offspring adiposity. Thus, if maternal glucose levels were carefully monitored and controlled during gestation, it might be possible to reduce the risk of later adiposity among offspring. The only evidence to date indicating whether directly reducing maternal glucose levels reduces offspring obesity is from a study conducted by Gillman et al.[42] This was a follow-up of a multicenter randomized trial of treatment of mild GDM that randomized mothers to a group that received dietary advice, blood glucose monitoring, and insulin therapy (~20% received insulin) or a control group. At birth, macrosomia was reduced in the treatment group compared to the control group, 5.3% to 21.9%, respectively. However, no significant differences in offspring BMI were observed at 4–5 years of age.[42] Since the EPOCH study found no differences in BMI growth trajectories by in utero exposure status at these ages, but only later in life, it is possible that longer follow-up of these offspring will show that reducing maternal glucose levels has an impact on offspring adiposity. However, such follow-up may require years before the answer is known. Another possible reason for the negative findings in the Gillman study may be the need to control the effect of other fuels that are elevated in obese pregnancies, such as FFA and triglycerides, which may have long-term programming consequences. For example, controlling gestational weight gain in pregnancies of obese women may reduce the levels of elevated maternal fuels and represent another potential avenue for prevention. Based on the observational evidence that breastfeeding is associated with less adiposity among offspring exposed to maternal diabetes, a study directly testing this hypothesis could be undertaken.

8.11 FUTURE RESEARCH DIRECTIONS

First and foremost, an improved understanding of the biologic mechanisms involving developmental overnutrition must be a priority. This can be obtained through animal studies, followed by rapid translation to studies in humans. Specific biologic mechanisms that need to be better understood include the effects of fuels on fetal target tissues, appetite regulation in exposed offspring, and the potential role of epigenetics. Additionally, large, longitudinal prebirth cohort studies need to be initiated with specific aims involving the interaction of intrauterine effects with postnatal life.

Subsequent to improving understanding of the mechanisms involved, randomized clinical trials of interventions prior to or during pregnancy, including reduction of gestational weight gain, as well as optimizing early life nutrition, and later eating behaviors and physical activity patterns, need to be conducted to determine how the transgenerational cycle may be broken. Preventing this cycle may not only provide direct health benefits to the offspring, but should provide a cumulative positive effect for succeeding generations.

8.12 CONCLUSION

It is clear that fetal overnutrition results in increased risk of obesity and T2D in exposed offspring. These associations appear to be above and beyond those that might be due to genetic susceptibility for diabetes and obesity. Of the potential mechanisms studied, it appears that the theory of fuel-mediated teratogenesis has substantial support. Maternal diabetes and obesity account for almost 50% of T2D in youth and likely trigger a transgenerational vicious cycle of obesity and diabetes. It appears likely that postnatal life can modify the long-term consequences of fetal overnutrition, though the observation that breastfeeding may reduce risks requires careful testing. It appears that adiposity risks are amplified during obesogenic and insulin-resistant periods such as puberty. There is an urgent need to better understand how best to reverse the long-term impact of developmental overnutrition and to develop effective interventions that promote healthier pregnancies and healthy children.

REFERENCES

1. Ogden CL, Carroll MD, Kit BK, et al. Prevalence of obesity and trends in body mass index among US children and adolescents, 1999–2010. JAMA. 2012;307:483–490.
2. Barker DJP. The fetal and infant origins of adult disease. BMJ. 1990;301:1111.
3. Curhan GC, Chertow GM, Willett WC, et al. Birth weight and adult hypertension and obesity in women. Circulation. 1996;94:1310–1315.
4. Rogers I. Birth weight and obesity and fat distribution in later life. Birth Defects Res A Clin Mol Teratol. 2005;73:485–486.

5. McMillen IC, Edwards LJ, Duffield J, et al. Regulation of leptin synthesis and secretion before birth: implications for the early programming of adult obesity. Reproduction. 2006;131:415–427.
6. Dabelea D, Hanson RL, Lindsay RS, et al. Intrauterine exposure to diabetes conveys risks for type 2 diabetes and obesity – a study of discordant sibships. Diabetes. 2000;49:2208–2211.
7. Lawlor DA, Fraser A, Lindsay RS, et al. Association of existing diabetes, gestational diabetes and glycosuria in pregnancy with macrosomia and offspring body mass index, waist and fat mass in later childhood: findings from a prospective pregnancy cohort. Diabetologia. 2010;53:89–97.
8. Patel S, Fraser A, Smith GD, et al. Associations of gestational diabetes, existing diabetes, and glycosuria with offspring obesity and cardiometabolic outcomes. Diabetes Care. 2012;35:63–71.
9. Drake AJ, Reynolds RM. Impact of maternal obesity on offspring obesity and cardiometabolic disease risk. Reproduction. 2010;140:387–398.
10. Hochner H, Friedlander Y, Calderon-Margalit R, et al. Associations of maternal prepregnancy body mass index and gestational weight gain with adult offspring cardiometabolic risk factors the Jerusalem Perinatal Family Follow-up Study. Circulation. 2012;125:1381–1389.
11. Fraser A, Tilling K, Macdonald-Wallis C, et al. Association of maternal weight gain in pregnancy with offspring obesity and metabolic and vascular traits in childhood. Circulation. 2010;121:2557–2564.
12. Mamun AA, O'Callaghan M, Callaway L, et al. Associations of gestational weight gain with offspring body mass index and blood pressure at 21 years of age: evidence from a birth cohort study. Circulation. 2009;119:1720–1727.
13. Oken E, Rifas-Shiman SL, Field AE, et al. Maternal gestational weight gain and offspring weight in adolescence. Obstet Gynecol. 2008;112:999–1006.
14. Dabelea D, Snell-Bergeon JK, Hartsfield CL, et al. Increasing prevalence of gestational diabetes mellitus (GDM) over time and by birth cohort – Kaiser Permanente of Colorado GDM screening program. Diabetes Care. 2005;28:579–584.
15. Pettitt DJ, Knowler WC. Diabetes and obesity in the Pima Indians: a crossgenerational vicious cycle. J Obes Weight Regul. 1988;7:61–65.
16. Fryar CD, Carroll MD, Ogden CL. Prevalence of Obesity Among Children and Adolescents: United States, Trends 1963–1965 Through 2009–2010. National Center for Health Statistics. Health E-Stat. 2012:1–6.
17. Pinhas-Hamiel O, Dolan LM, Daniels SR, et al. Increased incidence of non-insulin-dependent diabetes mellitus among adolescents. J Pediatr. 1996;128(5 Pt 1):608–615.
18. Dabelea D, Bell RA, D'Agostino RB, et al. Incidence of diabetes in youth in the United States. JAMA. 2007;297:2716–2724.
19. Dabelea D, Mayer-Davis EJ, Talton J, et al. Is prevalence of type 2 diabetes increasing in youth? The SEARCH for Diabetes in Youth Study (Abstract). Diabetes. 2012;61:A61.
20. Freinkel N. Banting Lecture 1980: of pregnancy and progeny. Diabetes. 1980;29:1023–1035.

21. Whitaker RC, Dietz WH. Role of the prenatal environment in the development of obesity. J Pediatr. 1998;132:768–776.
22. Ebbeling CB, Pawlak DB, Ludwig DS. Childhood obesity: public-health crisis, common sense cure. Lancet. 2002;360:473–482.
23. Pettitt DJ, Knowler WC, Bennett PH, et al. Obesity in offspring of diabetic Pima Indian women despite normal birth-weight. Diabetes Care. 1987;10:76–80.
24. Pettitt DJ, Bennett PH, Knowler WC, et al. Gestational diabetes mellitus and impaired glucose tolerance during pregnancy. Long-term effects on obesity and glucose tolerance in the offspring. Diabetes. 1985;2:119–122.
25. Crume TL, Ogden L, West NA, et al. Association of exposure to diabetes in utero with adiposity and fat distribution in a multiethnic population of youth: the Exploring Perinatal Outcomes among Children (EPOCH) Study. Diabetologia. 2011;54:87–92.
26. Boney CM, Verma A, Tucker R, et al. Metabolic syndrome in childhood: association with birth weight, maternal obesity, and gestational diabetes mellitus. Pediatrics. 2005;115:E290–E296.
27. Dabelea D, Hanson RL, Bennett PH, et al. Increasing prevalence of type II diabetes in American Indian children. Diabetologia. 1998;41:904–910.
28. Dabelea D, Mayer-Davis EJ, Lamichhane AP, et al. Association of intrauterine exposure to maternal diabetes and obesity with type 2 diabetes in youth – The SEARCH Case-Control Study. Diabetes Care. 2008;31:1422–1426.
29. Catalano PM, Kirwan JP, Haugel-de Mouzon S, et al. Gestational diabetes and insulin resistance: role in short- and long-term implications for mother and fetus. J Nutr. 2003;133(5 Suppl 2):S1674–S1683.
30. Hillier TA, Pedula KL, Schmidt MM, et al. Childhood obesity and metabolic imprinting – The ongoing effects of maternal hyperglycemia. Diabetes Care. 2007;30:2287–2292.
31. Schaefer-Graf UM, Graf K, Kulbacka I, et al. Maternal lipids as strong determinants of fetal environment and growth in pregnancies with gestational diabetes mellitus. Diabetes Care. 2008;31:1858–1863.
32. Zhang YY, Proenca R, Maffei M, et al. Positional cloning of the mouse obese gene and its human homolog. Nature. 1994;372:425–432.
33. Kieffer TJ, Habener JF. The adipoinsular axis: effects of leptin on pancreatic beta-cells. Am J Physiol Endocrinol Metab. 2000;278:E1–E14.
34. Trujillo ML, Spuch C, Carro E, et al. Hyperphagia and central mechanisms for leptin resistance during pregnancy. Endocrinology. 2011;152:1355–1365.
35. Mantzoros CS, Liolios AD, Tritos NA, et al. Circulating insulin concentrations, smoking, and alcohol intake are important independent predictors of leptin in young healthy men. Obes Res. 1998;6:179–186.
36. Reilly MP, Iqbal N, Schutta M, et al. Plasma leptin levels are associated with coronary atherosclerosis in type 2 diabetes. J Clin Endocrinol Metab. 2004;89:3872–3878.
37. Rodie VA, Caslake MJ, Stewart F, et al. Fetal cord plasma lipoprotein status in uncomplicated human pregnancies and in pregnancies complicated by pre-eclampsia and intrauterine growth restriction. Atherosclerosis. 2004;176:181–187.

38. Liese AD, D'Agostino RB Jr, Hamman RF, et al. The burden of diabetes mellitus among US youth: prevalence estimates from the SEARCH for Diabetes in Youth Study. Pediatrics. 2006;118:1510–1518.
39. Crume TL, Ogden L, Daniels S, et al. The impact of in utero exposure to diabetes on childhood body mass index growth trajectories: the EPOCH study. J Pediatr. 2011;158:941–946.
40. Taylor JS, Kacmar JE, Nothnagle M, et al. A systematic review of the literature associating breastfeeding with type 2 diabetes and gestational diabetes. J Am Coll Nutr. 2005;24:320–326.
41. Crume TL, Ogden L, Maligie M, et al. Long-term impact of neonatal breastfeeding on childhood adiposity and fat distribution among children exposed to diabetes in utero. Diabetes Care. 2011;34:641–645.
42. Gillman MW, Oakey H, Baghurst PA, et al. Effect of treatment of gestational diabetes mellitus on obesity in the next generation. Diabetes Care. 2010;33:964–968.

PART III

WHAT CAN WE DO TO END THE EPIDEMIC?

CHAPTER 9

PROTECTING CHILDREN FROM HARMFUL FOOD MARKETING: OPTIONS FOR LOCAL GOVERNMENT TO MAKE A DIFFERENCE

JENNIFER L. HARRIS AND SAMANTHA K. GRAFF

7.1 INTRODUCTION

The prevalence of childhood obesity in the United States imposes a major burden on society in health care costs and children's physical and mental health (1). Meanwhile, the food industry spends massive amounts of money marketing calorie-dense, nutrient-poor foods, and its marketing specifically targets children (2). The obesity crisis cannot be solved without dramatic changes to the obesogenic marketing environment that surrounds children (3).

The White House Task Force on Childhood Obesity has called for immediate action: "Key actors—from food and beverage companies, to restaurants, food retailers, trade associations, the media, government and others—all have an important role to play in creating a food marketing environment that supports, rather than undermines, the efforts of parents and

---

Reprinted with permission by the CDC. Harris JL and Graff SK. Protecting Children From Harmful Food Marketing: Options for Local Government to Make a Difference. Preventing Chronic Disease **8**,5 *(2011).*

other caregivers to encourage healthy eating among children and prevent obesity" (4). Given government's fundamental obligation to advance public health, lawmakers at all levels must take the lead to change this toxic environment and shield children from exposure to marketing of food products that contribute to the obesity crisis (3). Although the federal government has jurisdiction to regulate national media and the First Amendment to the US Constitution limits what government at any level can do to restrict advertising, municipalities do have constitutionally viable options to protect children from the harmful food marketing that permeates their communities.

In this article, we describe ways in which food companies market calorie-dense, nutrient-poor foods directly to children in national media and local communities. We present evidence that this marketing negatively affects children's diets, increases children's risk for obesity and obesity-related illness, and takes advantage of youths' unique vulnerabilities. We then discuss limitations in food industry self-regulatory initiatives that address these concerns. Next, we present the legal doctrine that balances government's obligation to promote public health against the liberty interests of individual citizens and organizations. Finally, we highlight potentially viable local policy options to restrict the marketing of obesogenic food to children.

9.2 FOOD MARKETING TARGETING CHILDREN

In 2006, the food industry spent more than $1.6 billion on marketing to youth, including $900 million in marketing aimed directly at children younger than 12 years and designed specifically to increase positive attitudes and preferences for its products (2). Approximately half ($514 million) was spent on television advertising and other forms of national media, including the Internet, print, and radio. Children's exposure to these advertisements is considerable. For example, the average child aged 6 to 11 years views 13 television food advertisements daily (5). Approximately 400,000 children spent more than 60 minutes per month playing games and viewing branded content promoting high-sugar cereals on General Mills's millsberry.com, which was closed down in April 2011 as a result of pressure from public health advocates (6).

Companies also spend considerable sums to reach children directly in their local communities, in stores, restaurants, schools, and almost anywhere children spend their time. These locally based food marketing practices include product packaging, signs, and promotions in stores that appeal specifically to children ($106 million spent in the United States in 2006), marketing to children in schools ($73 million), and local child-focused events ($30 million) (2). Additionally, food companies spend $127 million on premiums, cross-promotion licenses, athletic sponsorships, celebrity fees, and philanthropic tie-ins. These programs increase products' appeal to children by associating foods with popular cartoon characters, sports, and entertainment celebrities and events, and even charities (eg, Girl Scouts [Girl Scouts of the USA, New York, New York]) (7). Similarly, fast-food restaurants spent $360 million in the United States in 2006 on toy giveaways (2). In 2009, the average child viewed 262 television advertisements (5 per week) that encouraged them to visit their local fast-food restaurant for the toy or other promotion in children's meals (8).

Locally based marketing practices are more difficult to measure quantitatively because they vary widely by location; however, reports document the extent of child-targeted marketing in communities and schools. For example, in supermarkets, high-sugar cereals marketed directly to children are more likely to be placed on lower and middle shelves (ie, children's eye level) and be featured in special store displays and price promotions (6). Products featuring youth-oriented cross-promotions on packaging in the supermarket increased by 78% during 2006-2008 (7). In schools, where children provide a captive market for advertisers, examples of food marketing include sponsored incentives (eg, rewarding children with free pizza for reading books); fundraising programs in which schools receive funds when families purchase food products and give proof of purchase to the school; branded food items served in school cafeterias, stores, and vending machines; corporate logos on scoreboards, book covers, and team jerseys; and sponsored curricula with branded content (9). Although less overt than traditional media advertising, school-based marketing practices are designed specifically to increase children's affinity and desire for companies' products by increasing familiarity and positive associations with the brands (10).

Food companies expend these prolific marketing efforts almost exclusively to promote foods that children should consume only occasionally and in limited quantities. On television, 98% of food advertisements watched by children promote products high in fat, sugar, or sodium (11). In all forms of marketing targeted to children, calorie-dense, nutrient-poor foods predominate (3). Breakfast cereals are most frequently marketed directly to children, representing 25% of all child-targeted food marketing in 2006 (2). Moreover, cereal companies choose to market products to children that contain 85% more sugar, 60% more sodium, and 65% less fiber than the products they market to adults (6). Restaurants are the second most frequent food category marketed to children (2). In 2007, fast-food restaurants represented 22% of all television food advertisements viewed by children, an increase of 12% from 2003 (5). Child-targeted spending to market beverages—including carbonated beverages, fruit drinks, and juices—sweets and baked goods, and snack foods totaled $376 million in 2006 (2). In contrast, only 4% of all child-targeted food marketing ($38 million) promoted fruits, vegetables, and dairy products.

9.3 HARMFUL EFFECTS OF FOOD MARKETING

Food companies have traditionally argued that their advertising simply encourages children to prefer one brand over another and thus does not contribute to childhood obesity (3). Most research on the effects of television food advertising to children confirms that it increases children's preferences for advertised brands, choices of specific foods after advertisement exposure, and requests to parents for advertised foods (12). More recent research has demonstrated, however, that food marketing also has potentially profound effects on children's overall diet and health. For example, television food advertising increases consumption of any available snack foods during and immediately after exposure, and exposure to commercial television is associated with increased overall calorie consumption, higher body mass index, and reduced fruit and vegetable consumption 5 years later (10). Research has also demonstrated an association between exposure to soft drink advertising and consumption of all sugar-sweetened beverages (13). Marketing can even affect how much children like the taste of advertised foods: preschoolers indicated that snack foods presented in packages with licensed characters tasted better than the same foods in plain packages (14).

Research on the harmful effects of food marketing on broader health-related outcomes (beyond brand preference and attitudes) is in its early stages; however, potentially far-reaching and dangerous effects have been hypothesized (10). Because of its ubiquity, food marketing likely affects children's normative beliefs about the types of foods that are acceptable to eat regularly without adverse consequences, may affect how much children like the taste of advertised foods, and may automatically prime other unrelated goals and behaviors, including children's motivation to engage in unhealthful behaviors.

9.4 CHILDREN'S UNIQUE VULNERABILITY

Child advocates also question the ethics of marketing practices targeted to children who cannot yet defend against their influence (3). Research consistently demonstrates that until the age of 8 years, most children do not possess the necessary cognitive skills to understand that advertising is not just another source of information and presents a biased point of view (12). Although older children and adolescents understand the intent of advertising, they do not regularly act on that knowledge nor do they attempt to counteract its influence. Resisting advertisements for the highly tempting products commonly promoted also requires the ability to weigh long-term health consequences of consumption against short-term rewards, an ability that is not fully developed until the early 20s (15). Finally, marketing practices that persuade indirectly (eg, through logo placements, associations with popular characters and movies, and Internet games) are designed to create lifelong customers by imprinting brand meaning into the minds of young children (10). Before children know better, they have learned to love the products they encounter most frequently and associate with positive experiences.

Evidence also exists that food companies disproportionately target advertising for high-calorie, nutrient-poor foods to black and Hispanic communities, where youth are most vulnerable to obesity and obesity-related disease (16). For example, billboards for fast-food and sugar-sweetened beverages appear substantially more often in low-income black and Hispanic neighborhoods (17), and fast-food outlets in low-income black communities are more likely to promote less healthful menu items (18).

9.5 FOOD INDUSTRY INITIATIVES TO ADDRESS THESE PUBLIC HEALTH CONCERNS

The food industry appears to have heard concerns raised by the public health community about child-targeted marketing practices. In 2006, the Children's Food and Beverage Advertising Initiative (CFBAI), an industry-sponsored program purportedly designed to improve food-marketing practices, was launched (19). Sixteen of the largest food companies that market to children have joined CFBAI and implemented pledges to market only "better-for-you" foods in child-targeted media. However, exclusions and limitations demonstrate that these pledges are unlikely to produce substantial changes to existing marketing practices. For example, participating companies have created their own definitions of "better-for-you" foods that include products dietitians may regard as unhealthful, including high-sugar cereals, juice drinks made of 10% fruit juice with 16 grams of sugar per 6-ounce serving, and even certain flavors of toaster pastries. Similarly, participating companies have declared that widely used forms of marketing designed specifically to appeal to children are not child-targeted advertising and thus not subject to limitations, including product packaging and other types of marketing to children that occur in stores or restaurants, advertising on prime-time television shows popular with children but also viewed by a broader audience, and food and beverage displays in schools.

Recent evaluations of the effects of the CFBAI pledges on the volume and types of foods advertised to children demonstrate limited changes in the foods advertised to children (6,8,20). Public health professionals have suggested that industry self-regulatory efforts (eg, CFBAI) provide more public relations benefit to the food industry than real health benefits for children and that overreliance on such efforts could exacerbate the childhood obesity crisis (21-23).

TABLE 1: Local Policy Options to Restrict Marketing of Unhealthful Foods to Children[a]

Location	Policy Options
Supermarkets, convenience stores, and other retail outlets	Impose excise taxes or fees on sugar-sweetened beverages, and earmark a portion or all of the revenue to fund obesity prevention programs.
	Require "healthy checkout aisles," free of obesogenic food and beverages.
	Prohibit food sales in nonretail food outlets (eg, sporting goods stores, toy stores).
	Limit sales of obesogenic food and beverages near schools before, during, and immediately after the school day.
	Regulate the pricing of obesogenic food and beverages (eg, set minimum prices).
	Limit the total amount of store window space that can be covered by signs. To avoid potential First Amendment violations, the policy should apply to all signs no matter the message and should be based on non–speech-related considerations such as minimizing visual clutter.
	Require food retailers to obtain a license that comes with conditions limiting in some way the sale of obesogenic food and beverages.
Restaurants and other food service establishments	Set nutrition standards for children's meals that include a toy or other incentive item.
	Enact a menu labeling law that is identical to the federal law (thus enabling local enforcement) and/or that applies to food service establishments that are not covered under the federal law.
	Prohibit new fast-food restaurants from opening near schools.
	Restrict the number or density of fast-food restaurants.
	Ban drive-through windows.
	Prohibit use of trans fats in restaurant food.
	Set procurement standards for government-run food facilities.
	Implement a healthy restaurant certification program that encourages restaurants to reduce the sale and advertising of obesogenic food and beverages to children.
Schools[b]	Ban the sale of obesogenic food and beverages on school property.
	Ban all food advertising on school property or ban advertising on school property for foods that are not allowed to be sold on campus.
	Include provisions in vending contracts limiting the sale and advertising of obesogenic food and beverages on school property.
	Prohibit fundraisers that entail selling obesogenic food and beverages.
	Implement closed campus policies to reduce student exposure to obesogenic food marketing.

TABLE 1: *Cont.*

Location	Policy Options
Elsewhere in the community	Ban all commercial billboards except those located on the site of the advertised establishment. To avoid potential First Amendment violations, the ban should be based on non–speech-related considerations such as traffic safety or esthetics.
	Include provisions in vending contracts limiting the sale and advertising of obesogenic food and beverages in parks and other public venues that are frequented by children.

[a] *This list expands on a list originally developed by the members of the Food Marketing to Children Workgroup's local subcommittee, including Samantha Graff.* [b] *School districts, rather than local legislatures, usually have the authority to enact policies that restrict marketing of unhealthful foods in public schools.*

9.6 GOVERNMENT'S ROLE IN ADVANCING PUBLIC HEALTH

Because the food marketing environment contributes to the health crisis facing our nation's children and because members of the food industry appear unlikely to voluntarily make the considerable changes required to improve this environment, government at all levels has an obligation to intervene where it can. In our constitutional democracy, a core responsibility of government is to protect and promote public health—especially among vulnerable populations, including children. Public health is essential to civil society because it provides the general population with basic security and welfare that can be achieved only through collective action (24).

A common refrain among opponents of public health regulations is that government should not impede individual liberty to benefit the general public. The US Constitution addresses this concern: provisions of the Bill of Rights and the Fourteenth Amendment—including those regarding free speech, due process, equal protection, and property ownership—mandate that a balance be struck between the government's obligation to serve the general welfare and the interest of individual citizens and organizations in freedom, fairness, and self-determination (25). Therefore, when the government regulates food marketing to children, it must achieve a balance between public and private interests.

Congress and federal agencies (eg, the Federal Trade Commission, the Federal Communications Commission) have purview over media that cross state lines, including television, radio, the Internet, and other digital media. Consequently, policy efforts to limit food advertising in the national media must be initiated at the federal level. However, states and localities have power to take a regulatory stand against many forms of marketing for obesogenic food to youth that occur in their communities, including marketing in retail establishments, restaurants, and schools. In fact, states and their subdivisions have always borne primary responsibility for public health. In the constitutional compact, each state retains police power—the inherent authority to act in the interest of the public's health, safety, and welfare (24). Most states grant their localities a form of home rule, or the ability to legislate on the basis of the police power (26). Because regulating public health is a fundamental police power function, states and home-rule localities have the presumptive authority to pass public health laws as long as the laws do not overstep constitutional bounds and are not preempted (ie, trumped) by the law of a higher jurisdiction.

Accordingly, public health advocates have identified multiple policy proposals that localities can consider to reduce marketing of unhealthful food to children in stores, restaurants, schools, and elsewhere in the community (Table). A limited number of the policies listed have been tested in court, but in light of case law on analogous policies, these all have a reasonable chance of withstanding constitutional scrutiny. A community interested in pursuing any of these policies should involve government attorneys early in the process to ensure the proposal is legally sound in the jurisdiction.

An important role of local government is to serve as a testing ground for new and promising public health initiatives. One of the special features of our constitutional system is that, to paraphrase Justice Louis Brandeis, our states and localities serve as laboratories of democracy, testing new social and economic experiments that can be studied, adapted, and honed to benefit other jurisdictions. Given the recent attention to food marketing as a significant contributor to childhood obesity, many of the policies listed in the Table are untried or just starting to be tried. Therefore, we do not yet know which will be most effective at limiting marketing of unhealthful foods and ultimately improving children's health. As local governments develop and implement policies to address the marketing of unhealthful foods in their communities, it is critical that they form partnerships to conduct research and generate knowledge about the effectiveness of their policies and to transfer that knowledge to other municipalities (27). Protecting children from the harmful effects of food marketing requires a range of policy interventions at all levels of government—and ultimately a change in social norms of acceptable behavior.

9.7 CONCLUSION

Action must be taken to change the obesogenic environment that surrounds children, and food marketing is a key contributor to that environment. Initial actions by the food industry do not reflect a genuine commitment to reversing the effects of persistent and prolific marketing programs directly targeted to children, which continually reinforce the rewards of consuming nutrient-poor, calorie-dense foods. Accordingly, both the federal and local governments have an obligation to act. Municipalities can play a critical role in developing, implementing, and evaluating policies to improve the marketing environment for children in their own communities and across the country.

REFERENCES

1. 1. Kersh R, Stroup D, Taylor W. Prev Chronic Dis. 5. Vol. 8. overview and bioethical considerations. Prev Chronic Dis 2011; 2011. Childhood obesity and public policy: overview and bioethical considerations; p. A93. http://www.cdc.gov/pcd/issues/2011/sep/10_0273.htm.
2. 2. Marketing food to children and adolescents: a review of industry expenditures, activities, and self-regulation. A report to Congress. Federal Trade Commission; 2008. [Accessed October 4, 2010]. http://www.ftc.gov/os/2008/07/P064504foodmktingreport.pdf.
3. 3. Harris JL, Pomeranz JL, Lobstein T, Brownell KD. 2009. 30 211 225 A crisis in the marketplace: how food marketing contributes to childhood obesity and what can be done Annu Rev Public Health Harris JL, Pomeranz JL, Lobstein T, Brownell KD. A crisis in the marketplace: how food marketing contributes
4. 4. White House Task Force on Childhood Obesity. Report to the President: solving the problem of childhood obesity within a generation. Executive Office of the Presi-

dent of the United States; 2010. [Accessed October 4, 2010]. p. 28. http://www.letsmove.gov/sites/letsmove.gov/files/TaskForce_on_ Childhood_Obesity_May2010_ FullReport.pdf.
5. 5. Powell LM, Szczpka G, Chaloupka FJ. Trends in exposure to television food advertisements among children and adolescents in the United States. Arch Pediatr Adolesc Med. 2010;164(9):794–802.
6. 6. Harris JL, Schwartz MB, Brownell KD. Marketing foods to children and adolescents: licensed characters and other promotions on packaged foods in the supermarket. Public Health Nutr. 2010;13(3):409–417.
7. 7. Harris JL, Schwartz MB, Brownell KD, Sarda V, Ustjanauskus A, Javadizadeh J, et al. Fast food FACTS: evaluating fast food nutrition and marketing to youth. Yale University, Rudd Center for Food Policy and Obesity; http://www.fastfoodmarketing.org.
8. 8. Harris JL, Schwartz MB, Brownell KD, Sarda V, Weinberg ME, Speers S, et al. Cereal FACTS: evaluating the nutrition quality and marketing of children's cereals. Yale University, Rudd Center for Food Policy and Obesity; [Accessed October 4, 2010]. 2009. http://www.cerealfacts.org/media/Cereal_FACTS_Report.pdf.
9. 9. Molnar A, Garcia DR, Boninger F, Merrill B. Marketing of foods of minimal nutritional value to children in schools. Prev Med. 2008;47(5):504–507.
10. 10. Harris JL, Brownell KD, Bargh JA. The food marketing defense model: integrating psychological research to protect youth and inform public policy. Soc Issues Policy Rev. 2009;3(1):211–271.
11. 11. Powell LM, Szczpka G, Chaloupka FJ, Braunschweig CL. Nutritional content of television food advertisements seen by children and adolescents. Pediatrics. 2007;120(3):576–583.
12. 12. Institute of Medicine, Committee on Food Marketing and the Diets of Children and Youth . Food marketing to children and youth: threat or opportunity? Washington (DC): National Academies Press; 2006.
13. 13. Andreyeva T, Kelly IR, Harris JL. Exposure to food advertising on television: associations with children's fast food and soft drink consumption and obesity. Econ Hum Biol. 2011;9(3):221–233.
14. 14. Roberto C, Baik J, Harris JL, Brownell KD. Influence of licensed characters on children's taste and snack preferences. Pediatrics. 2010;126(1):88–93.
15. 15. Pechmann C, Levine L, Loughlin S, Leslie F. Impulsive and self-conscious: adolescents' vulnerability to advertising and promotion. Journal of Public Policy and Marketing 2005;24(2):202–221.
16. 16. Grier SA, Kumanyika SK. The context for choice: health implications of targeted food and beverage marketing to African Americans. Am J Public Health. 2008;98(9):1616–1629.
17. 17. Yancey AK, Cole BL, Brown R, Williams JD, Hillier A, Kline RS, et al. A cross-sectional prevalence study of ethnically targeted and general audience outdoor obesity-related advertising. Milbank Q. 2009;87(1):155–184.
18. 18. Lewis LB, Sloane DC, Nascimento LM, Diamant AL, Guinyard JJ, Yancey AK, et al. African Americans' access to healthy food options in South Los Angeles restaurants. Am J Public Health. 2005;95(4):668–673.

19. Peeler CL, Kolish ED, Enright M. The Children's Food and Beverage Advertising Initiative in action: a report on compliance and implementation during 2008. Council of Better Business Bureaus; 2009. [Accessed October 4, 2010]. http://www.bbb.org/us/storage/0/Shared%20Documents/finalbbbs.pdf.
20. Kunkel D, McKinley C, Wright P. The impact of industry self-regulation on the nutritional quality of foods advertised on television to children. Children Now; 2009. [Accessed October 4, 2010]. http://www.childrennow.org/uploads/documents/adstudy_2009.pdf.
21. Hawkes C. Regulating and litigating in the public interest: regulating food marketing to young people worldwide: trends and policy drivers. Am J Public Health. 2007;97(11):1962–1973.
22. Wilde P. Self-regulation and the response to concerns about food and beverage marketing to children in the United States. Nutr Rev. 2009;67(3):155–166.
23. Sharma LL, Teret SP, Brownell KD. The food industry and self-regulation: standards to promote success and to avoid public health failures. Am J Public Health. 2010;100(2):240–246.
24. Gostin LO. Public health law: power, duty, restraint. 2nd edition. Berkeley (CA): University of California Press; 2010.
25. Mermin T, Graff S. A legal primer for the obesity prevention movement. Am J Public Health. 2009;99(10):1799–1805.
26. Diller P, Graff S. J Law Med Ethics. 39 s1: 2011. pp. 89–93. Regulating food retail for obesity prevention: how far can cities go?
27. McKinnon RA, Orleans CT, Kumanyika SK, Haire-Joshu D, Krebs-Smith SM, Finkelstein EA, et al. Considerations for an obesity policy research agenda. Am J Prev Med. 2009;36(4):351–357.

CHAPTER 10

LIFE COURSE IMPACT OF SCHOOL-BASED PROMOTION OF HEALTHY EATING AND ACTIVE LIVING TO PREVENT CHILDHOOD OBESITY

BACH XUAN TRAN, ARTO OHINMAA, STEFAN KUHLE, JEFFREY A. JOHNSON, AND PAUL J. VEUGELERS

10.1 INTRODUCTION

Obesity affects the health of Canadians and costs the nation approximately $1.27 to 11.08 billion per year in health care [1]. A myriad of psychological and physical consequences hamper obese individuals to function as healthy and productive members of the society. The physical consequences include chronic and fatal diseases such as cardiovascular disease, type 2 diabetes, and various cancers [2], [3].

Poor eating habits and sedentary lifestyles are the established risk factors for obesity. Promotion of healthy eating and active living is considered to be most effective when targeting childhood years [4], [5]. In the Canadian province of Alberta, we recently demonstrated the feasibility and effectiveness of a school-based program in preventing childhood obesity [6]. This Alberta Project Promoting active Living and healthy Eating

---

Life Course Impact of School-Based Promotion of Healthy Eating and Active Living to Prevent Childhood Obesity. © Tran BX, Ohinmaa A, Kuhle S, Johnson JA, and Veugelers PJ. PLoS ONE 9,7 (2014), doi:10.1371/journal.pone.0102242. Licensed under Creative Commons Attribution 4.0 International License, http://creativecommons.org/licenses/by/4.0/.

in Schools (APPLE Schools) is a comprehensive school health program that started as a pilot in 2008 in 10 elementary schools. The intervention involved a full-time School Health Facilitator in each school for implementing healthy eating and active living policies, practices and strategies while engaging stakeholders, including parents, staff and the community. School Health Facilitators contributed to the schools' health curriculum, and organized nutrition programs such as cooking clubs and healthy breakfast, lunch and snack programs, after school physical activity programs, walk-to-school days, community gardens, weekend events and circulated newsletters. By 2010 the eating habits and physical activity levels of students attending APPLE Schools had significantly improved whereas the prevalence of obesity had declined relative to their peers attending other Albertan schools [6]. These findings are consistent with other school-based programs internationally that took a comprehensive approach to promoting healthy eating and active living [5], [7]–[9].

It is recognized that health status in early periods of life form the foundation for a healthier life course and that obesity in childhood often persists into adulthood. However, to date little is known about the long-term implications of successful prevention of childhood obesity [10]. Public health decision makers wish to be informed on the long-term health benefits and financial implications of these prevention programs. Guyer et al acknowledged the need for well-designed longitudinal studies to determine the importance of childhood interventions for health outcomes in adulthood, or in other words, to estimate the impact of early interventions on the life-course of the youngsters who had been subjected to these intervention (a life-course approach) [10]. The purpose of this study is to estimate the life course impact of the APPLE Schools program in terms of future body weight status and avoided health care costs.

10.2 MATERIALS AND METHODS

This study has been reviewed and approved by the Health Research Ethics Board of the University of Alberta, Edmonton, Alberta, Canada.

10.2.1 DATA SOURCE AND STATISTICAL ANALYSIS

We previously published that the prevalence of obesity among grade five students (typically 10 or 11 years of age) attending APPLE Schools reduced 2.2% between 2008 and 2010 as compared to a 2.8% increase in the prevalence of obesity among grade fivers attending other schools [6]. This difference is equivalent to reductions of 0.26 and 0.17 kg/m^2 in body mass index (BMI) per year among girls and boys, respectively, participating in APPLE Schools programs. These intervention benefits were used as the starting points of life course BMI trajectories to estimate the life course impact of the APPLE Schools intervention.

For the purpose of determining longitudinal BMI trajectories throughout the life course, we accessed longitudinal data of persons of all ages who participated in the Canadian National Population Health Surveys (NPHS). The NPHS included longitudinal assessment of 17,276 persons selected from each of the 10 Canadian provinces [11]–[13]. The data were anonymized and we accessed and analyzed the data at the Research Data Center of the University of Alberta, Edmonton, AB, Canada. The NPHS employed a stratified two-stage sample design based on the Labour Force Survey in all provinces except for the province of Québec, where the another survey, the Enquête Sociale et de Santé, was used. Participants were followed up and interviewed every two years (cycles) using a common set of health questions. Follow up response rates ranged from 92.8% in cycle 2 to 70.7% in cycle 8. Data collection continued when participants were institutionalized in a long-term care facility and included verification of vital status. Data collection at baseline (cycle 1 in 1994/1995) was through in-person interviews, and in subsequent cycles through telephone interviews [11]. To minimize systematic differences in data collection, we excluded cycle 1 from the present analysis. Cycle 2 to 8 provide longitudinal data for 1996 to 2008 that included self-reported heights and weights. We restricted our analyses to observations of individuals in the age range of 11 to 70 years, as 11 is the typical age students reach while in grade five (i.e., the grade level of the assessment of the APPLE Schools program effectiveness). Age 70 was set as the upper labour age in light of assessing potential economic implications. We used standards set by the World Health Organization to classify adult body weight categories; underweight (BMI <18.5), normal weight (BMI ≥18.5 to <25), overweight (BMI ≥25 to <30), and obesity (BMI ≥30).

We applied growth curve models to the longitudinal NPHS data to quantify individual changes in BMI over time. These BMI trajectories were estimated for 5 different age period: 11 to <23, 23 to <35, 35 to <47, 47 to <59, and 59 to 70 years of age. This staggered modeling approach provided flexibility to the full life course BMI trajectory and improved our ability to estimate the models since each NPHS participant was tracked for 14 years over 7 NPHS cycles. The growth curve models describe BMI changes in one age category as a function of the development of BMI in the previous age category. In other words, for each age category, the growth curve model estimates the changes in BMI based on the BMI starting value in that particular age category. For example, we estimated the BMI growth for the age 11 to less than 23 years using the BMI at age 11 years. This would provide a projected BMI at age 22.99 years, which would then be the starting value for the estimation of the BMI growth in the subsequent age category, 23 to less than 34 years, and so on.

The model selection was purposive, and we applied an analytical procedure that had been used in previous studies and shown to be robust in estimating trajectories of BMI of individuals using this data set [14], [15]. The models were adjusted for survey sampling weights, sex, body weight status, and calendar year. We further considered interaction terms of sex and age, and of sex and the quadratic form of age [14]. Body weight status (at the beginning of each age category) was considered as a random effect in these models, as were sex as well as intercept and linear slope [14]. The growth curve models were considered to have an unstructured covariance matrix [14]. We computed Bosker/Snijders and Bryk/Raudenbush R-square values for mixed models with two levels.

To project the life course BMI trajectories of grade five students in Alberta, we applied the parameters from the above described growth curve models to overweight and obesity prevalence rates of Alberta [6]. These prevalence rates originated from a population-based survey including 3,398 grade five students from 141 randomly selected schools from across Alberta in 2010 [6]. We then repeated the projection of the life course BMI trajectories adjusting the starting prevalence rates for the reduction in BMI resulting from the APPLE Schools program. The differences between the two models then represent the potential life course impact of the APPLE School program on the projected BMI status.

Projection of health care cost savings by reduction in the prevalence of overweight and obesity was estimated by multiplying the total direct health care cost for obesity by the proportion of overweight and obese cases prevented by the intervention. An updated estimation by Anis et al showed that the annual direct health care cost of overweight and obesity in Canada was $ 6 billion in 2006 [16]. We assumed that this cost remained unchanged overtime and for every overweight and obese case that we prevented, we avoided the costs for health conditions related to obesity.

10.3 RESULTS

Table 1 presents the parameter estimates for each of the 5 age-specific growth curve models used to project life course changes in BMI for grade five students in Alberta. Figure 1 presents the projected body weight status for grade five students with normal weight using the parameter estimates of Table 1. Approximately 40% of normal weight youth are estimated to progress to overweight by the time they turn 25 years of age. This percentage will further increase to 60% by the time they turn 35 years of age. Figure 2 depicts the projected body weight status for grade five students who were overweight and shows that 60% will progress to obesity by the time they turn 30 years of age. Very few overweight youth enter adulthood as normal weight (Figure 2). Lastly, figure 3 shows that nearly all obese youth progresses to obese adults.

When applying the grow curves to grade five students attending APPLE Schools, we estimated that for every unit increase in BMI at age 11, 23, 35, 47, and 59, the BMI growth rate over the five corresponding age-specific periods increased by 0.82, 0.890, 0.969, 0.930, and 0.863 kg/m^2 respectively ($p<0.05$). Comparing the estimates of the growth curves applied to students attending APPLE Schools and attending other Alberta schools, we quantified the benefits of the APPLE Schools program throughout the students' lifetime. This is presented in Figure 4. The lifetime prevalence of overweight (including obesity) was 1.2% to 2.8% (1.7 on average) less among students attending APPLE Schools relative to those attending other Alberta schools. The prevalence of obesity was 0.4% to 1.4% (0.8% on average) less among students attending APPLE Schools students relative to those attending other Alberta schools (Figure 4). We estimated that 2% to 5.5% of overweight cases and 3% to 6.5% of obesity cases could be prevented through the APPLE Schools program (Figure 5).

If this program were to be scaled up to Canada that spends approximately 6 billion dollars for health care for people with excess body weight, the potential cost savings would be 150 to 330 million dollars per year (Figure 6) [16]. Similarly, if this program were to be scaled up to Alberta, it could save 33–82 million dollars for obesity-related health care in Alberta (Figure 6). The avoided health care costs were in average higher at younger ages (Figure 6).

10.4 DISCUSSION

We projected of body weight trajectories of youth in Alberta and forecasted that more than two thirds is likely to develop excess body weight at some point in their lives. We further modeled the long-term benefits of the APPLE Schools intervention and forecasted that the prevalence of overweight (including obesity) among students attending APPLE Schools is 2% to 6% less relative to the prevalence among their peers who are attending other schools in Alberta. With a nationwide implementation of the APPLE Schools program, this could result in 150 to 330 million dollars per year in cost savings due to avoided health care services.

We forecasted that more than two thirds of current youth is likely to become overweight or obese at some point in their lives. This seems higher that the forecasts by Kuhle [17] who reported that 45% of youth would have excess body weight by 2006 and 55% by in 2026. Forecasts in the US had revealed that in 2010 the obesity prevalence of sex and racial subgroups ranges from 33 to 55% and that the national prevalence of obesity is expected to increase to 51% by 2030 [18], [19].

Impact of School-Based Promotion of Healthy Eating and Active Living 163

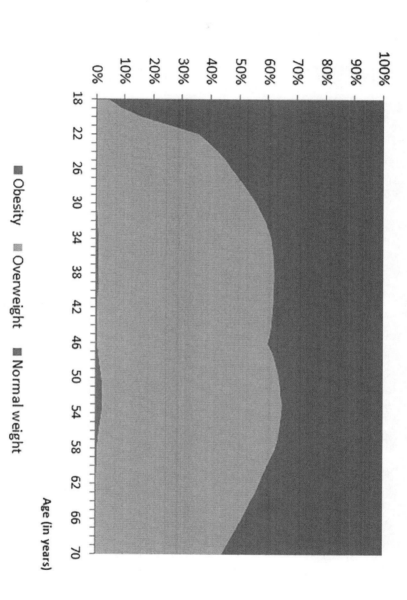

FIGURE 1: Life course weight status projections of normal weight grade five students.

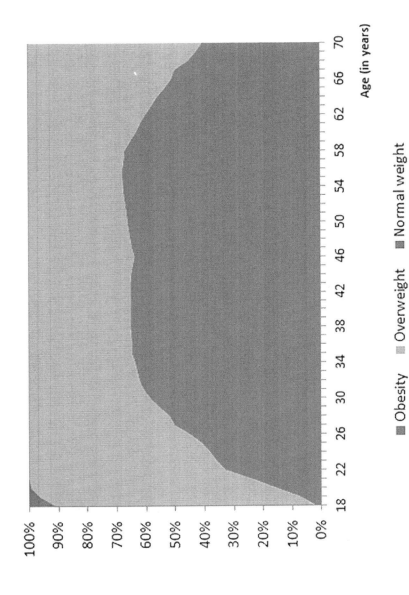

FIGURE 2: Life course weight status projections of overweight grade five students.

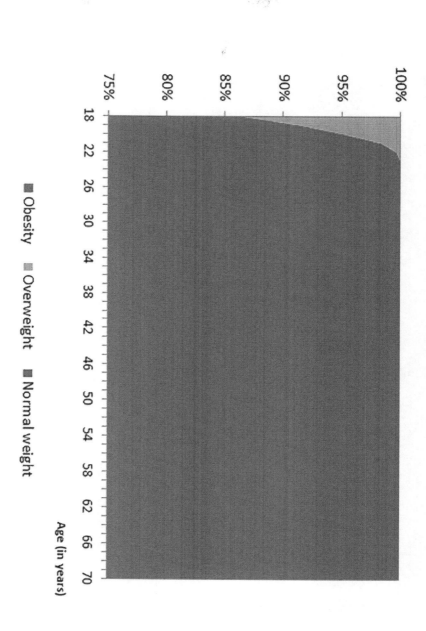

FIGURE 3: Life course weight status projections of obese grade five students.

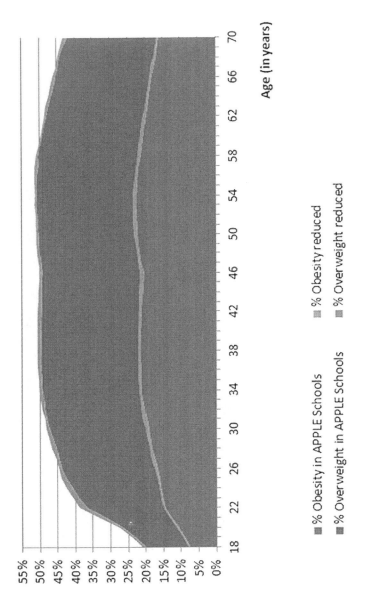

FIGURE 4: Life course weight status projections for the grade five students attending the APPLE Schools program and those who are not. Purple represents the percentage of students attending APPLE Schools who are projected to become overweight; Blue represents the percentage students attending other Alberta schools who are projected to become overweight; Red represents the percentage of students attending APPLE Schools who are projected to become obese; Orange represents the percentage students attending other Alberta schools who are projected to become obese.

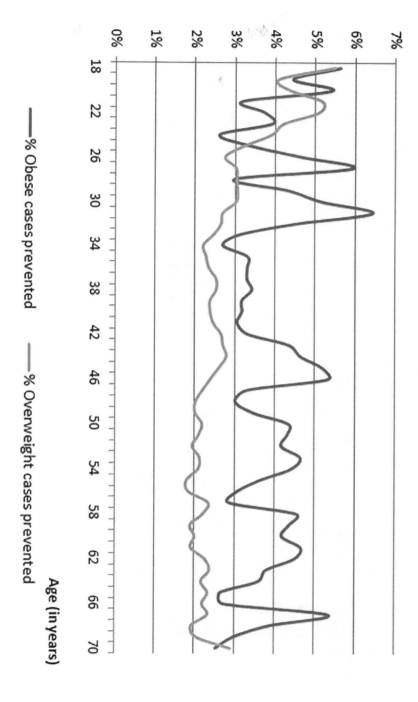

FIGURE 5: Life course projections of the percentage prevented overweight and obese cases.

168 The Childhood Obesity Epidemic

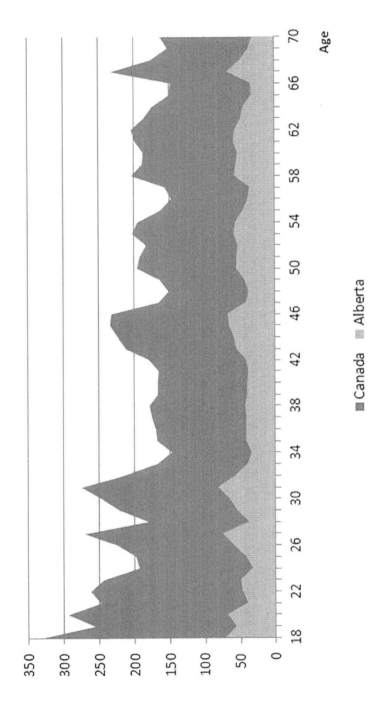

FIGURE 6: Life course projections of avoided health care costs for Canada and the province of Alberta (in million dollars).

TABLE 1: Growth curve modeling of BMI for five age categories of participants of the Canadian National Population Health Survey.

	Age: 11, <23	Age: 23, <35	Age: 35, <47	Age: 47, <59	Age: 59, <71
Boy	**7.767**	**15.442**	**29.673**	**2.766**	−0.300
Girl	**4.800**	**13.915**	**11.684**	9.631	−1.674
Boy × Age	**1.285**	**0.571**	−0.201	**0.903**	0.903
Girl × Age	**1.701**	0.569	**0.604**	0.562	0.903
Boy × Age^2	**−0.023**	−0.008	0.003	**−0.008**	−0.008
Girl × Age^2	**−0.040**	−0.008	−0.007	−0.005	−0.007
Year					
1996	reference	reference	reference	reference	reference
1998	−0.134	**0.207**	**0.220**	0.117	0.029
2000	−0.013	**0.358**	**0.589**	**0.380**	**0.328**
2002	0.162	**0.811**	**0.882**	**0.683**	**0.647**
2004	0.367	**0.911**	**0.978**	**0.643**	**0.673**
2006	0.058	**1.002**	**1.232**	**0.868**	**0.923**
2008	0.029	**1.139**	**1.299**	**1.011**	**1.082**
R2 coefficient	0.33	0.12	0.08	0.04	0.02

Note: Figures in bold represent statistically significant estimates ($p < 0.05$).

The present study is the first to follow a life course approach for the purpose of quantifying the impact on adulthood obesity of school-based promotion of healthy eating and active living. Our findings are consistent with the existing evidence that interventions at an early age are effective in influencing body weight status later in life and that school-based prevention programs may therefore be cost effective [5], [20]–[26]. In the United States, Wang et al. developed a progression model to project the long-term benefits of a school based intervention and reported a 1% reduction in overweight and obese and $586 million in cost savings [27]. We estimated direct health care costs savings of $150 to 330 million per year in Canada, based on the prevention of 2% to 6% of the projected cases of overweight and obesity. If these estimates hold true, it would seem that small reductions in childhood obesity prevalence translate into large costs savings at the population level, and thus school programs and other initiatives that can further reduce overweight prevalence rates will further contribute to program effectiveness and cost savings.

Body weight in childhood is an established predictor of body weight at a later age [20], [28]–[35]. For example, Magarey et al had tracked the weight status of Finnish children and identified weight status at age 6 as a strong predictor of weight status in adulthood [28], and Starc and Strel tracked 4,833 Slovenian children and found that those who were obese at age 18 years, 40% of males and 48.6% of females had been obese at 7 years [31]. It is for this reason that we had considered early body weight in our growth curves, and our analyses confirmed the importance of body weight for growth in body weight. However, reduction in the prevalence of excess body weight was not the only benefit reported for APPLE Schools. We had also reported benefits to healthy eating and active living [6], that were achieved throughout a comprehensive approach that improved students' knowledge levels, attitudes, self-efficacy and leadership skills related to making healthy choices. Where knowledge, attitudes and life skills may persist over the life course of APPLE Schools graduates, they may contribute to healthier choices later in life and herewith to more prevention of excess body weight. The health and costs benefits revealed in this study may therefore not have fully captured the potential impacts of the APPLE Schools program, and comprehensive school health programs in general.

A strength of the present study is that it was based on large established national and provincial studies as well as a feasible school-based intervention that will improve the generalizability of the findings. More over, we followed a life course approach to provide insight into the future health benefits and cost implications of interventions. Where students' heights and weights were measured in APPLE Schools and control schools, heights and weights in the longitudinal NPHS were obtained through self-report. Self-report of height and weight is prone to error which we acknowledge as a study limitation. Other study limitations may relate to the use of administrative health care databases for the purpose of estimating avoided health case costs. Furthermore, projections assume that future developments follow patterns similar to the patterns in the observations on which the projection models are based. We acknowledge that future patterns may deviate from observed patterns which, in turn, may affect our estimates.

To conclude, preventing childhood obesity during their school years is forecasted to reduce obesity in adulthood which may lead to substantial savings in future health care costs at population level. Youth with healthy weights are less likely to develop overweight and obesity through their lives. Also, healthy habits and skills acquired in childhood may lend for life long healthy behaviors that further reduce the likelihood of weight gain [36]. Potential cost savings should encourage the allocation of resources towards school-based promotion of healthy eating and active living.

REFERENCES

1. Tran BX, Nair AV, Kuhle S, Ohinmaa A, Veugelers PJ (2013) Cost analyses of obesity in Canada: scope, quality, and implications. Cost Eff Resour Alloc 11: 3. doi: 10.1186/1478-7547-11-3
2. Trasande L (2011) Quantifying the economic consequences of childhood obesity and potential benefits of interventions. Expert Rev Pharmacoecon Outcomes Res 11: 47–50. doi: 10.1586/erp.10.86
3. Saha AK, Sarkar N, Chatterjee T (2011) Health consequences of childhood obesity. Indian J Pediatr 78: 1349–1355. doi: 10.1007/s12098-011-0489-7
4. Zenzen W, Kridli S (2009) Integrative review of school-based childhood obesity prevention programs. J Pediatr Health Care 23: 242–258. doi: 10.1016/j.pedhc.2008.04.008
5. Veugelers PJ, Fitzgerald AL (2005) Effectiveness of school programs in preventing childhood obesity: a multilevel comparison. Am J Public Health 95: 432–435. doi: 10.2105/ajph.2004.045898
6. Fung C, Kuhle S, Lu C, Purcell M, Schwartz M, et al. (2012) From "best practice" to "next practice": the effectiveness of school-based health promotion in improving healthy eating and physical activity and preventing childhood obesity. Int J Behav Nutr Phys Act 9: 27. doi: 10.1186/1479-5868-9-27
7. Greening L, Harrell KT, Low AK, Fielder CE (2011) Efficacy of a school-based childhood obesity intervention program in a rural southern community: TEAM Mississippi Project. Obesity (Silver Spring) 19: 1213–1219. doi: 10.1038/oby.2010.329
8. Verstraeten R, Roberfroid D, Lachat C, Leroy JL, Holdsworth M, et al. (2012) Effectiveness of preventive school-based obesity interventions in low- and middle-income countries: a systematic review. Am J Clin Nutr 96: 415–438. doi: 10.3945/ajcn.112.035378
9. Khambalia AZ, Dickinson S, Hardy LL, Gill T, Baur LA (2012) A synthesis of existing systematic reviews and meta-analyses of school-based behavioural interventions for controlling and preventing obesity. Obes Rev 13: 214–233. doi: 10.1111/j.1467-789x.2011.00947.x

10. Guyer B, Ma S, Grason H, Frick KD, Perry DF, et al. (2009) Early childhood health promotion and its life course health consequences. Acad Pediatr 9: 142–149 e141–171. doi: 10.1016/j.acap.2008.12.007
11. Asakawa K, Senthilselvan A, Feeny D, Johnson J, Rolfson D (2012) Trajectories of health-related quality of life differ by age among adults: results from an eight-year longitudinal study. J Health Econ 31: 207–218. doi: 10.1016/j.jhealeco.2011.10.002
12. Orpana HM, Berthelot JM, Kaplan MS, Feeny DH, McFarland B, et al. (2010) BMI and mortality: results from a national longitudinal study of Canadian adults. Obesity (Silver Spring) 18: 214–218. doi: 10.1038/oby.2009.191
13. Katzmarzyk PT, Ardern CI (2004) Overweight and obesity mortality trends in Canada, 1985–2000. Can J Public Health 95: 16–20.
14. Ng C, Corey PN, Young TK (2012) Divergent body mass index trajectories between Aboriginal and non-Aboriginal Canadians 1994–2009–an exploration of age, period, and cohort effects. Am J Hum Biol 24: 170–176. doi: 10.1002/ajhb.22216
15. Pryor LE, Tremblay RE, Boivin M, Touchette E, Dubois L, et al. (2011) Developmental trajectories of body mass index in early childhood and their risk factors: an 8-year longitudinal study. Arch Pediatr Adolesc Med 165: 906–912. doi: 10.1001/archpediatrics.2011.153
16. Anis AH, Zhang W, Bansback N, Guh DP, Amarsi Z, et al. (2009) Obesity and overweight in Canada: an updated cost-of-illness study. Obes Rev 11: 31–40. doi: 10.1111/j.1467-789x.2009.00579.x
17. Kuhle S (2011) Forecasting the prevalence of overweight and obesity in Canada. Chapter 3 PhD thesis University of Alberta.
18. Wang YC, Colditz GA, Kuntz KM (2007) Forecasting the obesity epidemic in the aging U.S. population. Obesity (Silver Spring) 15: 2855–2865. doi: 10.1038/oby.2007.339
19. Finkelstein EA, Khavjou OA, Thompson H, Trogdon JG, Pan L, et al. (2012) Obesity and severe obesity forecasts through 2030. Am J Prev Med 42: 563–570. doi: 10.1016/j.amepre.2011.10.026
20. Wu JF (2013) Childhood obesity: a growing global health hazard extending to adulthood. Pediatr Neonatol 54: 71–72. doi: 10.1016/j.pedneo.2013.01.002
21. Lehnert T, Sonntag D, Konnopka A, Riedel-Heller S, Konig HH (2012) The long-term cost-effectiveness of obesity prevention interventions: systematic literature review. Obes Rev 13: 537–553. doi: 10.1111/j.1467-789x.2011.00980.x
22. Moodie M, Haby MM, Swinburn B, Carter R (2011) Assessing cost-effectiveness in obesity: active transport program for primary school children–TravelSMART Schools Curriculum program. J Phys Act Health 8: 503–515. doi: 10.1186/1479-5868-6-63
23. McAuley KA, Taylor RW, Farmer VL, Hansen P, Williams SM, et al. (2010) Economic evaluation of a community-based obesity prevention program in children: the APPLE project. Obesity (Silver Spring) 18: 131–136. doi: 10.1038/oby.2009.148
24. Carter R, Moodie M, Markwick A, Magnus A, Vos T, et al. (2009) Assessing cost-effectiveness in obesity (ACE-obesity): an overview of the ACE approach, economic methods and cost results. BMC Public Health 9: 419. doi: 10.1186/1471-2458-9-419

25. Wang LY, Gutin B, Barbeau P, Moore JB, Hanes J Jr, et al. (2008) Cost-effectiveness of a school-based obesity prevention program. J Sch Health 78: 619–624. doi: 10.1111/j.1746-1561.2008.00357.x
26. Brown HS 3rd, Perez A, Li YP, Hoelscher DM, Kelder SH, et al. (2007) The cost-effectiveness of a school-based overweight program. Int J Behav Nutr Phys Act 4: 47. doi: 10.1186/1479-5868-4-47
27. Wang LY, Denniston M, Lee S, Galuska D, Lowry R (2010) Long-term health and economic impact of preventing and reducing overweight and obesity in adolescence. J Adolesc Health 46: 467–473. doi: 10.1016/j.jadohealth.2009.11.204
28. Magarey AM, Daniels LA, Boulton TJ, Cockington RA (2003) Predicting obesity in early adulthood from childhood and parental obesity. Int J Obes Relat Metab Disord 27: 505–513. doi: 10.1038/sj.ijo.0802251
29. Dietz WH, Robinson TN (2005) Clinical practice. Overweight children and adolescents. N Engl J Med 352: 2100–2109. doi: 10.1056/nejmcp043052
30. Park MH, Falconer C, Viner RM, Kinra S (2012) The impact of childhood obesity on morbidity and mortality in adulthood: a systematic review. Obes Rev 13: 985–1000. doi: 10.1111/j.1467-789x.2012.01015.x
31. Starc G, Strel J (2011) Tracking excess weight and obesity from childhood to young adulthood: a 12-year prospective cohort study in Slovenia. Public Health Nutr 14: 49–55. doi: 10.1017/s1368980010000741
32. Herman KM, Craig CL, Gauvin L, Katzmarzyk PT (2009) Tracking of obesity and physical activity from childhood to adulthood: the Physical Activity Longitudinal Study. Int J Pediatr Obes 4: 281–288. doi: 10.1080/17477160802596171
33. Atkinson W (2008) Early intervention. Childhood obesity programs aim to put kids on a new, healthier path to adulthood. AHIP Cover 49: 26–28, 30, 32 passim.
34. Venn AJ, Thomson RJ, Schmidt MD, Cleland VJ, Curry BA, et al. (2007) Overweight and obesity from childhood to adulthood: a follow-up of participants in the 1985 Australian Schools Health and Fitness Survey. Med J Aust 186: 458–460.
35. Allman-Farinelli MA, King L, Bauman AE (2007) Overweight and obesity from childhood to adulthood: a follow-up of participants in the 1985 Australian Schools Health and Fitness Survey. Comment. Med J Aust 187: 314; author reply 314–315.
36. Lhachimi SK, Nusselder WJ, Lobstein TJ, Smit HA, Baili P, et al. (2013) Modelling obesity outcomes: reducing obesity risk in adulthood may have greater impact than reducing obesity prevalence in childhood. Obes Rev doi: 10.1111/obr.12029

CHAPTER 11

MODELING SOCIAL TRANSMISSION DYNAMICS OF UNHEALTHY BEHAVIORS FOR EVALUATING PREVENTION AND TREATMENT INTERVENTIONS ON CHILDHOOD OBESITY

LEAH M. FRERICHS, OZGUR M. ARAZ, AND TERRY T. K. HUANG

11.1 INTRODUCTION

The worldwide growth in overweight and obesity has created negative health, social and economic consequences for children, adults, and society as a whole [1]–[3]. In the US, alongside increasing adult overweight and obesity rates, the problem has grown among children [4], [5]. Some research indicates increases in US childhood overweight and obesity rates may be slowing [5], but we still need strategies to accelerate a downward trend in order to abate forthcoming obesity-related health and economic consequences [6]. Research that improves our understanding of the complex dynamics of social spread of obesity among children via both peer and

---

Modeling Social Transmission Dynamics of Unhealthy Behaviors for Evaluating Prevention and Treatment Interventions on Childhood Obesity. © Frerichs LM, Araz OM, Huang TTK. PLoS ONE 8,12 (2013); doi:10.1371/journal.pone.0082887. Licensed under Creative Commons Attribution 4.0 International License, http://creativecommons.org/licenses/by/4.0/.

adult influences may help identify key leverage points, and guide resource allocation to the most impactful combination of intervention strategies.

The immediate cause of overweight and obesity is energy imbalance, but complex interactions of multi-level factors including individual human biology, behavior, and environment give rise to the current worldwide epidemic [7]. Christakis and Fowler [8] found evidence that the adult obesity epidemic appears to be spreading through social ties, based on the clustering of surveyed individuals according to their BMIs and increased chance of becoming obese based on different ties. Social ties may transfer obesity and obesity-related behaviors through pathways of social norms, capital (i.e., resources, information and people accessible through a social network), and stress [9].

Additional evidence strengthens the role of social influence in both adult and child populations. Research continually uncovers adult-to-adult [8], adult-to-child [10]–[14], and child-to-child [14]–[18] associations and influence in terms of obesity and obesity-related attitudes, norms, and behaviors (i.e., nutrition and physical activity). Furthermore, a few recent obesity interventions found that targeting parents only may have a significant residual impact on children in regards to behavior and weight change [19]–[21].

The interdependencies among parent and peer influences on childhood obesity are difficult to understand using linear models. System dynamics modeling can help explore the complex multi-level social influences on child obesity risks, and identify potential research gaps and plausible intervention levers with policy implications by analyzing outcome patterns [22]. For example, system dynamics provides a methodology to test combinations of prevention and treatment intervention impact directed towards adults and children on childhood overweight and obesity trends, which can enhance our ability to understand the combination of strategies with potential for greatest impact.

11.1.1 OBESITY AND COMPLEX SYSTEMS MODELING BACKGROUND

Prior research has applied complex systems modeling to study obesity dynamics [23]–[29]. For our research we build upon several models that use mathematical and system dynamics methodologies to consider excess weight as a consequence of the transmission of unhealthy lifestyles from one individual to another [26], [29]–[31]; however, to our knowledge no models have simultaneously accounted for peer and adult transmission of behaviors for childhood overweight and obesity.

Computational and quantitative models of obesity have been used to understand the dynamics of energy regulation at the individual and biological level in order to understand issues such as weight cycling [23], [24], [32]–[34]. Research via system dynamics modeling has built upon these energy regulation models in order to capture these dynamics throughout the life course and simulate future population level trends [25], [28]. These models were also used to test and formulate information about policy interventions, but they do not explicitly account for the social transmission of obesogenic behaviors.

Karanfil et al's [27] agent-based framework provided value for understanding how opinions about nutrition and physical activity can be transferred through social ties. Other researchers have used mathematical models to understand the growth of obesity via social transmission [26], [29]–[31]. Evangelista et al [30] used peer pressure to become a fast food eater as a parameter in a model to simulate changes in overweight and obesity rates. Researchers in Spain built models with similar social transmission parameters to simulate population obesity rate growth for different age groups, including infants and adults, and used the models to test the impact of different combinations of prevention and treatment interventions [26], [29], [31]. Unfortunately, these models do not provide the functionality to understand different levels of influence on children from their peers and adults.

The aim of our research is to gain insight into potential research gaps and plausible levers for future childhood obesity prevention and treatment intervention and policy research. We hypothesize that the multi-level and dissimilar quantifications of social transmission of overweight and obesity from adult-to-adult, adult-to-child, and child-to-child create different patterns of overweight and obesity. In our research, we construct and parameterize a system dynamics model of the social transmission of behaviors that cause childhood overweight and obesity through adult and peer influence. Our objectives are: (1) to assess the sensitivity of childhood overweight and obesity prevalence to peer and adult social transmission rates, and (2) to test combinations of prevention and treatment interventions, with varying degrees of adult intervention impact on children and vice versa, on the prevalence of childhood overweight and obesity.

11.2 METHODS

We used Vensim PLE (Ventana Systems, Inc., Harvard, MA) to build and simulate the model and test the dynamic hypotheses and assumptions. We conducted two-way sensitivity analyses on social transmission rates from adult-to-child and from child-to-child. Alternative combinations of prevention and treatment interventions were tested by varying model parameters of social transmission and rates of overweight and obese individuals engaged in weight loss behaviors. We designed an experiment to explore the alternative combinations' impacts on childhood overweight and obesity prevalence using a set of scenarios, each with varying adult intervention impact on children and vice versa.

11.2.1 MODEL DESCRIPTION

A causal loop diagram illustrates the elements of the system we used to model and test hypotheses regarding child and adult social transmission of unhealthy behaviors causing overweight and obesity (Figure 1).

11.2.2 MODEL BOUNDARIES

The model boundary for our research included social transference of unhealthy behaviors at adult-to-adult, adult-to-child, and child-to-child levels. The transmission was assumed to occur through social influences on food consumption and physical activity behaviors via norms, attitudes, behaviors, and provision of interpersonal material and physical structures and resources. Previous similar mathematical models have used a broad interpretation of social encounters and have assumed factors of genetics and environment to be embedded within this social transmission factor [29]. For our research we considered these outside the system boundaries.

11.2.3 MODEL ELEMENTS

Figure 1 shows the elements of the system, which include an individual's health status related to weight (i.e., normal weight, overweight, and obese adults and similarly normal weight, overweight, and obese children). The levels of each of these elements influence the social transmission of overweight and obesity: adult levels influence adult-to-adult and adult-to-child transmission, and child levels influence child-to-child. We assumed child-to-adult transmission of these unhealthy behaviors was negligible.

Several elements were included in modeling intervention impact (Figure 1). Treatment intervention increases the level of overweight and obese children and adults actively engaging in dieting and physical activity to lose weight. Prevention intervention decreases the social transmission of obesity-related unhealthy behaviors. The obesity intervention influences both the targeted age group (e.g., adults) and opposite age group (e.g., children) based on the assumption that adults and children will model intervention-induced healthy behavior change for others. Rather than attempting to change individual behaviors only, obesity interventions may target psychosocial variables in order to encourage the intervention participant to actively model and encourage healthy behaviors among their social contacts. For example, a family centered model which was developed for addressing obesity would potentially include how parents may influence children through mechanisms of modeling, parenting practices of reinforcement and encouragement, and changes to the home environment [35]. Thus the model includes an explicit intervention impact parameter (apart from adult-to-child and child-to-child social transmission) to capture the potential to actively engage targeted individuals to model and encourage healthy behaviors among the other age group at varying degrees. However, the impact on the non-targeted age group is of a lesser magnitude. The line weights in Figure 1 indicate relative differences among the impact's magnitude.

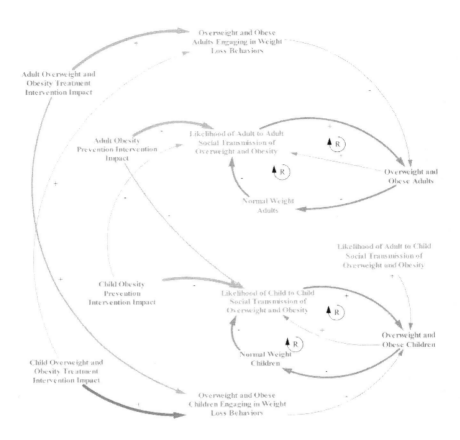

FIGURE 1: Causal Loop Diagram of Adult and Child Social Transmission of Obesity. This figure shows a causal loop diagram that illustrates the elements of the system we used for our research to model and test hypotheses regarding child and adult social transmission of unhealthy behaviors causing overweight and obesity. Adult level elements are shown in green and child level elements are shown in pink. Each element in the system is included with arrows drawn between elements to indicate relationships where they exist. The arrows are labeled with plus signs if a positive relationship exists between the elements and minus sign if an inverse relationship exists. The diagram includes adult-to-adult, adult-to-child, and child-to-child social transmission elements with arrows indicating how each increases overweight and obese individuals in the population for each respective age group. The overweight and obese individuals for each age group are shown with arrows to indicate its positive relationship with social transmission and inverse relationship with normal weight individuals. Finally normal weight individuals in each age group have arrows indicating an inverse relationship to social transmission of overweight and obesity. Within the elements and arrows described, circular arrows with a capital "R" are shown in the center to indicate

reinforcing feedback loops. Elements of intervention impact are also included with arrows and plus/minus signs indicating relationships. Treatment intervention impact for children and adults are shown with negative labeled arrows to overweight and obese children and adults actively engaging in weight loss behaviors. Prevention intervention impact for children and adult levels are shown with negatively labeled arrows to social transmission. Intervention impact lines are shown at different widths to indicate differences in relative magnitude of impact. The thickest lines are shown regarding adult-to-adult impact and child-to-child impacts. Lines of medium thickness are shown regarding adult-to-child impact. Finally the thinnest lines are shown regarding child to adult impact.

11.2.4 FEEDBACK LOOPS

Increased numbers of overweight and obese individuals raise the likelihood of social transmission of peer-to-peer unhealthy behaviors (i.e., greater contact of normal weight with overweight and obese individuals), which in turn increases the number of overweight and obese individuals. Additionally, increased numbers of overweight and obese individuals in a fixed population will decrease numbers of normal weight individuals, which also raises the likelihood of social transmission of peer-to-peer unhealthy behaviors (see Figure 1). Thus there are two reinforcing loops seen in both the adult and child populations: (1) a loop between the increase in overweight and obesity that leads to a rise in the likelihood of social transmission, and (2) a loop from the increase in overweight and obesity that leads to a decrease in normal weight population, which leads to a subsequent increase in the likelihood of maintained social transmission.

11.2.5 MATHEMATICAL MODEL

We built a stock and flow diagram to model the underlying structure, and governing equations of the model were adapted from previous models [26], [29]–[31]. The stock and flow diagram indicates stocks of normal, overweight, and obese adults and children respectively with flows in-between (Figure 2). In this section, we formulate the mathematical equations used to model the spread of obesity through multi-level transmission of obesity-related behaviors through the social environment.

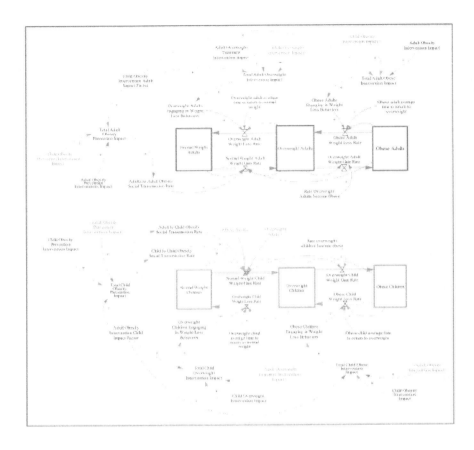

FIGURE 2: Stock Flow Diagram of Adult and Child Social Transmission of Obesity. This figure shows the stock flow diagram built in Vensim. Adult level influences are shown in green and child level influences in pink. The core model elements are shown in solid lines, and intervention variables are indicated in dotted lines. Stocks of normal weight, overweight and obese adults are shown in green and stocks of normal weight, overweight, and obese children are shown in pink. Variables are shown with arrows to the flow equation they are included in. For example, child-to-child and adult-to-child social transmission rates are included in the flow equation from normal weight children to overweight children stock. Intervention impact variables are also shown with arrows to the behavioral variable they impact. For example, the total child prevention intervention impact reduces the child-to-child and adult-to-child social transmission rates. Finally the adult intervention impact and child intervention impact factors are also indicated and arrows indicate the total intervention impact levels they influence.

To build the equations for the model, we made the following assumptions:

- We assume homogenous population mixing for behavioral transmission.
- We assume that unhealthy eating behaviors and low physical activity levels of individuals in the model increase the individual weight for both adults and children.
- Normal weight adults and children will become overweight over time because overweight and obese contacts transmit their unhealthy behaviors through social contacts (i.e., social transmission rates). Social contact is modeled proportionally to the number of contacts of normal weight with overweight and obese individuals. For children, this transmission is both in terms of proportional contacts with adults as well as their peers. For adults, the transmission occurs only through adult contacts, and children are assumed not to transmit unhealthy behaviors.
- Overweight adults and children are assumed to become obese proportionally to the total number of overweight adults and children over time.
- It is assumed that obese and overweight adults and children have potential to adopt behaviors that will lead to weight loss (i.e., diet and physical activity) if conditions and interventions are adequate. Obese and overweight adults and children can transition to overweight and normal weight, respectively, at a rate proportional to the respective stock, based on the extent of the subpopulation that engages in weight loss behaviors.

The model also includes several variables related to the potential for obesity prevention and treatment impact. The following assumptions were made for this purpose:

- Interventions are assumed to impact targeted behavioral variables by either increasing or decreasing them over time linearly.
- Obesity prevention intervention is assumed to fortify normal weight individuals against transmission of unhealthy behaviors of overweight and obese individuals. Thus prevention intervention impact is assumed to be a decrease to social transmission rates.
- Overweight and obesity intervention is assumed to help additional individuals in targeted subgroups to engage in weight loss behaviors. Thus treatment intervention impact is assumed to increase the rate of those engaging in weight loss behaviors.
- Adult obesity prevention intervention is assumed to decrease the adult-to-adult social transmission rate, and child obesity prevention intervention is assumed to decrease both child-to-child and adult-to-child transmission rates (i.e., children are fortified against social transmission from both peers and adults). However, the adult-to-child social transmission rate is assumed to decrease at a discounted rate of the child-to-child transmission rate given children's limited ability to change parental control around issues such as provision of healthy foods [36].

- Interventions are assumed to impact targeted subgroups as well as parallel subgroups with similar behaviors. Thus, adult intervention impact is assumed to also have an influence on child intervention impact and vice versa.
- The intervention impact on parallel subgroups is assumed to act through mechanisms that are different from social transmission rates alone due to the potential for interventions to actively engage targeted individuals to support and encourage others in their social environment in healthy behaviors.
- The subgroup impact is assumed to occur proportionally to the direct influence on the targeted subpopulation, modeled via an impact factor. For example, the total adult prevention intervention impact is assumed to be a function of both adult prevention intervention impact and a proportion of the child obesity prevention intervention impact. Similarly, the child obesity prevention intervention impact is assumed to be a function of both the child obesity prevention intervention impact and a proportion of the adult obesity prevention intervention impact. The same relationships are assumed for the overweight and obese child and adult intervention impacts as well.
- Regardless of prevention or treatment, for the impact of adults on children and vice versa, the impact factor is assumed to be the same.

11.2.5.1 STOCK VARIABLES

For the model, child and adult populations were each divided into three subpopulations of normal weight, overweight, and obese.

N_A, Normal weight adults, individuals with BMI<25 kg/m^2
S_A, Overweight adults, individuals with BMI≥25 and<30 kg/m^2
O_A, Obese adults, individuals with BMI≥30 kg/m^2
N_c, Normal weight children, children<85th percentile on BMI-for age growth charts
S_c, Overweight children, children between 85th to 95th percentile on BMI-for age growth charts
O_c, Obese children, children≥95th percentile on BMI-for age growth charts

10.2.5.2 BEHAVIORAL VARIABLES.

For this model, we included variables of behaviors related to overweight and obesity, including those of diet and physical activity. We also included social transmission rates.

ρ_{AWL} = proportion of overweight adults engaging in weight loss behaviors
ρ_{CWL} = proportion of overweight children engaging in weight loss behaviors
ε_{AWL} = proportion of obese adults engaging in weight loss behaviors
ε_{CWL} = proportion of obese children engaging in weight loss behaviors
P_{SA} = average time needed for overweight adult to return to normal weight
P_{SC} = average time needed for overweight child to return to normal weight
P_{OA} = average time needed for obese adult to return to overweight
P_{OC} = average time needed for obese child to return to overweight
γ_A = rate at which overweight adults become obese
γ_C = rate at which overweight children become obese
β_{AA} = adult-to-adult social transmission rate
β_{CC} = child-to-child social transmission rate
β_{AC} = adult-to-child social transmission rate

11.2.5.3 TRANSITION EQUATIONS

Given the assumptions, the transitions from one state to another are described by the following differential equations of (1)–(6) with the initial conditions of $N_A(0) = N_{A0}$, $S_A(0) = S_{A0}$, $O_A(0) = O_{A0}$, $N_C(0) = N_{C0}$, $S_C(0) = S_{C0}$, $O_C(0) = O_{C0}$.

Normal Weight Adult Stock

$$\frac{dN_A(t)}{dt} = -(\beta_{AA} * N_A(t) * S_A(t) + O_A(t) + (\rho_{AWL} * P_{SA} * S_A(t))$$

(1)

Overweight Adult Stock

$$\frac{dS_A(t)}{dt} = -(\beta_{AA} * N_A(t) * (S_A(t) + O_A(t))) + (\varepsilon_{AWL} * P_{OA} * O_A(t)) - (\rho_{AWL} * p_{SA} * S_A(t)) - (\gamma_A * S_A(t))$$

(2)

Obese Adult Stock

$$\frac{dO_A(t)}{dt} = (\gamma_A * S_A(t)) - (\varepsilon_{AWL} * P_{OA} * O_A(t)) \qquad (3)$$

Normal Weight Children Stock

$$\frac{dN_C(t)}{dt} = (\rho_{CWL} * p_{SC} * S_C(t)) - (\beta_{AC} * N_C(t) * (S_A(t) + O_A(t))) - (\beta_{CC} * N_C(t) * (S_C(t) + O_C(t)))$$

(4)

Overweight Children Stock

$$\frac{dS_C(t)}{dt} = (\varepsilon_{CWL} * p_{OC} * O_C(t)) - (\gamma_C * N_C(t)) - (\rho_{CWL} * p_{SC} * S_C(t)) + (\beta_{AC} * N_C(t) * (S_A(t) + O_A(t)) + \beta_{CC} * N_C(t) * (S_C(t) + O_C(t))$$

(5)

Obese Children Stock

$$\frac{dO_C(t)}{dt} = (\gamma_C * S_C(t)) - (\varepsilon_{CWL} * P_{OC} * O_C(t)) \qquad (6)$$

11.2.5.4 INTERVENTION VARIABLES

For this model, we included variables of intervention impact for each potential subgroup that could be targeted.

η_{oc}, childhood obesity treatment intervention impact
η_{sc}, childhood overweight treatment intervention impact
η_{NC}, childhood prevention treatment intervention impact
η_{OA}, adult obesity treatment intervention impact
η_{SA}, adult overweight treatment intervention impact
η_{NA}, adult obesity prevention treatment intervention impact
ψ_A, adult obesity intervention impact factor (impact of adult interventions on children)
ψ_c, child obesity intervention impact factor (impact of child interventions on adults)
, discount factor (accounts for resistance of adult-to-child social transmission to respond to child prevention interventions)

11.2.6 INTERVENTION EQUATIONS

Total childhood obesity prevention intervention impact

$$= \eta_{NC} + \psi_A * \eta_{NA} \tag{7}$$

Total childhood overweight treatment intervention impact

$$= \eta_{SC} + (\psi_A * \eta_{SA}) \tag{8}$$

Total childhood obesity treatment intervention impact

$$= \eta_{OC} + (\psi_A * \eta_{OA}) \tag{9}$$

Total adult obesity prevention intervention impact

$$= \eta_{NA} + (\psi_C * \eta_{NC}) \tag{10}$$

Total adult overweight treatment intervention impact

$$= \eta_{SA} + (\psi_C * \eta_{SC}) \quad (11)$$

Total adult obesity treatment intervention impact

$$= \eta_{OA} + (\psi_C * \eta_{OC}) \quad (12)$$

11.2.7 BEHAVIORAL IMPACT EQUATIONS

Given the assumptions, the impact of interventions on targeted behavioral-related variables can be described by the following equations of (13)–(19).

$$\beta_{AA}(t) = \beta_{AA0} - \sum_{t=0}^{t}(\eta_{NA} + (\psi_C + \eta_{NC})) \quad (13)$$

$$\beta_{CC}(t) = \beta_{CC0} - \sum_{t=0}^{t}(\eta_{NC} + (\psi_A * \eta_{NA})) \quad (14)$$

$$\beta_{AC}(t) = \beta_{AC0} - \sum_{t=0}^{t}\lambda(\eta_{NC} + (\psi_A * \eta_{NA})) \quad (15)$$

$$\rho_{AWL}(t) = \rho_{AWL0} + \sum_{t=0}^{t}(\eta_{SA} + (\psi_C * \eta_{SC})) \quad (16)$$

$$\rho_{CWL}(t) = \rho_{CWL0} + \sum_{t=0}^{t}(\eta_{SC} + (\psi_A * \eta_{SA})) \qquad (17)$$

$$\varepsilon_{AWL}(t) = \varepsilon_{AWL0} + \sum_{t=0}^{t}(\eta_{OA} + (\psi_C * \eta_{OC})) \qquad (18)$$

$$\varepsilon_{CWL}(t) = \varepsilon_{CWL0} + \sum_{t=0}^{t}(\eta_{OC} + (\psi_A * \eta_{OA})) \qquad (19)$$

11.2.8 PARAMETERS ESTIMATION

Model parameters were identified using existing US surveillance system data and research literature (Table S1). Stock variables were parameterized with 2009–2010 data from NHANES [37] to identify rates of normal, overweight and obesity in adults and children using current BMI and percentile guidelines. NHANES data in combination with recent research data were used to identify needed trends of flow between overweight and obese status (e.g., rates of dieting, exercise, and average time to lose weight). Finally, existing literature was used to provide coefficients for adult-to-adult, adult-to-child, and child-to-child social transmission. The details of parameter identification and estimation follow.

11.2.8.1 ENGAGING IN WEIGHT LOSS BEHAVIORS

Experts recommend both dietary changes and physical activity for obese and overweight children and adult weight loss [38], [39]. For clinically significant weight loss, recommendations include both a reduced calorie diet and a minimum of moderate-intensity physical activity for 250 minutes per week. For our parameters, we defined engaging in weight loss behaviors to apply to individuals who follow the recommended guidelines at a minimum, and calculated rates using data from the 2009–2010 NHANES dietary interview and the physical activity questionnaire [37]. Individuals who responded yes to following a "weight loss or low calorie diet" on the dietary interview were considered engaging in dieting for weight loss. Total minutes of weekly moderate and vigorous physical activity were calculated from the physical activity questionnaire by summing each respondent's typical number of days per week of moderate and vigorous recreational activity multiplied by time spent in minutes on a typical day in moderate and vigorous activity, respectively. Individuals who engaged in 250 minutes or more moderate and vigorous recreational activity per week were considered engaging in physical activity for weight loss. The proportion of individuals by stock variables (i.e., overweight adults, obese adults, overweight children, obese children) who were both dieting and doing physical activity for weight loss was calculated.

11.2.8.2 OBESE AND OVERWEIGHT ADULT AVERAGE TIME TO RETURN TO OVERWEIGHT AND NORMAL WEIGHT

These parameters were estimated using body measures from the 2009–2010 NHANES Anthropometry Examination [37] and a systematic review regarding expected weight loss for adults engaged in treatment programs involving diet and physical activity for weight loss [40]. The average amount of weight (in kg) obese and overweight adults needed to lose to transition to overweight or normal weight, respectively, was calculated using 2009–2010 NHANES data [37]. A review of overweight and obesity treatment indicated that adults can expect to lose an average of 5.5 kg in 12 months while engaged in behavioral modification for weight loss [40]. Thus, the average time overweight and obese adults needed to return to normal and overweight, respectively, was calculated by multiplying the average weight loss in proportion to the weight loss expected by the amount of time required for expected weight loss.

11.2.8.3 OBESE AND OVERWEIGHT CHILD AVERAGE TIME TO RETURN TO OVERWEIGHT AND NORMAL WEIGHT

The average BMI decrease obese and overweight children need to transition to overweight or normal weight, respectively, was calculated using 2009–2010 NHANES Anthropometry Examination data [37]. The needed BMI decrease was calculated with respect to BMI-percentiles by age and gender with adjustment for time needed to decrease weight (one year for overweight to return to normal weight and two years for obese to return to overweight). A review of overweight and obesity treatment indicated that effective treatment interventions were shown to decrease children's BMI by 1.7 in one year while engaging in behavioral modification for weight loss [41]. Thus the average time overweight and obese children needed to return to normal and overweight, respectively, was calculated by multiplying the average BMI decrease needed in proportion to the BMI decrease expected by the amount of time required for expected BMI decrease.

11.2.8.4 ADULT AND CHILD OVERWEIGHT RATE OF BECOMING OBESE

The overweight adult and child rates of becoming obese were calculated using longitudinal data. The four year incidence of obesity of adult individuals in the Framingham longitudinal cohort study (data collected from 1979–2001) was found to be approximately 16% [42]. Thus, the rate for adults was calculated as: γ_A = 0.16/(4 years *52 weeks per year) = 0.000769 week^{-1}. The incidence of obesity in children who began as non-obese in a longitudinal study was found to be approximately 4.3% in 28 months [43]. Thus the rate for children was calculated as: γ_C = 0.043/(28 months * 4.333 weeks per month) = 0.000354 week^{-1}.

11.2.8.5 SOCIAL TRANSMISSION RATES

The adult-to-adult social transmission rate, β_{AA}, was identified from numerical simulations reported from a study in Spain [29]. This value was used to define an appropriate range for sensitivity analysis for our research. In our experiments for the second objective, this value was assumed for the adult-to-adult social transmission rate and the child-to-child social transmission rate. The adult-to-child parameter was assumed to be 50% higher than the child-to-child social transmission rate due to evidence that child food intake is significantly higher in association with their parent's than peer's food intake [44]–[46].

11.2.9 SIMULATION EXPERIMENTS AND ANALYSIS

The first research objective was to conduct a sensitivity analysis on social transmission rates to determine their potential influence on childhood overweight and obesity prevalence. The second objective was to test alternative combinations of prevention and treatment intervention impacts at adult and child levels in order to determine where were the most impactful, based on varying degrees of adult intervention impact on children and vice versa. We used the combined childhood overweight and obesity prevalence as the decision criteria.

We defined a range of adult-to-child and child-to-child social transmission rates near reported values from the literature [29]. We conducted two-way sensitivity analyses using a set of 5 values each for adult-to-child and child-to-child social transmission rates in .0002 increments between 0.0011 and 0.0019. This range evaluated an adult-to-child social transmission rate that was between 0.58 to 1.73 times the child-to-child social transmission. A total of 25 total simulations using each potential combination of adult-to-child and child-to-child social transmission rates were run over a 10 year period. Baseline values of parameters were used and no interventions were applied.

We then defined 15 different combinations of adult and child obesity prevention and treatment interventions (Table 1), and tested a set of six scenarios that varied the adult obesity intervention impact factor at 25%, 50%, and 75%; and the child obesity intervention impact factor at 10% and 25% (Table 2). Quantification of these impact factors is limited, but research suggests a wide potential range for adult impact on children. For example, review studies note that a majority of research finds correlations between parents and child physical activity and food intake levels, but they range from weak to moderate levels [47], [48]. Knowledge regarding child impact on adults is also limited; however, a relatively weak influence is implied from awareness that child weight and behavioral interventions have minimal impact unless parents and home environments are also targeted [36], [49], [50]. Thus we chose to use scenarios to include a wide range of adult obesity intervention impact factors (i.e., 25%, 50%, and 75%), and a relatively low and smaller range of child obesity intervention impact factors (i.e., 10%, 25%), resulting in a total of 6 scenarios.

For each simulation, the targeted behavioral parameter was changed by 50% (social transmission rates were decreased and overweight and obese individuals engaging in weight loss behaviors was increased). The behavioral parameters were modeled to occur in a continuous linear change over a period of 10 years.

A lack of comprehensive data regarding weight loss behaviors and treatment and prevention interventions applied over the past several decades limited our ability to conduct formal statistical tests for model validation. As an alternative, we used a behavioral pattern testing approach [51] to compare our model simulations with US surveillance data trends. Our estimated and assumed baseline parameters produced an appropriate pattern and range of relative outcomes. From the early to mid-90s, US childhood overweight and obesity prevalence increased approximately 1.5 times [52]–[54] with recent evidence of potentially leveling rates [55]. Similarly, across our simulations (see results section), the childhood overweight and obesity prevalence increased from 1.45 to 1.97 across ten years, and in some scenarios a leveling to slight reduction is apparent.

TABLE 1: Description of the Obesity Prevention and Treatment Intervention Alternatives.

	Alternatives	Description*
AP	Adult Obesity Prevention Interventions Only	Decrease in the adult-to-adult social transmission rate
CP	Child Obesity Prevention Interventions Only	Decrease in the child-to-child social transmission rate
AT	Adult Overweight & Obese Treatment Interventions Only	Decrease in the overweight and obese adults engaging in weight loss behaviors
CT	Child Overweight & Obese Treatment Interventions Only	Increase in overweight and obese adults engaging in weight loss behaviors
APCP	Adult Obesity Prevention AND Child Obesity Prevention Interventions	Decrease in the adult-to-adult social transmission rate, and decrease in the child-to-child social transmission rate
ATCT	Adult and Child Overweight AND Obesity Treatment Interventions	Increase in overweight and obese adults and children engaging in weight loss behaviors
ATCP	Adult Overweight & Obesity Treatment AND Child Obesity Prevention Interventions	Increase in the overweight and obese adults engaging in weight loss behaviors and decrease in the child-to-child and adult-to-child social transmission rates
APCT	Adult Obesity Prevention AND Child Overweight & Obese Treatment Interventions	Decrease in the adult-to-adult social transmission rate, and an increase in the overweight and obese children engaging in weight loss behaviors
CPCT	Child Obesity Prevention AND Child Overweight & Obese Treatment Interventions	Decrease in the child-to-child and adult-to-child social transmission rates, and increase in the overweight and obese children engaging in weight loss behaviors.
APAT	Adult Obesity Prevention AND Adult Overweight & Obese Treatment Interventions	Decrease in the adult-to-adult social transmission rate, and an increase in the overweight and obese adults engaging in weight loss behaviors
APCPCT	Adult Obesity Prevention AND Child Obesity Prevention AND Child Overweight & Obesity Treatment Interventions	Decrease in the adult-to-adult social transmission rate, and a decrease in the child-to-child and adult-to-child social transmission rates, and an increase in the overweight and obese children engaging in weight loss behaviors
ATCPCT	Adult Overweight & Obesity Treatment AND Child Obesity Prevention AND CHild Overweight & Obesitry Treatment Interventions	Increase in the overweight and obese adults and children engaging in weight loss behaviors, and a decrease in the child-to-child and adult-to-child social transmission rates.
APATCP	Adult Obesity Prevention AND Adult Overweight & Obesity Treatment Interventions AND Child Obesity Prevention	Decrease in the adult-to-adult social transmission rate, and an increase in the overweight and obese adults engaging in weight loss behaviors, and decrease in the child-to-child and adult-to-child social transmission rates

TABLE 1: *Cont.*

	Alternatives	Description*
APATCT	Adult Obesity Prevention AND Adult Overweight & Obesity Treatment Interventions AND Child Overweight & Obesity Treatment	Decrease in the adult-to-adult social transmission rate, and an increase in the overweight and obese adult engaging in weight loss behaviors, and an increase in the overweight and obese children
ALL	Adult Obesity Prevention AND Adult Overweight & Obese Treatment Interventions AND Child Obesity Prevention AND Child Overweight & Obese Treatment Interventions	Decreases in the adult-to-adult social transmission rate, and an increase in the overweight and obese adults and children engaging in weight loss behaviors, and decrease in the child-to-child and adult-to-child social transmission rates

All interventions were modeled with a 50% continuous linear increase or decrease in designated paramters over the course of 10 years.

TABLE 2: 3×2 Table of Defined Scenario Sets for Simulation Experiments.

	Adult Intervention Impact on Child (Ψ_A, Adult Obesity Intervention Child Impact Factor)		
Child Intervention Impact on Adult (Ψ_c, Child Obesity Intervention Adult Impact Factor)	25%	50%	75%
10%	Scenario 1	Scenario 2	Scenario 3
25%	Scenario 4	Scenario 5	Scenario 6

11.3 RESULTS

Figure 3 provides the results from the two-way sensitivity analysis. The prevalence rate was slightly more sensitive to the adult-to-child social transmission rate. For example, holding the converse rate constant, reducing the adult-to-child social transmission rate from .0019 to .0011 resulted in a 1.8% lower childhood overweight and obesity prevalence than the same reduction in the child-to-child social transmission rate.

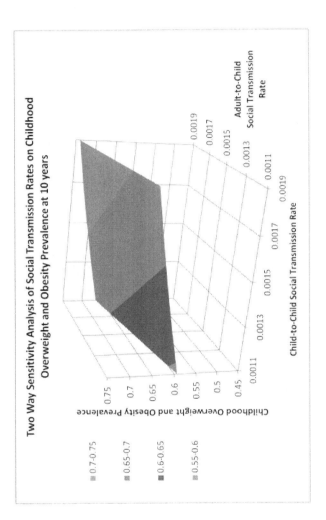

FIGURE 3: Two Way Sensitivity Analysis of Social Transmission Rates on Childhood Overweight and Obesity Prevalence at 10 years. This figure shows the results of the two-way sensitivity analysis of adult-to-child and child-to-child social transmission rates. The graph presents a three dimensional depiction of the childhood overweight and obesity prevalence at 10 years for each combination of adult-to-child and child-to-child social transmission rates tested. The chart indicates that the lowest childhood overweight and obesity prevalence is realized when both adult-to-child and child-to-child social transmission are at their lowest levels in each range. The change in overweight and obesity prevalence is greater across the adult-to-child than the child-to-child social transmission rate axis indicating slightly more sensitivity to the adult-to-child social transmission rate.

Modeling Social Transmission Dynamics of Unhealthy Behaviors 197

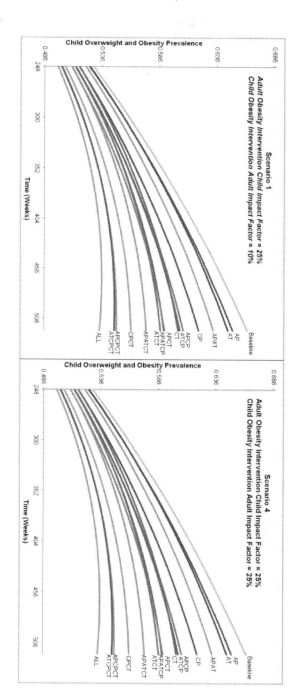

FIGURE 4: Alternatives Impact on Childhood Overweight and Obesity Prevalence from Scenarios 1 and 4. This figure shows the charts for each alternative from Scenario 1 and 4 influence on childhood overweight and obesity prevalence. The time frame charted is from 248 to 520 weeks. All alternatives are labeled and indicate that the ranking did not change between Scenario 1 or 4, nor was prevalence of each alternative greatly affected. The final childhood overweight and obesity prevalence ranges from approximately 53% with the intervention that included all intervention types and levels to 66% for baseline (no intervention).

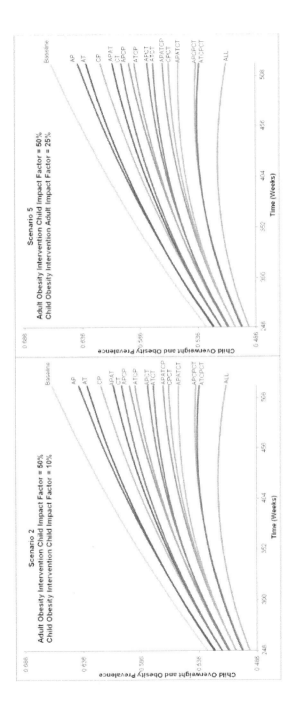

FIGURE 5: Alternatives Impact on Childhood Overweight and Obesity Prevalence from Scenarios 2 and 5. This figure shows the charts for each alternative from Scenarios 2 and 5 influence on childhood overweight and obesity prevalence. The time frame charted is from 248 to 520 weeks. All alternatives are labeled and indicate that the ranking did not change between Scenario 2 or 5, nor was prevalence of each alternative greatly affected. The final childhood overweight and obesity prevalence ranges from approximately 51% with the intervention that included all intervention types and levels to 66% for baseline (no intervention).

Modeling Social Transmission Dynamics of Unhealthy Behaviors 199

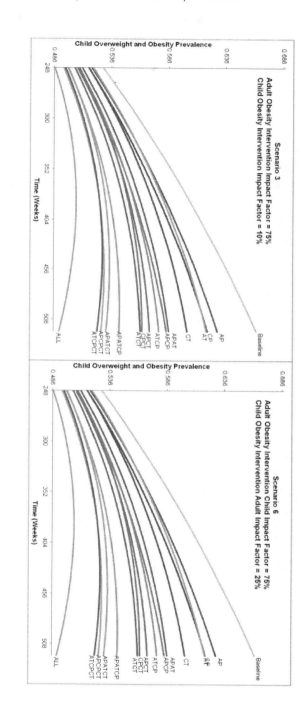

FIGURE 6: Alternatives Impact on Childhood Overweight and Obesity Prevalence from Scenarios 3 and 6. This figure shows the charts for each alternative from Scenario 3 and 6 influence on childhood overweight and obesity prevalence. The time frame charted is from 248 to 520 weeks. All alternatives are labeled and indicate that the ranking did not change between Scenario 3 or 6, nor was prevalence of each alternative greatly affected. The final childhood overweight and obesity prevalence ranges from approximately 49% with the intervention that included all intervention types and levels to 66% for baseline (no intervention).

Figures 4, 5, 6 provide the childhood overweight and obesity prevalence trends for each prevention and treatment intervention alternative from the six scenarios. Overall, many alternatives resulted in continued increase of childhood overweight and obesity prevalence, and only a few of the most comprehensive strategies (combining all or most treatment and prevention options) led to a downward trend by the end of the 10 years. Variation between the alternatives was not significantly apparent until after approximately 5 years (260 weeks).

As would be expected, the alternative that included all treatment and prevention options at both adult and child levels was the most impactful. Excluding this, the combination of adult treatment with child prevention and treatment interventions resulted in the lowest prevalence at the end of 10 years in all scenarios. Adult prevention alone resulted in the highest end prevalence at the end of 10 years. In each scenario, alternatives with treatment alone (targeted at either adults or children) reduced prevalence more than prevention alone (1.2–1.8% when targeted at children and 0.2 to 1.0% when targeted at adults).

Scenarios that compared different child intervention impact factors (10% versus 25%) with the same adult intervention impact factor did not result in large differences in childhood overweight and obesity prevalence. Comparing Scenarios 1 and 4; 2 and 5; and 3 and 6, the ranking of alternatives remained the same and the difference of the final prevalence was less than a tenth of a percent for each (Figures 4, 5, 6).

Conversely, the ranking of alternatives changed among scenarios that varied the adult intervention impact factor, and differences were seen in the final prevalence rates. Table 3 provides the ranking of alternatives and final childhood overweight and obesity prevalence for Scenarios 4–6. As the impact of adult interventions on children was increased, the rank of six alternatives that included adults became better (i.e., resulting in lower 10 year childhood overweight and obesity prevalence) than alternatives that only involved children. For example, in Scenario 4 (with an adult intervention impact factor of 25%), childhood treatment intervention only was ranked ninth best, better than adult prevention and treatment intervention combined (ranked thirteenth best). These alternatives' ranks changed in

Scenario 6 (with adult intervention impact factor of 75%), where the childhood treatment intervention only was ranked twelfth, worse than adult prevention and treatment combined (ranked at eleventh). In Scenario 6, the adult treatment and child prevention alternative ranked as ninth.

TABLE 3: Ranking and Final Childhood Overweight and Obesity Prevalence for Scenarios 4–6.

	Adult-to-child Impact Factor*					
	25% (Scenario 4)		50% (Scenario 5)		75% (Scenario 6)	
	Alternative	Final Childhood Overweight and Obesity Prevalence	Alternative	Final Childhood Overweight and Obesity Prevalence	Alternative	Final Childhood Overweight and Obesity Prevalence
Highest Final Childhood Overweight and Obesity Prevalence	AP	65.01%	AP	63.97%	AP	62.91%
	AT	64.60%	AT	63.26%	CP	62.01%
	APAT	63.34%	CP	62.01%	AT	61.94%
	CP	62.01%	APAT	60.98%	CT	60.21%
	APCP	60.67%	CT	60.21%	APAT	58.65%
	ATCP	60.37%	APCP	59.55%	APCP	58.41%
	CT	60.21%	ATCP	59.07%	ATCP	57.78%
	APATCP	59.05%	APCT	57.97%	APCT	56.95%
	APCT	58.97%	ATCT	57.48%	ATCT	56.30%
	ATCT	58.67%	APATCP	56.66%	CPCT	56.11%
	APATCT	57.45%	CPCT	56.11%	APATCP	54.30%
	CPCT	56.11%	APATCT	55.28%	APATCT	53.14%
	APCPCT	54.81%	APCPCT	53.75%	APCPCT	52.68%
	ATCPCT	54.62%	ATCPCT	53.47%	ATCPCT	52.33%
Lowest Final Childhood Overweight and Obesity Prevalence	APATCPCT	53.35%	APATCPCT	51.17%	APATCPCT	49.03%

*Child to Adult Impact Factor is 25% for all scenarios

Alternatives with greater numbers of intervention types (prevention and treatment at adult and child levels) did not directly correspond to better ranking. For example, in Scenarios 1 and 4 five alternatives with fewer intervention types had better rankings than alternatives with more intervention types. For example, including two intervention types (child prevention and child treatment) resulted in a better ranking than several alternatives that included three intervention types but were more adult focused (i.e., adult prevention and treatment combined with child prevention only or adult prevention and treatment combined with child treatment only). Conversely, in Scenarios 3 and 6 any alternative that included three intervention types (regardless of adult or child focus) was better ranked than any with only two.

11.4 DISCUSSION AND CONCLUSIONS

This research provides new insight that has implications on future policies and decision-making regarding prevention versus treatment intervention combinations and adult versus peer levers of social influence. Childhood obesity prevalence may be more sensitive to changes in adult-to-child social transmission rates compared to child-to-child rates. Similar to previous modeling research [29], our experiments found that combinations of prevention and treatment generally have greater impact than either alone. However, the additional complexity of adult and child influences and social transmission resulted in changes to an alternative's impact depending on varying influence of adult and child interventions on each other.

The two-way sensitivity analyses revealed that childhood obesity and overweight prevalence is sensitive to changes in social transmission rates from both adult and peer levels. Using current surveillance data from the US for baseline values and no interventions, changes to the adult-to-child transmission rate had slightly greater impact than child-to-child on childhood overweight and obesity. Current research strongly suggests the presence of social influences on obesity and obesity-related health behaviors [9]. However, the quantification of social transmission is limited in current research. Compared to infectious disease, the complexities of issues such as longer exposure timeframes and nuanced social protective and risk factors make exploration of such quantification more difficult. Research that attempts to intervene on social transmission at adult-to-child and child-to-child levels may help to elucidate the mechanisms and improve the target within interventions.

Our findings also indicate that the combination of prevention and treatment interventions may need to consider the social transmission context for optimum impact. Within any of our scenarios, alternatives that included treatment intervention impact (especially targeted at child levels) versus a prevention intervention impact, resulted in lower childhood overweight and obesity prevalence after 10 years. Santonja et al [29] found that for adults in Spain, prevention alone strategies resulted in greater reductions of overweight and obesity. The difference in our findings is possibly due to the higher initial prevalence of overweight and obesity found in the US and used for our model parameters. Determining priorities regarding prevention or treatment interventions for obesity and chronic diseases is a source of ongoing debate, though, most concede a blend of both approaches are needed [56]–[60]. Our research does not minimize the importance or potential of obesity prevention interventions, but challenges us to consider how a society with high prevalence of overweight and obesity and noted obesogenic socio-cultural environments [61] might respond to prevention interventions that simply seek to educate and change attitudes about healthy lifestyles.

Furthermore, evidence that combinations of prevention and treatment interventions are most influential encourage thoughtful consideration of how both strategies should address mechanisms of social transmission. The role of social-cultural environments is evident in multilevel and systems-oriented models for obesity intervention [7], [61] and can be useful to conceptualize and define targets for both prevention and treatment interventions at population-levels. For example, interventions should consider how to target social norms regarding the desire and advocacy for environments that support healthy behaviors for both prevention and weight loss.

Our research also tested the potential for interventions to act through targeted mechanisms of adult influence on children and vice versa (e.g., actively engaging individuals to support and encourage others in their social environment in healthy behaviors).The results indicated childhood overweight and obesity prevalence is sensitive to adult influence. The ranking of alternative interventions at child and adult levels changed based on the degree of influence adult interventions had on children. Intervention combinations that focus more heavily on adults may result in greater reductions in childhood obesity than those that target children only if adult interventions have higher residual impact on children. Targeting children has been noted as advantageous due to issues such as political expediency [62] and relative ease of shifting behavior [63]; however, our results indicate that if effective interventions are available, targeting adults may be more efficient. A recent intervention study found that a parent-only intervention resulted in equal impact on child weight loss as compared to those that included both parents and children [64], and that parent weight loss was slightly better for the parent only intervention group. Research should seek to expand and strengthen this type of intervention.

The results of our research indicate the potential for such methodologies to aid in intervention planning and finite resource allocation by determining the potential impact of different intervention combinations. It is noted that public health policy makers can be overwhelmed by the complicated task of using data, evidence, reviews and summaries to determine best practices [65]. Our model provides evidence about the impact of different combinations, which could be combined with decision making models that includes factors such as adult influence and cost, to assist with resource allocation decisions.

This research does have its limitations. The current model and research is deterministic and was not built for predictive purposes. It does not allow testing for statistical significance between the intervention combinations. Another key constraint of the model is the assumption of homogenous mixing. Research has indicated that social transmission is likely to occur through clustering effects and spreads differently through various types of social ties [8], [66]. Regardless, the model does allow consideration of patterns and outcomes that point to potential gaps in current research and new hypotheses about plausible intervention levers.

System dynamics modeling provides a tool that can strengthen the connections between generation, synthesis, and translation of evidence. Our results highlight areas of research that could provide beneficial information to inform future modeling and enhance decision making. Better quantification of the relative impact of adult-to-adult, adult-to-child, and child-to-child social influences in terms of transference of both unhealthy and healthy behaviors would strengthen our ability to answer questions regarding optimum combinations of interventions. However, in the absence of such information the model can still provide valuable insight into potential patterns and trends.

Future research can use and expand this model to answer additional research questions. This model established the core structure for modeling the child and adult dynamic social transmission of unhealthy obesity-related behavior, but future work is needed to expand the model boundaries to include elements of intervention implementation (i.e., intervention resources, cost, demand, and supply) (Figure S1). The model should also be considered in combination with agent-based models to explore the influence of networks and clustering in different population structures. Finally, future studies should use this model to explore important leverage points in order to harness impact and target the different combinations of interventions dynamically. For example, the rate of change in childhood overweight and obesity prevalence may be greater with certain alternative policy combinations. Thus, points of inflection can be identified to improve our understanding when and how alternatives should be planned and implemented through time.

REFERENCES

1. Wolf AM, Colditz GA (2012) Current estimates of the economic cost of obesity in the united states. Obes Res 6: 97–106. doi: 10.1002/j.1550-8528.1998.tb00322.x
2. Wang YC, McPherson K, Marsh T, Gortmaker SL, Brown M (2011) Health and economic burden of the projected obesity trends in the USA and the UK. The Lancet 378: 815–825. doi: 10.1016/s0140-6736(11)60814-3
3. Reilly J, Kelly J (2010) Long-term impact of overweight and obesity in childhood and adolescence on morbidity and premature mortality in adulthood: Systematic review. Int J Obes 35: 891–898. doi: 10.1038/ijo.2010.222
4. Flegal KM, Carroll MD, Ogden CL, Curtin LR (2010) Prevalence and trends in obesity among US adults, 1999–2008. JAMA 303: 235–241. doi: 10.1001/jama.2009.2014
5. Ogden CL, Carroll MD, Kit BK, Flegal KM (2012) Prevalence of obesity and trends in body mass index among US children and adolescents, 1999–2010. JAMA 307: 483–490. doi: 10.1001/jama.2012.40

6. Institute of Medicine (IOM), Committee on Accelerating Progress in Obesity Prevention. (2012) Accelerating progress in obesity prevention: Solving the weight of the nation. Washington, DC: The National Academies Press.
7. Huang TT, Drewnowski A, Kumanyika SK, Glass TA (2009) A systems-oriented multi-level framework for addressing obesity in the 21st century. Prev Chronic Dis 6(3): A82.
8. Christakis NA, Fowler JH (2007) The spread of obesity in a large social network over 32 years. N Engl J Med 357: 370–379. doi: 10.1056/nejmsa066082
9. Hammond RA (2010) Social influence and obesity. Curr Opin Endocrinol Diabetes Obes 17: 467–471. doi: 10.1097/med.0b013e32833d4687
10. Van Der Horst K, Oenema A, Ferreira I, Wendel-Vos W, Giskes K, et al. (2007) A systematic review of environmental correlates of obesity-related dietary behaviors in youth. Health Educ Res 22: 203–226. doi: 10.1093/her/cyl069
11. Wagner A, Klein-Platat C, Arveiler D, Haan M, Schlienger J, et al. (2004) Parent-child physical activity relationships in 12-year old french students do not depend on family socioeconomic status. Diabetes Metab 30: 359–366. doi: 10.1016/s1262-3636(07)70129-5
12. Franzini L, Elliott MN, Cuccaro P, Schuster M, Gilliland MJ, et al. (2009) Influences of physical and social neighborhood environments on children's physical activity and obesity. Am J Public Health 99(2): 271–278. doi: 10.2105/ajph.2007.128702
13. Gable S, Lutz S (2004) Household, parent, and child contributions to childhood obesity. Fam Relat 49: 293–300. doi: 10.1111/j.1741-3729.2000.00293.x
14. Koehly LM, Loscalzo A (2009) Peer reviewed: Adolescent obesity and social networks. Prev Chronic Disease 6(3): A99.
15. Ali MM, Amialchuk A, Gao S, Heiland F (2012) Adolescent weight gain and social networks: Is there a contagion effect? Appl Econ 44: 2969–2983. doi: 10.1080/00036846.2011.568408
16. De la Haye K, Robins G, Mohr P, Wilson C (2010) Obesity-related behaviors in adolescent friendship networks. Soc Networks 32: 161–167. doi: 10.1016/j.socnet.2009.09.001
17. Renna F, Grafova IB, Thakur N (2008) The effect of friends on adolescent body weight. Econ Hum Biol 6: 377–387. doi: 10.1016/j.ehb.2008.06.005
18. Salvy S, De La Haye K, Bowker JC, Hermans RC (2012) Influence of peers and friends on children's and adolescents' eating and activity behaviors. Physiol Behav 106(2): 369–378. doi: 10.1016/j.physbeh.2012.03.022
19. Wrotniak BH, Epstein LH, Paluch RA, Roemmich JN (2004) Parent weight change as a predictor of child weight change in family-based behavioral obesity treatment. Arch Pediatr Adolesc Med 158: 342–347. doi: 10.1001/archpedi.158.4.342
20. Golley RK, Magarey AM, Baur LA, Steinbeck KS, Daniels LA (2007) Twelve-month effectiveness of a parent-led, family-focused weight-management program for prepubertal children: A randomized, controlled trial. Pediatrics 119: 517–525. doi: 10.1542/peds.2006-1746
21. Boutelle KN, Cafri G, Crow SJ (2011) Parent-only treatment for childhood obesity: A randomized controlled trial. Obesity (Silver Spring) 19: 574–580. doi: 10.1038/oby.2010.238
22. Forrester JW (1994) System dynamics, systems thinking, and soft OR. System Dynamics Review 10: 245–256. doi: 10.1002/sdr.4260100211

23. Abdel-Hamid TK (2002) Modeling the dynamics of human energy regulation and its implications for obesity treatment. System Dynamics Review 18: 431–471. doi: 10.1002/sdr.240
24. Goldbeter A (2006) A model for the dynamics of human weight cycling. J Biosci 31: 129–136. doi: 10.1007/bf02705242
25. Homer J, Milstein B, Dietz W, Buchner D, Majestic D. (2006) Obesity population dynamics: Exploring historical growth and plausible futures in the US. Proceedings from the 24th International System Dynamics Conference Proceedings.
26. 26. Jódar L, Santonja FJ, González-Parra G (2008) Modeling dynamics of infant obesity in the region of valencia, spain. Comput Math Appl 56: 679–689. doi: 10.1016/j.camwa.2008.01.011
27. Karanfil Ö, Moore T, Finley P, Brown T, Zagonel A, et al.. (2011) A multi-scale paradigm to design policy options for obesity prevention: Exploring the integration of individual-based modeling and system dynamics. Sandia National Laboratories. Available online: http://www.sandia.gov/casosengineering/docs/SD%202011%20Obesity_2011-6146.pdf. Accessed 2013 Nov 10.
28. Rahmandad H, Sabounchi NS. (2011) Building and estimating a dynamic model of weight gain and loss for individuals and populations. Proceedings from The 29th International Conference of the System Dynamics Society.
29. Santonja F, Morales A, Villanueva R, Cortés J (2012) Analysing the effect of public health campaigns on reducing excess weight: A modelling approach for the spanish autonomous region of the community of valencia. Eval Program Plann 35: 34–39. doi: 10.1016/j.evalprogplan.2011.06.004
30. Evangelista AM, Ortiz AR, Rios-Soto K, Urdapilleta A. (2004) USA the fast food nation: Obesity as an epidemic. Accessible online: http://mtbi.asu.edu/downloads/Obesity.pdf . Accessed 2013 Oct 12.
31. Gonzalez-Parra G, Jodar L, Santonja FJ, Villanueva RJ (2010) An age-structured model for childhood obesity. Math Pop Studies 17: 1–11. doi: 10.1080/07481180903467218
32. Hall KD (2006) Computational model of in vivo human energy metabolism during semistarvation and refeeding. Am J Phys-End Metab 291: E23–E37. doi: 10.1152/ajpendo.00523.2005
33. Flatt J (2004) Carbohydrate–Fat interactions and obesity examined by a two-compartment computer Model. Obes Res 12: 2013–2022. doi: 10.1038/oby.2004.252
34. Chow CC, Hall KD (2008) The dynamics of human body weight change. PLoS computational biology 4: e1000045. doi: 10.1371/journal.pcbi.1000045
35. Davison KK, Lawson HA, Coatsworth JD (2012) The family-centered action model of intervention layout and implementation (FAMILI) the example of childhood obesity. Health Prom Pract 13: 454–461. doi: 10.1177/1524839910377966
36. Golan M, Crow S (2004) Parents are key players in the prevention and treatment of weight-related problems. Nutr Rev 62: 39–50. doi: 10.1111/j.1753-4887.2004.tb00005.x
37. Centers for Disease Control and Prevention (CDC) National center for health statistics (NCHS). National Health and Nutrition Examination Survey Questionnaire. Hyattsville, MD: U.S. Department of Health and Human Services, Centers for Disease Control and Prevention, (2009–2010) Available: http://wwwn.cdc.gov/nchs/nhanes/search/nhanes09_10.aspx.Accessed 2013 Nov 10.

38. Division of Nutrition Physical Activity and Obesity National Center for Chronic Disease Prevention and Health Promotion.(2011) Losing weight. Available online: http://www.cdc.gov/healthyweight/physical_activity/index.html July 20, 2013. Accessed 2013 Nov 10.
39. Panel, NHLBI Obesity Education Initiative Expert (1998) On the identification, evaluation, and treatment of overweight and obesity in adults. Clinical guidelines on the identification, evaluation, and treatment of overweight and obesity in adults—the evidence report. Obes Res 6: 51S–209S.
40. LeBlanc E, O'Connor E, Whitlock EP, Patnode C, Kapka T. (2011) Screening for and management of obesity and overweight in adults. Rockville (MD): Agency for Healthcare Research and Quality. Report No.: 11–05159-EF-1.
41. Whitlock EP, O'Connor EA, Williams SB, Beil TL, Lutz KW (2010) Effectiveness of weight management interventions in children: A targeted systematic review for the USPSTF. Pediatrics 125: e396–e418. doi: 10.1542/peds.2009-1955
42. Vasan RS, Pencina MJ, Cobain M, Freiberg MS, D'Agostino RB (2005) Estimated risks for developing obesity in the framingham heart study. Ann Intern Med 143: 473–480. doi: 10.7326/0003-4819-143-7-200510040-00005
43. Williamson DA, Han H, Johnson WD, Stewart TM, Harsha DW (2010) Longitudinal study of body weight changes in children: Who is gaining and who is losing weight. Obesity 19: 667–670. doi: 10.1038/oby.2010.221
44. Feunekes GI, de Graaf C, Meyboom S, van Staveren WA (1998) Food choice and fat intake of adolescents and adults: Associations of intakes within social networks. Prev Med 27: 645–656. doi: 10.1006/pmed.1998.0341
45. Ali MM, Amialchuk A, Heiland FW (2011) Weight-related behavior among adolescents: The role of peer effects. PloS one 6: e21179. doi: 10.1371/journal.pone.0021179
46. Fortin B, Yazbeck M. (2011) Peer effects, fast food consumption and adolescent weight gain. CIRANO-Scientific Publications 2011s-20 http://thema.u-cergy.fr/IMG/pdf/seminaire_du_02-02-12.pdf.
47. Gustafson SL, Rhodes RE (2006) Parental correlates of physical activity in children and early adolescents. Sports Med 36: 79–97. doi: 10.2165/00007256-200636010-00006
48. Rasmussen M, Krolner R, Klepp K, Lytle L, Brug J, et al. (2006) Determinants of fruit and vegetable consumption among children and adolescents: A review of the literature. part I: Quantitative studies. Int J of Behav Nutr Phys Act 3: 22 doi:10.1186/1479-5868-3-22.
49. Birch L, Ventura A (2009) Preventing childhood obesity: What works. Int J Obes 33: S74–S81. doi: 10.1038/ijo.2009.22
50. Golan M, Weizman A, Apter A, Fainaru M (1998) Parents as the exclusive agents of change in the treatment of childhood obesity. Am J Clin Nutr 67: 1130–1135.
51. Barlas Y (1989) Multiple tests for validation of system dynamics type of simulation models. Eur J Oper Res 42: 59–87. doi: 10.1016/0377-2217(89)90059-3
52. Ogden CL, Flegal KM, Carroll MD, Johnson CL (2002) Prevalence and trends in overweight among US children and adolescents, 1999–2000. JAMA 288: 1728–1732. doi: 10.1001/jama.288.14.1728
53. Hedley AA, Ogden CL, Johnson CL, Carroll MD, Curtin LR, et al. (2004) Prevalence of overweight and obesity among US children, adolescents, and adults, 1999–2002. JAMA 291: 2847–2850. doi: 10.1001/jama.291.23.2847

54. Ogden C, Carroll M. (2010) Prevalence of obesity among children and adolescents: United states, trends 1963–1965 through 2007–2008. Atlanta: Centers for Disease Control and Prevention. National Center for Health Statistics: 201.
55. Flegal KM, Carroll MD, Ogden CL, Curtin LR (2010) Prevalence and trends in obesity among US adults, 1999–2008. JAMA 303: 235–241. doi: 10.1001/jama.2009.2014
56. Rein AS, Ogden LL (2012) Public health: A best buy for america. J Public Health Manag Pract 18: 299–302. doi: 10.1097/phh.0b013e31825d25dd
57. Rappange DR, Brouwer WB, Rutten FF, van Baal PH (2010) Lifestyle intervention: From cost savings to value for money. J Public Health 32: 440–447. doi: 10.1093/pubmed/fdp079
58. Goetzel RZ (2009) Do prevention or treatment services save money? the wrong debate. Health Aff 28: 37–41. doi: 10.1377/hlthaff.28.1.37
59. McDermott R, Chancellor PV (2008) Why primary prevention is (mostly) a better bet than clinical prevention. Public Health Bulletin SA 6: 14.
60. Kumanyika SK, Obarzanek E, Stettler N, Bell R, Field AE, et al. (2008) Population-based prevention of obesity the need for comprehensive promotion of healthful eating, physical activity, and energy balance: A scientific statement from american heart association council on epidemiology and prevention, interdisciplinary committee for prevention (formerly the expert panel on population and prevention science). Circulation 118: 428–464. doi: 10.1161/circulationaha.108.189702
61. Kirk SF, Penney TL, McHugh T (2010) Characterizing the obesogenic environment: The state of the evidence with directions for future research. Obes Rev 11: 109–117. doi: 10.1111/j.1467-789x.2009.00611.x
62. Brownell KD, Kersh R, Ludwig DS, Post RC, Puhl RM, et al. (2010) Personal responsibility and obesity: A constructive approach to a controversial issue. Health Aff 29: 379–387. doi: 10.1377/hlthaff.2009.0739
63. Steinbeck KS (2001) The importance of physical activity in the prevention of overweight and obesity in childhood: A review and an opinion. Obesity reviews 2: 117–130. doi: 10.1046/j.1467-789x.2001.00033.x
64. Boutelle KN, Cafri G, Crow SJ (2011) Parent-Only treatment for childhood obesity: A randomized controlled trial. Obesity 19: 574–580. doi: 10.1038/oby.2010.238
65. Waters E (2009) Evidence for public health decision-making: Towards reliable synthesis. Bull World Health Organ 87: 164–164. doi: 10.2471/blt.09.064022
66. Bahr DB, Browning RC, Wyatt HR, Hill JO (2009) Exploiting social networks to mitigate the obesity epidemic. Obesity 17: 723–728. doi: 10.1038/oby.2008.615

There are several supplemental files that are not available in this version of the article. To view this additional information, please use the citation on the first page of this chapter.

CHAPTER 12

EFFECTS OF AN INTERVENTION AIMED AT REDUCING THE INTAKE OF SUGAR-SWEETENED BEVERAGES IN PRIMARY SCHOOL CHILDREN: A CONTROLLED TRIAL

VIVIAN M. VAN DE GAAR, WILMA JANSEN, AMY VAN GRIEKEN, GERARD JJM BORSBOOM, STEF KREMERS, AND HEIN RAAT

12.1 BACKGROUND

Weight gain and subsequent overweight in children is a growing problem worldwide. One of the contributions to this problem is thought to be the consumption of sugar-sweetened beverages (SSB) [1]–[6]. Indeed, small reductions in daily SSB servings have been shown to potentially improve health [7],[8]; for example De Ruyter et al. showed that over a period of 18 months, children who replaced one SSB serving per school day with a non-caloric drink gained less weight, with an average difference of 1.0 kg [7]. Several other intervention studies with water as an alternative drink

---

Effects of an Intervention Aimed at Reducing the Intake of Sugar-Sweetened Beverages in Primary School Children: A Controlled Trial. © van de Gaar VM, Jansen W, van Grieken A, Borsboom GJJM, Kremers S, and Raat H. International Journal of Behavioral Nutrition and Physical Activity **11**,98 *(2014), doi:10.1186/s12966-014-0098-8. Licensed under Creative Commons Attribution 4.0 International License, http://creativecommons.org/licenses/by/4.0/.*

have demonstrated successful behavioural changes, weight loss and other health benefits [9]–[13].

As the number of obese children is not declining—at best it is levelling off [14]–[16]—effective interventions aimed at supporting a healthy lifestyle are needed. Schools are a relevant setting in which to improve healthy lifestyles among children, not only because most children attend school, but also because it allows an intervention to reach children with varied ethnicities and socio-economic backgrounds [17]–[26]. Nevertheless, schools are not the only setting that needs to be addressed. Parents also play an essential role in establishing healthy habits in children [24],[27]–[31]. In addition, the wider environment outside schools contains many so-called obesogenic determinants that should be targeted to promote a healthy environment. This means that interventions are needed at multiple levels [32]–[34]. As an example, Bleich et al. showed that community-based interventions that have a school component are more effective at preventing childhood overweight than interventions that are only school-based or only community-based [35]. Community involvement may also contribute to more sustainable programmes with higher reach and more impact [18],[32],[36]–[38]. It has therefore been suggested that childhood obesity must be addressed in multiple settings, i.e. at the individual, family, school and community level [17],[18],[24],[33],[35],[39],[40]. This advice with regard to multiple settings has led to initiatives such as the European EPODE network (where EPODE is a French acronym that stands for "Together let's prevent childhood obesity") and its Dutch version JOGG, which are both using an approach that incorporates social marketing techniques [41]–[43]. These techniques are expected to enhance the outcomes of integrated approaches since many other social marketing-based programmes throughout the world have been successful [18],[36],[44]–[51].

Recently, within the JOGG city network in Rotterdam an intervention was developed aimed at reducing SSB intake. This water promotion intervention, called the 'water campaign', is school- and community-based and applies social marketing. The water campaign is an intervention tailored to children (aged 6-12 years) and their families who live in multi-ethnic, socially more deprived neighbourhoods; populations who remain disproportionately affected by childhood overweight [15],[52]–[54].

In this study, we evaluate the effectiveness of the water campaign. We hypothesized that after one year of intervention, children in the intervention group would have a lower SSB intake than children in the control group.

TABLE 1: Overview of activities in the water campaign and regular health promotion programme

Activities	Aimed at	Water campaign	Regular programme
Three physical education lessons per week by professional physical education teacher	Children	☐	☐
School sport clubs	Children	☐	☐
Education in choosing healthy food and sports	Children & parents	☐	☐
School dietician	Children & parents	☐	☐
Annual height and weight measurements (for BMI tracking) and fittest	Children & parents	☐	☐
Additional non-compulsory play and sports activities outside school hours	Children	☐	☐
Special event: water campaign kick-off 'Drinking water is fun!'	Children & parents	☐	
Use of promotional material: posters 'Water is the best thing I can give to my child!'	Children & parents	☐	
Activity	Children & parents	☐	
For children: Pimp up your water bottle		☐	
For parents: Pimp up your water jug		☐	
Provision of free water bottles by community organizations during summer activities	Children	☐	
Provision of free water at school throughout the day	Children	☐	
Taking a water break during physical education lessons; parents responsible for giving the child his/her water bottle to school	Children & parents	☐	
Water theme week, including activities	Children & parents	☐	

For children: special educational water lessons, fun games such as happy families, board and card games involving water consumption, and a special water show provided by children's role models

For parents: storytelling about promoting water consumption, different fun games involving water consumption and other aspects of water, including a water magazine for mothers; and promotion by water ambassadors

12.2 METHODS

12.2.1 INTERVENTION CONDITION

The water campaign consists of lessons at school combined with integrated community activities that promote water consumption in various ways. Table 1 provides an overview of the water campaign activities. The intervention was developed by the local government using health promotion tools—intervention mapping [55]—in combination with social marketing. According to French et al., social marketing aims to change voluntary behaviour by taking the needs and wishes of the target audience as the starting point and from there trying to understand how best to promote the desired behaviour using an integrated, tailored approach [43].

Following the social marketing guidelines, desk research and focus-group interviews were applied to identify specific risk groups and risk behaviours. Based on these results, the local government intervention-development team decided to focus the water campaign on Turkish and Moroccan families [52]. These families form a large group of non-Western immigrants in the study area, a group disproportionately affected by childhood overweight [15],[53],[54]. Although the intervention was tailored to, pre-tested in and developed for children and mothers from these ethnic minorities, the water campaign was delivered to all children (and their families) attending the intervention schools and/or living in these neighbourhoods. By encouraging the children to consume more water, the water campaign intended to reduce children's SSB intake [5],[7],[8],[10]–[13],[20],[23].

12.2.2 CONTROL CONDITION

The intervention and control schools continued with their regular health promotion programme, the effective school-based curriculum 'Enjoy Being Fit' (EBF). Initiated in 2006, this multi-component programme for primary school children encourages a healthy lifestyle by educating children and providing additional extracurricular physical activity lessons (see Table 1) [56]. This programme addresses behavioural and environmental determinants based on elements of the "Environmental Research Framework for Weight Gain Prevention" [33]. A more detailed description of the EBF programme and a study describing its effects is provided elsewhere [57].

12.2.3 STUDY DESIGN

To evaluate the water campaign, we conducted a controlled trial with baseline measures collected prior to the intervention and follow-up measures after one year of intervention. A controlled design was chosen for practical reasons that were related to the spread of intervention activities throughout the community. Four schools were included, which were randomly allocated to either intervention or control condition. The Medical and Ethical Review Committee of the Erasmus Medical Centre issued a "declaration of no objection" (i.e. formal waver) for this study (reference number MEC-2011-183). Parents and children were informed about the study and were free to refuse participation without giving any explanation.

The outcome measure was children's SSB consumption, which was estimated by means of parent and child questionnaires and observations of drinks brought to school. Blinding of participants and data collectors was not possible since the water campaign's activities were visible at the intervention schools and throughout the neighbourhoods.

12.2.4 SAMPLE AND PARTICIPANTS

Two intervention schools were assigned to the water campaign. A total of four schools, located in four different non adjacent neighbourhoods in Rotterdam, the Netherlands, were matched in pairs of two. The matched schools had a roughly equal number of pupils, had pupils of similar socioeconomic status, and had a similar prevalence of overweight. On the basis of these criteria, we were able to select only six school pairs from the 80 schools that were eligible for the study. These pairs were then approached based on convenience, in the knowledge that a school pair could only be included in the study if both schools in the pair provided consent and a maximum of two school pairs in total could be included in the study. One of the schools in the school pair was then allocated to either the intervention or control condition by the flip of a coin. Figure 1 provides an overview of study enrollment and participant flow. At the four participating schools, all children in grades 2 to 7 (aged 6-12 years) were invited to participate, as were their parents.

12.2.5 POWER

The study was powered to detect a difference in SSB servings of 0.50 per day between the intervention and control groups. We hereby assumed a standard deviation of 1.00 serving, with a power of 0.80 and an alpha of 0.05 (two-sided), taking into account adjustment of baseline values and loss to follow-up (assuming a correlation of 0.80 between baseline and follow-up measurements).

12.2.6 MEASUREMENTS

Data on children's SSB consumption and socio-demographic characteristics were collected at baseline and after one year of intervention, using parent and child questionnaires (assessed separately) and observations at school.

The parents of all children in grades 3 to 7 (aged 6-12 years) received the questionnaire at two time points: at baseline (April 2011) and after one year of intervention (June 2012). Children in grades 5 to 7 (aged 9-12 years) were invited to complete child questionnaires at two time points: at baseline (April 2011-September 2011) and after one year of intervention (June 2012). The observations of children in grades 2 to 7 took place at two time points: at baseline (April 2011-September 2011) and after one year of intervention (June 2012).

Since the intervention was implemented over two school years, it was necessary to combine the baseline measurements for the child questionnaire and the observations. Children in grades 6 and 7 completed the baseline questionnaire in April 2011; children in grade 5 (and children in grades 6 and 7 who were absent during the April measurement) completed their baseline questionnaire in September 2011. Children in grades 3-7 were observed for baseline measurement in April 2011 and children in grade 2 (and children grades 3-7 who were absent during the April measurement) were observed for baseline measurement in September 2011. Hypothetically, the fact that we used a combined baseline could have led to underestimation of effect because some children had already been exposed to the intervention. However, when we repeated the analyses using only the April 2011 data as baseline measurement we found similar results (data not shown). An overview of the data collection is presented in Figure 2.

12.2.7 SSB CONSUMPTION

The following definition of SSB was used: beverages containing added sugar, sweetened dairy products (e.g. chocolate milk), fruit juice (e.g. apple juice), soft drinks (e.g. cola) and energy drinks (e.g. sport energy drinks).

The consumption of SSB was assessed using similar questionnaire items for both parents and children (an overview of several items used in the parent and child questionnaire to assess child's SSB intake are shown in Additional file 1: Table S1). Examples of SSB were provided, based on our definition of SSB. First, we asked whether the child consumed SSB on a daily basis. Answer categories were "yes, every day"; "no, not every day"; and "never", except for the baseline parent questionnaire, where the answer categories were only "yes, every day" or "no, not every day". At follow-up, this outcome measure was recoded into "yes, every day" and "no, not every day" (including "never").

Average SSB intake was measured by asking the child or parent to indicate how many glasses (250 ml), cans (330 ml) or bottles (500 ml) the child consumed on an average day on which the child drank SSB. Answer categories ranged from "none" to "5 or more". The total SSB intake per day, converted to litres, was calculated by summing up the multiplications of the number of glasses, cans or bottles with their volume. The average number of SSB servings was measured using the same question, adding up the number of glasses, cans or bottles that were reported to be consumed (under the assumption that a child would not consume multiple SSB drinks at once, e.g. consuming a glass and a can SSB simultaneously).

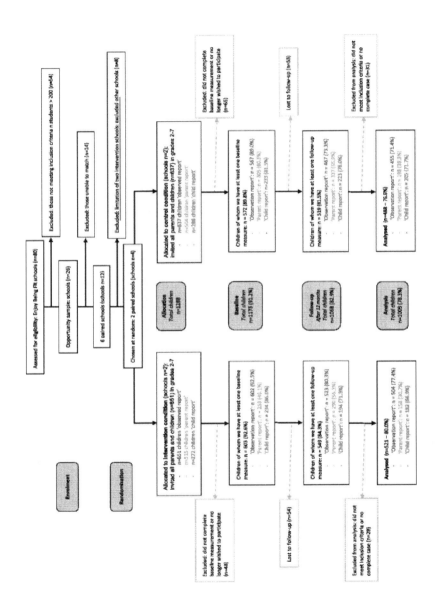

FIGURE 1: Overview of the course of the study.

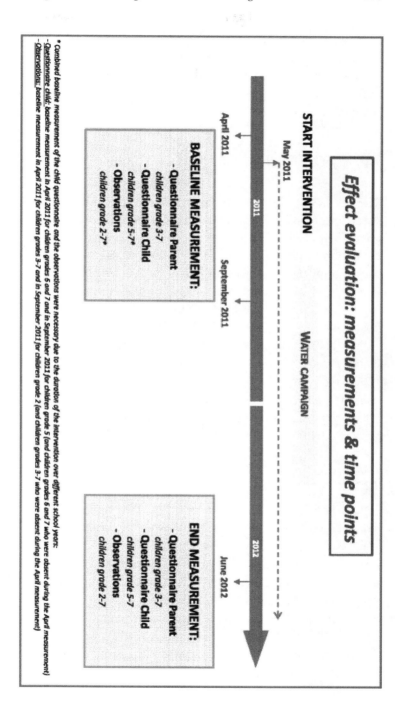

FIGURE 2: Overview of the data collection.

Observations at school were conducted by trained observers, who objectively recorded one morning on a random school day the drinks that the children brought to consume at school during morning break (10:00 am). Before analysis, the beverages were classified as "SSB" or "not SSB" based on the definition provided above.

12.2.8 SOCIO-DEMOGRAPHIC FACTORS

The parent and child questionnaires included items on child's gender, age, grade and ethnic background. Ethnic background was determined by the country of birth of the parents according to definitions given by Statistics Netherlands [58]. The child's ethnic background was defined as Dutch only if both parents had been born in the Netherlands; if one of the parents had been born in another country, ethnic background was defined according to that country; and if both parents had been born in different foreign countries, ethnic background was defined as the mother's country of birth. Ethnic background was categorized as either Dutch, Surinamese/Antillean, Moroccan/Turkish or other/unknown.

Gender, age and educational level of the caregiver were also recorded using the parent questionnaire. The caregiver's highest educational level was categorized as either "high" (high/mid-high); "low" (mid-low/low); or "unknown", based on standard Dutch cut-off points [59].

12.2.9 WEIGHT STATUS

Trained personnel measured height and weight at baseline. Weight status was determined by calculating the Body Mass Index (BMI) in kg/m^2 with height measured to the nearest 0.1 cm and weight measured to the nearest 0.2 kg, in light clothing or gym clothes, according to a national standardized protocol for youth health care taking into account the child's age and gender [60]. Children were categorized as being either "non-overweight" or "overweight/obese", based on cut-off points published by the International Obesity Task Force [61].

12.2.10 DATA ANALYSIS

To evaluate the water campaign's effects on SSB consumption, we used the following three data sets: (1) data collected using parent questionnaires, from now on referred to as the "parent report"; (2) data collected using child questionnaires, from now on referred to as the "child report"; and (3) data collected using observations, from now on referred to as the "observation report". All statistical analyses were performed using SPSS, version 21.0 (IBM Corp., NY, USA).

In all data sets, outliers were checked and implausible recordings were recoded as missing. For children lost to follow-up, we performed additional analyses that compared their data with that of children for whom follow-up data was complete. T-tests and Pearson Chi-square tests were used for comparisons at baseline.

To evaluate the intervention's effectiveness, regression analyses were applied with a significance level of $p<0.05$. Multi-level analyses were not possible due to the low number of clusters (i.e. four schools) [62]. Only complete case analyses were performed, meaning we analysed data only from children whose data from both time points was complete. The dependent variable was defined as the SSB measurement after one year of intervention. This meant that for the "parent report" and "child report" the outcome measures were "daily SSB consumption (yes/no)" and "average SSB intake (in litres and number of servings)"; and for the "observation report" the outcome measure was "daily SSB intake (yes/no)". The condition (intervention/control) was entered as the independent variable. In all analyses, outcome measures were adjusted for baseline SSB values, several socio-demographic characteristics (grade, gender and ethnic background of the child and educational level of the caregiver) and child's weight status at baseline. This was done by also entering them as independent variables. For the "parent report", the caregiver's age and gender were added to the analyses as a potential confounder if these variables differed at baseline between the intervention and control group. No imputations were performed for these potential confounders given the relatively small number of missing data points (range $n=3$-35). Additionally, the analyses were corrected with the variable "school pair" to adjust for the matching of schools. We explored interaction effects of "condition" on the socio-demographic variables, child's weight status at baseline and school pair (p<0.10) [63].

12.3 RESULTS

In total, 1288 children were invited to participate in this study. At baseline, response was 54.8% among parents, 83.7% among children, and 90.8% for the observations. At follow-up, response was 61.5% among parents, 74.7% among children, and 76.9% for the observations.

We were able to conduct non-response analyses for the variables gender, grade and ethnic background of the child. Parents of children who participated in the study were more often parents of children in the lower grades (p<0.001) and of children with a Dutch ethnic background (p<0.001) as compared to parents lost to follow-up. Children who completed a questionnaire were more often children in the lower grades (p<0.001) and children with a Dutch ethnic background (p=0.007) as compared to children lost to follow-up. Children who were observed were more often children with a non-Dutch ethnic background (p<0.001) as compared to children lost to follow-up.

Non-response analyses were also conducted for the condition variable. Here we saw a difference between the intervention and control conditions in parents of children who participated in the study compared to parents lost to follow-up (p=0.006) and for children who underwent observation compared to children lost to follow-up (p=0.014).

As shown in the flowchart depicted in Figure 1, the population for analysis comprised of 356 children using the data from the "parent report" (34.9%); of 387 children using the data from the "child report" (69.4%); and of 959 children using the data from the "observation report" (74.5%). This meant that at least one complete case analysis could be performed for 1009 children (78.3%). In Additional file 1: Figure S1, a diagram is depicted to provide information on the combinations of responses between the three data reports.

12.3.1 BASELINE CHARACTERISTICS

Baseline measures of child and caregiver characteristics in both conditions are shown in Table 2. Children in the intervention condition were more often children in the higher grades ("observation report" $p<0.016$), more often children with a non-Dutch ethnic background ("parent report" $p=0.033$; "child report" $p=0.001$; "observation report" $p<0.001$), more often children of caregiver with lower educational levels ("child report" $p=0.001$; "observation report" $p<0.001$), and more often children of younger caregivers ("parent report" $p<0.001$) as compared to children in the control condition.

12.3.2 INTERVENTION EFFECTS

Table 3 describes child's SSB consumption at baseline, with only the "observation report" showing the frequency of SSB being brought to school to be significantly lower in the intervention group than in the control group ($p<0.001$).

Table 3 also shows the unadjusted and adjusted results of the regression analyses. Given the unadjusted and adjusted results are very similar, only the results based on the fully adjusted model are described. Based on the "parent report", no intervention effects were found for the outcome measure daily SSB consumption. Intervention effects were found on the outcome measure average SSB intake (SSB consumed in litres and number of SSB servings). Average SSB consumption in the intervention group was significantly lower than that in the control group (B -0.19 litres per day, 95% CI -0.28;-0.10, $p<0.001$). The decrease in the number of SSB servings was also significantly higher in the intervention group than in the control group (B -0.54 servings per day, 95% CI -0.82;-0.26, $p<0.001$). On the basis of the "child report" we found no significant intervention effects for any of the outcome measures ($p>0.05$ for daily SSB consumption and average SSB intake in litres or servings). On the basis of the "observation report", we found the increase in SSB brought to consume at school to be significantly smaller in the intervention group than in the control group (OR 0.51, 95% CI 0.36;0.72, p<0.001).

When we evaluated interactions between condition and socio-demographic characteristics, child's weight status at baseline or school pair, we found no significant results on the basis of the "parent report" or "child report" (p>0.10). However, on the basis of the "observation report", caregiver's educational level and school pair appeared to be significant as effect modifiers (p<0.10).

After conducting stratified analyses, we found no significant effect of the intervention for children of caregivers with a low educational level (high educational level OR 0.43, 95% CI 0.25;0.77, p=0.004; and unknown educational level OR 0.45, 95% CI 0.22;0.91, p=0.027).

The intervention effect was found only within one school pair (OR 0.37, 95% CI 0.22;0.64, p<0.001). Regarding the other school pair, children at the intervention school did not differ significantly from the children at the control school with respect to bringing SSB to school.

12.4 DISCUSSION

This study evaluated the "water campaign" programme. We found an effect on SSB on the basis of two of the three sources of information that were used to assess SSB consumption (i.e. "parent report" and "observation report").

Although the intervention had no effect on whether or not children consumed SSB on a daily basis, their average SSB consumption did change: after one year of intervention, on the basis of information gathered using the "parent report", both average SSB consumption and average SSB servings were lower for children in the intervention group than for children in the control group. On the basis of information gathered using the "child report", no significant differences in average SSB intake (in litres or servings) were found between children in the intervention and control group. An explanation for this discrepancy is lacking, but the lack of effect seen with the "child report" can most likely be attributed to the fact that children are still too young to properly estimate their behaviour. Children's inability to conceptualize—not only SSB but also the concepts of frequency and averaging—make it debatable whether these young children provide valid responses to food questionnaires that have items covering periods greater than one day [64]–[66]. In addition, research has shown that parents are more prone to reporting socially desirable answers compared to children [67]. This could also partly explain the fact that SSB consumption reported by children was higher than that reported by parents. On the basis of the "parent report", no differences in intervention effect were found between the younger children (grades 2 to 4) and the older children (grades 5 to 7) ($p > 0.05$, data not shown). The parent-reported SSB consumption is probably more reliable and is supported by similar findings in the observations.

After one year of intervention, the number of children bringing SSB to school was lower in the intervention condition than in the control condition. Although the observations did not measure total daily SSB consumption, merely what children brought along to school for break time, they were the most objective measure of SSB consumption in our study. Furthermore, what children bring along to school is most probably largely dependent on their parents' decisions.

The stratified analyses performed on the basis of the "observation report" demonstrated that intervention effects are limited to subgroups. Differences in intervention effect were found between the two school pairs. Replication of the study with more clusters is recommended to confirm or reject our findings. Also, the effect of the intervention differed according to caregiver's educational level in a manner that contradicted our expectations. Because the intervention schools are located in socially more deprived neighbourhoods, we expected to see an intervention effect among children of caregiver's who have lower levels of education. This contradictory finding could be due to some degree of response bias: we may have had higher responses from caregivers with a higher level of education. It could also be explained by the large group of caregivers with an 'unknown' educational level that we found in the "observation report".

A number of studies have been published on interventions that aimed to reduce SSB consumption by promoting water. These studies found similar but smaller intervention effects: for example, Tate et al. found a 80.7 ml decrease in SSB intake after a 6-month intervention and Sichieri et al. found a 55.0 ml SSB decrease after a one-year intervention [11],[13]. The study of Muckelbauer et al. found a significant increase in water consumption, but no effects on the consumption of juice or soft drinks were observed after adjustment for ethnic background and baseline intake [12]. Compared with these other studies the intervention effects in our study are thus encouraging.

Although the intervention was aimed at reducing the intake of children's SSB consumption by promoting the intake of water, water consumption was not an outcome measure of our study. Despite this, we did explore the average intake of water, measured in litres, as reported in the parent and child questionnaires. On the basis of the "parent report", there was a significant overall increase in water intake over time in both the intervention and control groups (respectively $p<0.001$ and $p=0.015$). However, on the basis of the "parent report" and the "child report" we found the intervention to have no effect on children's water consumption ($p>0.05$; see Additional file 1: Table S2). When we also explored whether the decrease in SSB consumption could be explained by an increase in water intake, we found that children with reduced SSB consumption did not differ in their water consumption at follow-up ($p>0.05$; data not shown). These findings correspond with those of Veitch et al. [68]. However, since the mechanisms underlying the decrease in SSB consumption still remain unclear, further research is required.

The fact that we found an effect on SSB consumption does not necessarily imply a decrease in total energy intake or weight gain. However, a number of studies have indicated that a reduction in SSB consumption can have beneficial effects on total energy intake and weight status/BMI. For instance, Daniels and Popkin demonstrated that replacing SSB with water reduced total energy intake, implying less weight gain which may well contribute to preventing overweight [9]. In addition, the study by De Ruyter et al. demonstrated that replacing SSB with sugar-free alternatives resulted in reduced weight gain [7]. We explored the effects of the intervention on child's BMI and weight status which are shown in Additional file 1: Table S3. Children in the intervention group had a significant higher increase of BMI compared to children in the control group (0.26BMI, 95% CI 0.11;0.40, $p=0.001$). According the effect size criteria by Cohen, this can be regarded as a negligible effect ($d=0.03$) [69].

The intervention in our study was a school- and community-targeted intervention, developed using social marketing. Our results suggest that a combined school and community approach may be beneficial for children to successfully develop healthier intake of drinks, supporting Bleich's et al. findings [35]. Furthermore, the use of social marketing meant that it was also possible to aim the intervention at a specific population (i.e. Turkish and Moroccan families) within a specific setting (i.e. socially more deprived neighbourhoods). However, when we explored whether such tailoring of the water campaign specifically to these minorities improved the effects seen among these children, we were unable to detect significant differences in intervention effect between children of Turkish and Moroccan background and children from other ethnic backgrounds ($p > 0.05$ in all three data sets; data not shown). However, the fact that the intervention had similar effects among all ethnic groups could be an indication that the reach and participation among this hard-to-reach target audience has improved, possibly due to the application of social marketing. We recommend that future studies should include a larger sample to increase the power for detecting behavioural changes within such a varied population.

12.4.1 STRENGTHS AND LIMITATIONS

The main strengths of this study are the setting and the duration (i.e. activities in daily practice at primary schools and in neighbourhoods for over a year). The study's pragmatic setting means that the effects can be generalized to similar settings. A further strength of this study is that we used observations as well as questionnaires to determine the children's SSB consumption.

A limitation of this study is the fact that randomization on the individual level was not possible. A further limitation is the small number of clusters (i.e. four), which inhibited multi-level analyses but was countered by adding the 'school pair' variable in the analyses. Since the use of self-report questionnaires to assess behavioural change is subject to limitations (e.g. misreporting of behaviour and providing socially desirable answers), we used different methods (i.e. observations and questionnaires) and assessed questionnaires from both parents and children. The non-response of parents to the parent questionnaire (complete case analyses only possible for 35%) is another limitation of this study. Our study included a diverse group of children with different ethnic backgrounds; between the three data reports the child's ethnic backgrounds differed in distribution. Although no intervention effect of ethnic background and intervention condition was found, the intervention effects should be interpreted and generalized with caution (especially our findings based on the "parent report"). We assessed SSB intake "on average a day" with the parent and child questionnaires and observed SSB consumption "on a random school day". Further research is recommended to gain insight into different patterns of the child's SSB consumption (e.g. on weekdays vs. weekend-days). It may be debatable whether some beverages should be in- or excluded from the definition "SSB". We recognize that some beverages may have additional nutritional benefits for children; however, we defined SSB in this study based on the amount of sugar within the beverages. A next step in altering the child's consumption intake could be to give attention to and differentiate even more between SSB's with and without nutritional value for the child's diet. Finally, the water campaign consists of several components that promote water consumption. However, when applying such a multicomponent intervention, it remains unclear which intervention activities are essential for obtaining the observed effects. We were unable to gather detailed implementation information as it was impossible to register the delivery of components at an individual level. Further research is therefore needed to understand the pathways of the behaviour changes that seem to have occurred.

12.5 CONCLUSIONS

The findings of this study support the effectiveness of the water campaign in reducing the consumption of SSB, adding to evidence from other studies. Further studies are required to replicate the findings and to elucidate the possible mechanism underlying this intervention effect, the impact on BMI and the effectiveness in different subgroups. We also suggest that the water campaign be evaluated in other settings, using larger samples and with longer follow-up.

In the meantime, we recommend that schools and communities be aware of water as thirst-quencher, and as an alternative for SSB.

REFERENCES

1. Ludwig DS, Peterson KE, Gortmaker SL: Relation between consumption of sugar-sweetened drinks and childhood obesity: a prospective, observational analysis. Lancet 2001, 357:505-508.
2. Mrdjenovic G, Levitsky DA: Nutritional and energetic consequences of sweetened drink consumption in 6- to 13-year-old children. J Pediatr 2003, 142:604-610.
3. Vartanian LR, Schwartz MB, Brownell KD: Effects of soft drink consumption on nutrition and health: a systematic review and meta-analysis. Am J Public Health 2007, 97:667-675.
4. Malik VS, Willett WC, Hu FB: Sugar-sweetened beverages and BMI in children and adolescents: reanalyses of a meta-analysis. Am J Clin Nutr 2009, 89:438-439. author reply 439-440
5. Deboer MD, Scharf RJ, Demmer RT: Sugar-sweetened beverages and weight gain in 2- to 5-year-old children. Pediatrics 2013, 132:413-420.
6. Hu FB: Resolved: there is sufficient scientific evidence that decreasing sugar-sweetened beverage consumption will reduce the prevalence of obesity and obesity-related diseases. Obes Rev 2013, 14:606-619.
7. de Ruyter JC, Olthof MR, Seidell JC, Katan MB: A trial of sugar-free or sugar-sweetened beverages and body weight in children. N Engl J Med 2012, 367:1397-1406.
8. Ebbeling CB, Feldman HA, Chomitz VR, Antonelli TA, Gortmaker SL, Osganian SK, Ludwig DS: A randomized trial of sugar-sweetened beverages and adolescent body weight. N Engl J Med 2012, 367:1407-1416.
9. Daniels MC, Popkin BM: Impact of water intake on energy intake and weight status: a systematic review. Nutr Rev 2010, 68:505-521.
10. Pan A, Malik VS, Schulze MB, Manson JE, Willett WC, Hu FB: Plain-water intake and risk of type 2 diabetes in young and middle-aged women. Am J Clin Nutr 2012, 95:1454-1460.
11. Tate DF, Turner-McGrievy G, Lyons E, Stevens J, Erickson K, Polzien K, Diamond M, Wang X, Popkin B: Replacing caloric beverages with water or diet beverages for weight loss in adults: main results of the Choose Healthy Options Consciously Everyday (CHOICE) randomized clinical trial. Am J Clin Nutr 2012, 95:555-563.
12. Muckelbauer R, Libuda L, Clausen K, Toschke AM, Reinehr T, Kersting M: Promotion and provision of drinking water in schools for overweight prevention: randomized, controlled cluster trial. Pediatrics 2009, 123:e661-e667.
13. Sichieri R, Paula Trotte A, de Souza RA, Veiga GV: School randomised trial on prevention of excessive weight gain by discouraging students from drinking sodas. Public Health Nutr 2009, 12:197-202.
14. Olds T, Maher C, Zumin S, Peneau S, Lioret S, Castetbon K, Bellisle de Wilde J, Hohepa M, Maddison R, Lissner L, Sjöberg A, Zimmermann M, Aeberli L, Ogden C, Flegal K, Summerbell C: Evidence that the prevalence of childhood overweight is plateauing: data from nine countries. Int J Pediatr Obes 2011, 6:342-360.
15. Schonbeck Y, Talma H, van Dommelen P, Bakker B, Buitendijk SE, Hirasing RA, van Buuren S: Increase in prevalence of overweight in Dutch children and adoles-

cents: a comparison of nationwide growth studies in 1980, 1997 and 2009. PLoS ONE [Electronic Resource] 2011, 6:e27608.
16. Wabitsch M, Moss A, Kromeyer-Hauschild K: Unexpected plateauing of childhood obesity rates in developed countries. BMC Med 2014, 12:17.
17. Roseman MG, Riddell MC, Haynes JN: A content analysis of kindergarten-12th grade school-based nutrition interventions: taking advantage of past learning. J Nutr Educ Behav 2011, 43:2-18.
18. Romon M, Lommez A, Tafflet M, Basdevant A, Oppert JM, Bresson JL, Ducimetiere P, Charles MA, Borys JM: Downward trends in the prevalence of childhood overweight in the setting of 12-year school- and community-based programmes. Public Health Nutr 2009, 12:1735-1742.
19. Gonzalez-Suarez C, Worley A, Grimmer-Somers K, Dones V: School-based interventions on childhood obesity: a meta-analysis. Am J Prev Med 2009, 37:418-427.
20. Singh AS, Chin APMJ, Brug J, van Mechelen W: Dutch obesity intervention in teenagers: effectiveness of a school-based program on body composition and behavior. Arch Pediatr Adolesc Med 2009, 163:309-317.
21. Katz DL, O'Connell M, Njike VY, Yeh MC, Nawaz H: Strategies for the prevention and control of obesity in the school setting: systematic review and meta-analysis. Int J Obes 2008, 32:1780-1789.
22. Kropski JA, Keckley PH, Jensen GL: School-based obesity prevention programs: an evidence-based review. Obesity (Silver Spring) 2008, 16:1009-1018.
23. James J, Thomas P, Kerr D: Preventing childhood obesity: two year follow-up results from the Christchurch obesity prevention programme in schools (CHOPPS). BMJ 2007, 335:762.
24. Warren JM, Henry CJ, Lightowler HJ, Bradshaw SM, Perwaiz S: Evaluation of a pilot school programme aimed at the prevention of obesity in children. Health Promot Int 2003, 18:287-296.
25. Johnston CA, Moreno JP, El-Mubasher A, Gallagher M, Tyler C, Woehler D: Impact of a school-based pediatric obesity prevention program facilitated by health professionals. J Sch Health 2013, 83:171-181.
26. Story M, Kaphingst KM, French S: The role of schools in obesity prevention. Future Child 2006, 16:109-142.
27. Sleddens EF, Gerards SM, Thijs C, de Vries NK, Kremers SP: General parenting, childhood overweight and obesity-inducing behaviors: a review. Int J Pediatr Obes 2011, 6:e12-e27.
28. West F, Sanders MR, Cleghorn GJ, Davies PS: Randomised clinical trial of a family-based lifestyle intervention for childhood obesity involving parents as the exclusive agents of change. Behav Res Ther 2010, 48:1170-1179.
29. Golley RK, Hendrie GA, Slater A, Corsini N: Interventions that involve parents to improve children's weight-related nutrition intake and activity patterns - what nutrition and activity targets and behaviour change techniques are associated with intervention effectiveness? Obes Rev 2011, 12:114-130.
30. Hebden L, Hector D, Hardy LL, King L: A fizzy environment: availability and consumption of sugar-sweetened beverages among school students. Prev Med 2013, 56:416-418.

31. Ferreira I, van der Horst K, Wendel-Vos W, Kremers S, van Lenthe FJ, Brug J: Environmental correlates of physical activity in youth - a review and update. Obes Rev 2007, 8:129-154.
32. Swinburn B, Egger G, Raza F: Dissecting obesogenic environments: the development and application of a framework for identifying and prioritizing environmental interventions for obesity. Prev Med 1999, 29:563-570.
33. Kremers SP, de Bruijn GJ, Visscher TL, van Mechelen W, de Vries NK, Brug J: Environmental influences on energy balance-related behaviors: a dual-process view. Int J Behav Nutr Phys Act 2006, 3:9.
34. Brug J, van Lenthe FJ, Kremers SP: Revisiting Kurt Lewin: how to gain insight into environmental correlates of obesogenic behaviors. Am J Prev Med 2006, 31:525-529.
35. Bleich SN, Segal J, Wu Y, Wilson R, Wang Y: Systematic review of community-based childhood obesity prevention studies. Pediatrics 2013, 132:e201-e210.
36. Mathews LB, Moodie MM, Simmons AM, Swinburn BA: The process evaluation of It's Your Move!, an Australian adolescent community-based obesity prevention project. BMC Public Health 2010, 10:448.
37. Barlow SE, Expert C: Expert committee recommendations regarding the prevention, assessment, and treatment of child and adolescent overweight and obesity: summary report. Pediatrics 2007, 120(Suppl 4):S164-S192.
38. National Collaborating Centre for Primary Care. Obesity: The Prevention, Identification, Assessment and Management of Overweight and Obesity in Adults and Children. National Institute for Health and Clinical Excellence, London; 2006.
39. Robertson W, Friede T, Blissett J, Rudolf MC, Wallis M, Stewart-Brown S: Pilot of "Families for Health": community-based family intervention for obesity. Arch Dis Child 2008, 93:921-926.
40. Birch LL, Ventura AK: Preventing childhood obesity: what works? Int J Obes 2009, 33(Suppl 1):S74-S81.
41. EPODE European Network [http://www.epode-european-network.com]
42. "Youth on Healthy Weight" (Jongeren Op Gezond Gewicht) [http://www.jogg.nl/]
43. French JB-SC, McVey D, Merritt R: Social Marketing and Public Health – Theory and Practice. Oxford University Press, Oxford; 2010.
44. Evans WD, Christoffel KK, Necheles JW, Becker AB: Social marketing as a childhood obesity prevention strategy. Obesity (Silver Spring) 2010, 18(Suppl 1):S23-S26.
45. Evans WD: How social marketing works in health care. BMJ 2006, 332:1207-1210.
46. Gracia-Marco L, Vicente-Rodriguez G, Borys JM, Le Bodo Y, Pettigrew S, Moreno LA: Contribution of social marketing strategies to community-based obesity prevention programmes in children. Int J Obes 2011, 35:472-479.
47. Rayner M: Social marketing: how might this contribute to tackling obesity? Obes Rev 2007, 8(Suppl 1):195-199.
48. Evans WD, Necheles J, Longjohn M, Christoffel KK: The 5-4-3-2-1 go! Intervention: social marketing strategies for nutrition. J Nutr Educ Behav 2007, 39:S55-S59.
49. Huhman ME, Potter LD, Nolin MJ, Piesse A, Judkins DR, Banspach SW, Wong FL: The Influence of the VERB campaign on children's physical activity in 2002 to 2006. Am J Public Health 2010, 100:638-645.

50. Wong FL, Greenwell M, Gates S, Berkowitz JM: It's what you do! Reflections on the VERB campaign. Am J Prev Med 2008, 34:S175-S182.
51. Government HM: Change 4 Life - One Year On. HM Government, London; 2010.
52. Krul C, Blanchette L, Jansen W, Meima B: "City of Rotterdam: Scoping Enjoy Being Fit Family Approach" (Scoping Rapport: Gezinsaanpak Lekker Fit!). City of Rotterdam, Department of Sport and Culture, Rotterdam; 2012.
53. Fredriks AM, Van Buuren S, Sing RA, Wit JM, Verloove-Vanhorick SP: Alarming prevalences of overweight and obesity for children of Turkish, Moroccan and Dutch origin in The Netherlands according to international standards. Acta Paediatr 2005, 94:496-498.
54. Rotterdam-Rijnmond MHS: "Youth Rijnmond 2011" (GGD Rotterdam: Jeugd Rijnmond in Beeld 2011, Gemeenterapport Rotterdam). In Book "Youth Rijnmond 2011" (GGD Rotterdam: Jeugd Rijnmond in Beeld 2011, Gemeenterapport Rotterdam) (Editor ed.^eds.). City, Department of Youth and Education, Municipal Health Service Rotterdam-Rijnmond; 2012.
55. Bartholomew LK, Parcel GS, Kok G: Intervention mapping: a process for developing theory- and evidence-based health education programs. Health Educ Behav 1998, 25:545-563.
56. Jansen W, Raat H, Zwanenburg EJ, Reuvers I, van Walsem R, Brug J: A school-based intervention to reduce overweight and inactivity in children aged 6-12 years: study design of a randomized controlled trial. BMC Public Health 2008, 8:257.
57. Jansen W, Borsboom G, Meima A, Zwanenburg EJ, Mackenbach JP, Raat H, Brug J: Effectiveness of a primary school-based intervention to reduce overweight. Int J Pediatr Obes 2011, 6:e70-e77.
58. Swertz O, Duimelaar P, Thijssen J: Statistics Netherlands. Migrants in the Netherlands 2004. In Book Statistics Netherlands. Migrants in the Netherlands 2004. (Editor ed.^eds.). City, Statistics Netherlands; 2004.
59. Netherlands S: Dutch Standard Classification of Education 2003. In Book Dutch Standard Classification of Education 2003 (Editor ed.^eds.). City, Statistics Netherlands; 2004.
60. Bulk-Bunschoten AMW, Renders CM, Leerdam FJM, Hirasing RA: Protocol for detection of overweight in preventive youth health care. [Signaleringsprotocol overgewicht in de jeugdgezondheidszorg]. In Book Protocol For Detection Of Overweight In Preventive Youth Health Care. [Signaleringsprotocol overgewicht in de jeugdgezondheidszorg] (Editor ed.^eds.). City, VUMC; 2004.
61. Cole TJ, Bellizzi MC, Flegal KM, Dietz WH: Establishing a standard definition for child overweight and obesity worldwide: international survey. BMJ 2000, 320:1240-1243.
62. Campbell MK, Piaggio G, Elbourne DR, Altman DG, Group C: Consort 2010 statement: extension to cluster randomised trials. BMJ 2012, 345:e5661.
63. Sun X, Briel M, Walter SD, Guyatt GH: Is a subgroup effect believable? Updating criteria to evaluate the credibility of subgroup analyses. BMJ 2010, 340:c117.
64. Smith AF, Baxter SD, Hardin JW, Guinn CH, Royer JA: Relation of Children's Dietary reporting accuracy to cognitive ability. Am J Epidemiol 2011, 173:103-109.

65. McPherson RS, Hoelscher DM, Alexander M, Scanlon KS, Serdula MK: Dietary assessment methods among school-aged children: Validity and reliability. Prev Med 2000, 31:S11-S33.
66. Livingstone MB, Robson PJ: Measurement of dietary intake in children. Proc Nutr Soc 2000, 59:279-293.
67. Bornhorst C, Huybrechts I, Ahrens W, Eiben G, Michels N, Pala V, Molnar D, Russo P, Barba G, Bel-Serrat S, Moreno LA, Papoutsou S, Veidebaum T, Loit HM, Lissner L, Pigeot I: Prevalence and determinants of misreporting among European children in proxy-reported 24 h dietary recalls. Br J Nutr 2013, 109:1257-1265.
68. Veitch J, Singh A, van Stralen MM, van Mechelen W, Brug J, Chinapaw MJ: Reduction in sugar-sweetened beverages is not associated with more water or diet drinks. Public Health Nutr 2011, 14:1388-1393.
69. Cohen J: Statistical power analysis for the behavioural sciences. Academic, New York; 1977.

There are two tables and several supplemental files that are not available in this version of the article. To view this additional information, please use the citation on the first page of this chapter.

CHAPTER 13

LISTENING TO THE EXPERTS: IS THERE A PLACE FOR FOOD TAXATION IN THE FIGHT AGAINST OBESITY IN EARLY CHILDHOOD?

ERIN PITT, ELIZABETH KENDALL, ANDREW P. HILLS AND TRACY COMANS

13.1 BACKGROUND

The incidence and prevalence of overweight and obesity has been escalating around the world over the past few decades, including in the early childhood years [1]–[3]. The most recent data from the 2011–2012 Australian Health Survey indicates that 25.1% of children aged 2 to 17 years were overweight or obese, including 18.2% overweight and 6.9% obese based on Body Mass Index (BMI) [4]. Although some recent literature suggests childhood obesity may be starting to plateau in parts of Australia [5],[6], the condition continues to be a global public health priority [7] and there is consensus regarding an urgent need for government to take rapid action [8].

Listening to the Experts: Is There a Place for Food Taxation in the Fight Against Obesity In Early Childhood?. © *Pitt E, Kendall E, Hills AP, and Comans T.* BMC Obesity **1***,15 (2014);* doi:10.1186/ s40608-014-0015-3. *Licensed under Creative Commons Attribution 4.0 International License, http:// creativecommons.org/licenses/by/4.0/.*

Eating habits are established early in life and many dietary behaviours are maintained during the growing years and throughout adulthood [9]–[11]. Hence obesity and poor eating behaviours in childhood are potential risk factors for adult overweight and obesity [12]. It is therefore of utmost importance to direct obesity interventions towards the very early years of life [1],[13].

Many researchers in public health have attributed the increase in obesity rates to an increasingly obesogenic environment [14],[15]. If we agree that the environment, including the food environment, has a major impact on childhood obesity, there are several potential policy levers available to influence food choices; some of which include price, availability and marketing. Taxation has been suggested and investigated as a strategy to influence price and therefore modify food purchasing behaviour [16] and subsequent consumption, and is a growing area of interest in the prevention of obesity [17],[18]. The interest in taxation to combat obesity is warranted given other public health successes such as the reduction of tobacco and alcohol consumption [19],[20].

Various countries have implemented food taxation on certain groups of foods including soft drinks, snack foods and fat [21]. While it has been demonstrated that price increases on food negatively affect consumption [22], evidence on the real world effectiveness of taxation to reduce obesity rates is limited and the feasibility of taxing some food groups is unclear, particularly in the light of strong industry opposition and repeals of taxes that have occurred in the United States and Denmark [20],[23].

In the presence of insufficient, inadequate or conflicting evidence, it is useful to turn to expert opinion for clarity. Obtaining expert opinion through methods of consensus also derives first-hand accounts from researchers and clinicians, enabling decisions that capitalise on their experience and expertise [24],[25]. Consensus methods are useful in determining research priorities through the generation of priority qualitative information that is both relevant and reliable [26]. Consensus building methods can address individual discrepancies and reach shared or collective agreement about a way forward but still retain the diversity of different perspectives [27].

This paper describes a consensus-based investigation of Australian experts aimed at identifying foods that are most problematic in terms of consumption during early childhood and those that might also be amenable to taxation as a strategy to reduce consumption. Our research addresses a gap in the literature around the understanding of the relative importance of particular food groups to obesity development in early childhood and the responsiveness of these foods to taxation from the unique perspective of academics, researchers, clinicians and policy makers. This paper also reports on the use of a systematic consensus-building method—the nominal group technique—as a tool for identifying priority foods with the potential to respond to taxation.

13.2 METHODS

We applied the nominal group technique [28] which enables a selected group of participants to generate and share ideas, undertake discussion to clarify those ideas and then rank ideas to identify the top priorities for all group members [29]. This process permits effective group decision-making and builds consensus by allowing contentious issues to be addressed collectively. It enables the simplification of complex areas and establishment of priorities at the same time as fostering in-depth discussion of issues surrounding the topic [28],[30].

13.2.1 PARTICIPANTS

A list of potential expert panel members was constructed by Chief Investigators and team members and was achieved using a combination of methods. Prominent publications and literature were reviewed as identified through literature searches relating to childhood obesity, nutrition, taxation and public policy in the Australian context. Snowballing and purposive sampling was also used to ensure inclusion of key organizations (e.g. Food Standards Australian and New Zealand (FSANZ)) as well as government public health departments and universities. Criteria for inclusion as a member of the panel included holding a position in Australia as a researcher, teaching academic or clinician with significant experience, contribution and public presence in a combination of areas of areas including nutrition, public policy and childhood obesity. Experience and contribution was deemed significant based on a track record of international journal publications, speaker invitations or involvement in relevant professional organisations.

Participants were purposively sampled to ensure that the final mix of invited experts represented both clinical and research fields. Fifteen experts were invited to attend, with three people unable to participate. The final panel was comprised of twelve Australian experts, including five clinicians, two researchers and five people with dual roles in both research and academia. Ethics approval for this research was obtained through the Griffith University Human Research Ethics Committee (HREC—MED/32/12/HREC). Written informed consent to participate was obtained from all members of the panel.

13.2.2 PROCEDURE

Experts were provided with pre-reading material during the week prior to the panel discussion. The material summarised the epidemiology of childhood obesity, trends in expenditure, consumption and commercial sales of key categories of foods; particularly beverages (e.g. sugar-sweetened and artificially sweetened) and unhealthy foods (e.g. take-away foods, snacks and confectionary). No interpretation or discussion of the facts was provided.

The expert panel was a closed event held at a hotel near to Brisbane airport to accommodate travel arrangements of inter-state panel members. The panel convened for 3.5 hours which commenced with a welcome and introduction session followed by a presentation of background information, a summary of the evidence and an outline of the purpose of the meeting. Four members of the research team were present to record and manage the process. The panel discussion was facilitated and all sessions were audio recorded with written consent of participants.

The first stage of the nominal group technique required panel members to individually identify key foods that they considered to be the strongest contributors to obesity in early childhood. Panel members then individually presented their top idea to the larger group. Members each presented a single idea without significant discussion. The technique requires participants to present only one idea and not to engage in discussion about each idea until later. However in reality it is necessary to accommodate the flow of the discussion, subsequently minor discussion was allowed and other relevant ideas of importance that were nominated out of sequence were recorded. Each idea was written on large format paper and placed around the room for later clarification. The clarification process involved group discussion about the nature of the idea, the overlap amongst ideas and any definitions that needed to be refined.

Once all the ideas were exhausted and clarified they remained on display around the room for panel members to view. Panel members were then asked to vote for their top priorities. Members were each given five stickers numbered one to five which they were asked to place alongside their top priorities (i.e. the foods that they believed would most impact on obesity if consumption was reduced), with five representing the most important idea (i.e. the most points). Multiple points could be allocated to a single idea if desired.

Votes given to each idea were totalled to identify the ideas that were considered most important to the entire group. The top priorities were then described in more detail and subjected to a group discussion about how influential and feasible implementation of taxation would be in relation to the identified food items. The discussion focused on price elasticity for each of the top priorities (i.e. how much would consumption of this food item change if price increased), substitution (i.e. is there a close substitute that may be more or less healthy) and practicality (i.e. what would be the barriers to, or facilitators of, taxation).

13.2.3 DATA ANALYSIS

The panel discussion was transcribed verbatim and stored in NVivo 10.0. Identification of key themes from transcripts was undertaken with qualitative analysis software by one author (E.P.). Coding of themes was validated through cross checking by a second author (T.C.) with additional discussion to resolve discrepancies.

TABLE 1: Key foods and other relevant issues/factors contributing to obesity in 0 to 5 year old children

Number of votes[a]	Identified key foods, issues and factors
Total: 66 votes	Sweetened drinks
Soft drinks: 25 votes	• Soft drinks (carbonated beverages)
Sweet drinks: 41 votes	• Cordials
	• Other sugar-sweetened beverages
	• High fat and sweetened flavoured milks
	• Fruit juice, fruit drinks and vitamin waters
Total: 32 votes	Portion-packed snacks and portion sizes
Portion-packed snacks: 16 votes	• Tiny Teddies
	• Individually wrapped packs
Portion sizes: 9	• Sweet and savoury snacks such as cake bars, chocolates and muffins
Chips: 7 votes	• Packets of chips
26 Votes	Increase consumption of fruit, vegetables, legumes, whole grain cereals and milk, yoghurt and cheese
	• Remove tax deduction on advertising and subsidizing freight or removing tax on freight of healthy foods
	• Tax particular foods in order to subsidize fruit and vegetables
	• Position fruit and vegetables as healthy alternatives through use of subsidies to increase equity of access
Total: 20 votes	Fast foods
Fast food: 13 votes	• Well known icons such as McDonald's Hungry Jack's, Red Rooster and Subway etc.
'Red foods': 7 votes	• Drive through, up-sizing and 24 hour operation
	• Serving size
	• Advertising
	• Energy fat, sugar and sodium content
	• Provision of 'meals'
15 votes	Infant formula
	• High protein infant formula products
	• Follow on formula for toddlers
13 votes	Processed meats and meat alternatives
	• Chicken nuggets and sausages
	• High fat and sodium content

a12 experts had a total of 15 votes each to allocate. The total votes should add to 180, thus there are 8 votes that cannot be accounted for.

13.3 RESULTS

13.3.1 IDENTIFYING AND PRIORITISING KEY FOODS

"What is it that causes obesity? Well, any drink, which contains calories, any food, which contains calories."

Through the Nominal Group Technique, a number of problem foods and other important factors associated with childhood obesity were identified. The outcome of voting can be seen in Table 1. The first column contains the number of votes allocated to each category of food, with larger votes indicating higher priority based on the perceived importance to childhood obesity.

The voting process revealed a clear consensus among the experts that the most problematic food group was sweetened beverages. The experts agreed that reducing consumption of sugar-sweetened drinks would impact most significantly on childhood obesity. Although achieving less than half the votes allocated to sugar-sweetened drinks, portion-packed snacks and take-away foods were also considered problematic for childhood obesity. Of slightly lower importance were high protein infant formula products and processed meats. Experts believed that an important strategy was to increase consumption of fresh foods with high nutrient content.

13.3.2 DETERMINING THE ABILITY TO INFLUENCE CONSUMPTION

Following the initial voting, panel members discussed the amenability of each food group to influences on consumption such as taxation. In discussing the potential influence of taxation, panel members considered the extent to which price influenced consumption. Additionally, the panel unanimously agreed that food taxation efforts should also consider means to increase the consumption of healthy foods consistent with the Australian Dietary Guidelines and The Australian Guide to Healthy Eating. Particularly through means such as subsidies, increasing consumption of healthy foods was viewed by the panel as a potentially acceptable strategy to society that would enable equity regardless of financial means and might facilitate a greater level of impact in reducing consumption of problem foods in early childhood.

The notion of product substitution was also raised by the panel when contemplating how food consumption is influenced by price (i.e. the extent to which a particular product would be replaced by another product of either greater or lower health value). The panel noted that increasing the price of some food and beverage items through taxation could successfully reduce consumption, but in many cases they identified alternative products that could potentially be less healthy.

The panel agreed that sugar-sweetened drinks could be amenable to taxation as most drinks represented relatively distinct products that could be easily defined; however, they noted some complexity in relation to the impact of taxation. They provided examples of the way in which the beverage industry actively promoted product substitution in response to price fluctuations. For example, as 100% fruit juice increased in price, beverage companies began marketing substantially cheaper sweetened fruit drinks with lower percentages of juice content.

> *"...substitution has been shown in juices and juice drinks so that juice drinks have had increases in sales...and some of the juice drinks that have 25-50% juice have gone up [in price] and the pure fruit juices haven't so the people have been substituting those because they are a lot cheaper..."*

They also noted that taxation on sugar-sweetened drinks may have no effect on product substitution depending on the nature of the product or brand. Some expensive brands of soft drink, for instance, are so popular that preferences may not be substantially altered by price increases. Aside from product substitution, another perspective provided by a panel member raised the notion that consumers should either be having less of unhealthy foods or having nothing, instead of substituting:

> *"...we talk about...substituting food, when ultimately, from my perspective, another message is actually having less. It seems to*

be lost in this whole thing about what should we be having instead of something, well, the answer is nothing."

The panel discussed the role of high protein infant formula in contributing to obesity. They mentioned this particular group of products is usually of lower quality and is an unnecessary product for young children in the general population above the age of 12 months, who can gain all nutritional requirements from a regular adult diet. Thus the panel felt this distinct group of products would be amenable to taxation to reduce consumption. Panel members mentioned the potentially regressive nature of tax on this particular product however this was not discussed in detail, nor were comment made on the influence of taxation for lower income groups.

TABLE 2: Final consensus

1.	Prepared foods consumed outside the home
2.	High protein infant formula products
3.	Sugar-sweetened drinks
4.	Subsidizing fresh fruit and vegetables; whole and unprocessed foods

13.3.3 CONSENSUS OUTCOMES

Final voting resulted in consensus on four dominant foods and concepts. Consensus outcomes can be seen in Table 2. Sugar-sweetened drinks and low quality infant and toddler formula products were identified as reasonable and practical to apply taxation. In addition to this, the panel unanimously felt subsidizing healthy foods was of utmost importance. In terms of prepared foods consumed outside the home and other food groups discussed, panel members agreed that they would not be amenable to taxation; not because they were insensitive to price fluctuations, but because the application of taxation was complicated by a number of fundamental issues. These complications included (1) problems associated with definitions, (2) lack of consensus about the evidence supporting a focus on these foods, (3) significant complexity around the energy or nutrient density of these foods and how this content would be taxed, (4) the power of specific companies and the food industry, (5) equity issues associated with food security for those on low incomes, and (6) the increasing presence of unhealthy foods in society.

A member of the panel provided a different perspective on food taxation complexities by saying:

"People get this analogy with smoking but it is not like smoking. There is no benefit at all in smoking, just pure danger, but with food, it's not like that. It's a gradient so therefore what do you tax?"

13.3.4 ISSUES AND BARRIERS ASSOCIATED WITH TAXATION

13.3.4.1 FOOD CATEGORY AND PRODUCT DEFINITIONS

The expert panel frequently discussed problems with definitions of certain food products when considering taxation. For example, what constitutes a snack or treat? How do we define fast food? It was thus identified that the ambiguity regarding definitions associated with particular food categories makes it difficult to conceptualise how a strategy such as taxation might be effective in reducing unhealthy food consumption. In relation to "fast food", panel members discussed iconic fast food chains as most representative of typical fast food. On the other hand, they were unsure whether purchasing a salad-laden burger from a hamburger shop or franchises selling healthier options would still be considered as fast food. Discussion was held around whether foods and beverages should be defined based on attributes such as their nutrient content or portion size.

In terms of portion sizes of food items, a major concern is the relationship between energy density and nutrient value. Thus in relation to childhood food intake, not only does the type of food need to be considered but also the serving size provided. The panel discussed the importance of identifying where the bulk of the energy intake is coming from in the 0–5 years age group. It was highlighted that sweet snacks is what partly drives the energy density increase in young children. Overall, energy-dense and

Listening to the Experts: Is There a Place for Food Taxation 245

nutrient-poor foods provide a substantial portion of children's energy intake. This raised the notion of how taxation could be considered using energy density as a potential criterion, yet no easy solutions were conceivable.

> *"...the little cake bars that come portion packed and are easy to buy as a snack. They are incredibly difficult to define so to actually write some sort of regulation to tax them as a group would be nigh on impossible..."*

Food category and product definitions were deemed to be very complex topic and the panel found it very difficult to define majority of food and drink items for the purposes of taxation. The only exception to this was sugar-sweetened drinks which were seen as potentially easier to target in terms of definition and that the public generally understand they are not a healthy choice of beverage. Furthermore, it was deemed easier to separate out soft drinks from other sugar-sweetened beverages as it is a defined product and usually marketed separately.

Apart from the challenge associated with defining various foods and beverages, the panel raised the concept of labelling foods as either 'good' or 'bad'. Some members of the panel considered it problematic to refer to foods in this manner. For example, they felt it could potentially contribute to stigma, discrimination and social alienation for people consuming such food items:

> *"...you're bad for eating that food..."*

In addition to this, the panel mentioned that the public often change their reporting of food consumption, particularly under-reporting their usual intake when responding to national or state nutrition surveys; again, potentially as a result of perceptions associated with consuming less healthy food options or "bad" foods.

13.3.4.2 EVIDENCE

The availability of scientific evidence regarding food and health was considered of utmost importance during the panel's discussions, particularly when contemplating and proposing foods that may be potentially amenable to taxation. The panel felt all discussion should be defensible and based on evidence. It was mentioned that soft drink consumption had received considerable attention in the recent past with an increasing evidence base for the potential impact of high consumption levels on health. However, evidence is not always conclusive regarding all sugar-sweetened beverage consumption and there is insufficient evidence for other food and beverage items. In a response to a lack of evidence between some foods and health, panel members noted there is a need to continually contribute to the evidence base through best practice and novel solutions to address the complexities of obesity in the early childhood years. The panel highlighted the importance of looking at consumption data and agreed this could help inform the evidence base for areas that currently do not have strong evidence.

> *"...I think there needs to be some action...perhaps before the conclusive evidence is there..."*

13.3.4.3 VESTED INTERESTS OF INDUSTRY PLAYERS

The panel raised the role of food companies and industry more broadly as a potential barrier to facilitation of population level policy change and regulation of unhealthy foods. For example, there was particular discussion around food companies paying exorbitant fees for shelf space in supermarkets to promote their products:

> *"Companies already pay for particular shelf space or pay for particular shelves and they're more than willing to do it...It works beautifully. ...the shelf that's most expensive is for the small child sitting in the shopping trolley..."*

The concept of industry 'loopholes' and 'tactics' was identified in relation to companies readily changing product ingredients to meet changing food standards and requirements, thereby demonstrating efficiency in their ability to constantly adjust and adapt. Taking action to reduce unhealthy food consumption essentially means taking on some of the largest companies in the world. The panel discussed the extremely influential role of the food industry and their ability to influence eating practices of some members of society. A more appropriate balance is needed between the business imperative of industry and social responsibility, including a stronger engagement with the industry sector to effect population level policy. This is particularly challenging in the context of potential changes to taxation.

13.3.4.4 EQUITY ISSUES

Members of the panel expressed concern about ensuring equity for all Australians, particularly disadvantaged populations, when considering taxation initiatives. Some panel members conveyed it would be more important for the health of disadvantaged people to subsidize healthy foods rather than increase the tax on less valuable foods:

> *"Poor people are the ones who are obese and we're going to tax them more. It seems very inequitable unless you then reduce the price of fruit and veg..."*

13.3.4.5 THE INCREASING PRESENCE OF UNHEALTHY FOOD IN SOCIETY

The panel discussed that serving sizes or portion sizes have been changing over time and are generally becoming much larger. This demonstrates that the perception of what is 'normal' in society has been re-defined over time and has had a profound effect on food intake and how we think about food. Members of the panel expressed comments such as:

> *"We have redefined treats as something you have any time you want but that's not the right definition and at the same time this redefines what is normal."*

Although it is feasible to investigate taxation as a means to reduce unhealthy food consumption in the early childhood years, a notion that was frequently raised during the panel discussions was the importance of promoting nutrient rich food choices for children as opposed to simply thinking about how to steer children away from foods that are detrimental to their health. The panel considered that taxation of unhealthy foods and promotion of nutrient rich food sources in combination could potentially help influence perceptions as well as social and cultural norms regarding the presence and availability of less healthy food options.

13.4 DISCUSSION

Panel discussion resulted in a positive consensus regarding taxation of sugar-sweetened beverages. However, the overall task of identifying foods potentially amenable to taxation was evidently not an easy decision for the experts, particularly given the contribution of discussion to a significant number of barriers and issues, which subsequently played a central part in reaching consensus. Barriers such as lack of definitions for food items, portion sizes and the nutrient density of foods were deemed to hinder support for taxation methods to reduce unhealthy food consumption in the early childhood years. The effective conceptualisation of taxation is a barrier in itself [21]. This and a number of other barriers such as the role of food industry are corroborated with previous research outcomes [31]. Moreover, subsidizing fresh foods was a dominant theme in the expert panel discussions and ultimately became one of the key outcomes of consensus. Previous research however, is inconsistent regarding the effectiveness of subsidies in reducing obesity rates [21],[32].

The discussion about positively impacting population health through implementation of taxation was very insightful. The expert panel contributed a range of diverse individual opinions, allowing insight to those who were supportive or against the idea of implementing food taxation. Moreover, panel members were careful in their rigorous discussion around making the assumption that introduction of food taxation would causally result in change in consumption, however there is evidence to suggest that this might be so [21].

Panel discussion highlighted that taxation should be considered in relation to overall health, rather than taxing food solely to address the obesity crisis. A panel member went on to elaborate that there is an interest in food for many reasons other than the link to obesity and that many of the topics discussed by the panel will have an impact on disease outcomes in general. In addition to this, the panel thought it would be best to make broad consensus statements to highlight multiple health benefits to consumers in general, rather than specifically for young children and also highlight taxation as a package of complementary measures to make it even more effective. Thus there was unanimous agreement and acknowledgement that taxation should not occur in isolation to a suite of other strategies [33].

This research concentrates on dietary elements, specifically consumption of unhealthy or 'non-core' foods in contributing to early childhood obesity. The breadth of discussion on early childhood dietary intake continues to highlight and support the complexity of early childhood obesity with no easy answers or solutions [34]. The array of childhood obesity determinants is a dynamic interplay of genetic, perinatal and early life factors, physical inactivity, environmental factors and family factors [35]. Panel members reiterated that obesity is an extremely complex health state when considering types of foods, particular age ranges as well as the context of energy intake, energy expenditure and growth.

We believe this is the first study that explores expert opinions considering population level taxation to reduce childhood obesity. This article represents a summary of professional opinion from the unique perspective of experts in the field. Strengths of this research include utilising the nominal group technique which is still a relatively new method, particularly in the health field. The benefit is in the purpose of the technique to force a decision, no matter how hard it might be. The forced decision does not mean a correct answer has been identified [25], but in line with consensus methodology, has identified a number of potentially feasible priorities regarding food and beverage taxation and new evidence as to where public health and policy efforts could be directed.

The current research is not without its limitations. The complexity of the topic along with undertaking specific, sequential tasks meant that panel members needed to seek clarification on the process and activities on several occasions to ensure clarity and understanding. Another limitation is that although lack of definitions of food groups or items was continually identified by the panel as a significant barrier to food taxation, it was out of the scope and purpose of this research to define some of the problematic categories. Further to the research scope, this research only considered the contribution of whole foods and food items in contributing to early childhood obesity and did not delve into macro or micronutrients or a multitude of other diverse factors associated with obesity. Finally, the panel process was convened over a period of three and a half hours due to travel arrangements of experts. Regardless, a panel of longer duration may or may not have altered the outcomes of this process, given the intended purpose of forcing a decision and outcome.

One particular area for ongoing research would be to investigate the price elasticity of proposed taxable foods. In the Australian context, only broad categories of foods have been explored such as dairy, meat, fruits and vegetables [36], rather than the specific foods identified in this study and work has not focussed on the impact of changes in price in the food intake of children. This would help to theoretically identify the likely impact of taxation on consumer food choices and consumption for a range of different food and beverage items. Evidence synthesising U.S. studies [22] suggests that take away or restaurant food, soft drinks, juice, and meats are the most sensitive to price changes with a 10% increase in soft drink prices likely to decrease consumption by 8-10%.

As suggested by the panel, increasing only soft drink prices however, may lead to substitution of fruit juice or other sweetened drinks thereby not having the desired outcome of reducing obesity rates. The impact of this substitution is unclear and Andreyeva and Colleagues [22] suggest that further studies are required to investigate cross-price elasticities to determine what the substitution rates will be in order to target strategies to reduce obesity effectively. Even if these foods are shown to not be particularly price sensitive or substitution occurs, taxation may still be a useful public health strategy if used to cross-subsidize healthy food options or education.

It seems imperative to generate consistent definitions or criteria to distinguish between particular food items or groups. Definitional issues are problematic for a range of different sub-disciplines of nutrition. Contribution to clarification of definitions would provide enormous benefit to a number of research endeavours within the field of health and nutrition. Finally, although we know energy-dense nutrient-poor food choices comprise a significant proportion of early childhood energy intake, it is suggested to investigate particular dietary patterns and trends of children to identify the bigger picture of diet consumption, rather than just the contribution of individual foods.

13.5 CONCLUSION

Results of this research highlight priority areas regarding food and beverage taxation which have applicability and relevance to developed and developing countries alike. The outcomes indicate taxation should not be dismissed in endeavours to reduce childhood obesity and could have a wider impact than just in the early childhood years. This research has contributed unique expert opinion from researchers, academics and clinicians around Australia. The expert panel explicitly identified foods contributing most to early childhood obesity and have proposed potential leverage points in the form of consensus outcomes where taxation may have its best chance of success—for example, taxing sugar-sweetened beverages. Future work should rigorously explore the feasibility of each individual consensus outcome in further detail.

REFERENCES

1. Hesketh KD, Campbell KJ: Interventions to prevent obesity in 0–5 year olds: an updated systematic review of the literature. Obesity 2010, 18:S27-S35.
2. Lobstein T, Baur L, Uauy R, TaskForce IIO: Obesity in children and young people: a crisis in public health. Obes Rev 2004, 5(Suppl 1):4-104.
3. Wang Y, Lobstein T: Worldwide trends in childhood overweight and obesity. Int J Pediatr Obes 2006, 1(1):11-25. [http://www.abs.gov.au/ausstats/abs@.nsf/Lookup/4364.0.55.001main+features12011-12]
4. Australian health survey: first results, 2011–12. []
5. Olds TS, Tomkinson GR, Ferrar KE, Maher CA: Trends in the prevalence of childhood overweight and obesity in Australia between 1985 and 2008. Int J Obes 2010, 34(1):57-66.
6. Booth ML, Dobbins T, Okely AD, Denney-Wilson E, Hardy LL: Trends in the prevalence of overweight and obesity among young Australians, 1985, 1997, and 2004. Obesity (Silver Spring, Md) 2007, 15(5):1089-1095.

7. Population-based approaches to childhood obesity prevention. World Health Organization Press, Geneva, Switzerland; 2012.
8. Waters E, de Silva-Sanigorski A, Hall BJ, Brown T, Campbell KJ, Gao Y, Armstrong R, Prosser L, Summerbell CD: Interventions for preventing obesity in children. Cochrane Database Of Systematic Reviews (Online) 2011., 12
9. Campbell K, Crawford D: Family food environments as determinants of preschool-aged children's eating behaviours: implications for obesity prevention policy. A review. Australian Journal of Nutrition & Dietetics 2001, 58(1):19-25.
10. Grieger JA, Scott J, Cobiac L: Dietary patterns and breast-feeding in Australian children. Public Health Nutr 2011, 14(11):1939-1947.
11. Birch LL, Fisher JO: Development of eating behaviors among children and adolescents. Pediatrics 1998, 101(3 Pt 2):539-549.
12. Whitaker RC, Wright JA, Pepe MS, Seidel KD, Dietz WH: Predicting obesity in young adulthood from childhood and parental obesity. New Engl J Med 1997, 337(13):869-873.
13. van der Horst K, Oenema A, Ferreira I, Wendel-Vos W, Giskes K, van Lenthe F, Brug J: A systematic review of environmental correlates of obesity-related dietary behaviors in youth. Health Educ Res 2007, 22(2):203-226.
14. Gortmaker SL, Swinburn BA, Levy D, Carter R, Mabry PL, Finegood DT, Huang T, Marsh T, Moodie ML: Changing the future of obesity: science, policy, and action. Lancet 2011, 378(9793):838-847.
15. Swinburn BA, Sacks G, Hall KD, McPherson K, Finegood DT, Moodie ML, Gortmaker SL: The global obesity pandemic: shaped by global drivers and local environments. Lancet 2011, 378(9793):804-814.
16. Epstein LH, Raja S, Daniel TO, Paluch RA, Wilfley DE, Saelens BE, Roemmich JN: The built environment moderates effects of family-based childhood obesity treatment over 2 years. Ann Behav Med 2012, 44(2):248-258.
17. Faith MS, Fontaine KR, Baskin ML, Allison DB: Toward the reduction of population obesity: macrolevel environmental approaches to the problems of food, eating, and obesity. Psychol Bull 2007, 133(2):205-226.
18. Cash SB, Sunding DL, Zilberman D: Fat taxes and thin subsidies: Prices, diet, and health outcomes. Acta Agriculturae Scand 2005, 2:167-174.
19. [http://www.abs.gov.au/AUSSTATS/abs@.nsf/allprimarymainfeatures/2A1907FD31D727FCA257AD0000F29D2?op endocument] Australian Social Trends September 2012. []
20. Stafford N: Denmark cancels "fat tax" and shelves "sugar tax" because of threat of job losses. BMJ 2012, 345:e7889.
21. Mytton OT, Clarke D, Rayner M: Taxing unhealthy food and drinks to improve health. BMJ 2012, 344:e2931.
22. Andreyeva T, Long MW, Brownell KD: The impact of food prices on consumption: a systematic review of research on the price elasticity of demand for food. Am J Public Health 2010, 100(2):216-222.
23. Brownell KD, Warner KE: The perils of ignoring history: big tobacco played dirty and millions died. How similar is Big Food? Milbank Q 2009, 87(1):259-294.
24. Harvey N, Holmes CA: Nominal group technique: an effective method for obtaining group consensus. Int J Nurs Pract 2012, 18(2):188-194.

25. Jones J, Hunter D: Consensus methods for medical and health services research. BMJ: British Medical Journal 1995, 311(7001):376-380.
26. Ven A, Delbecq AL: Nominal versus interactinf group processes for committee decision-making effectiveness. Acad Manag J 1971, 14(2):203-212.
27. Susskind L, McKearnan S, Thomas-Larmer J: The consensus building handbook: a comprehensive guide to reaching agreement. Sage Publications, United Kingdom; 1999.
28. Van de Ven AH, Delbecq AL: The nominal group as a research instrument for exploratory health studies. Am J Public Health 1972, 62(3):337-342.
29. Gallagher M, Hares T, Spencer J, Bradshaw C, Webb I: The nominal group technique: a research tool for general practice? Fam Pract 1993, 10(1):76-81.
30. Carney O, McIntosh J, Worth A: The use of the Nominal Group Technique in research with community nurses. J Adv Nurs 1996, 23(5):1024-1029.
31. Powell LM, Chaloupka FJ: Food prices and obesity: evidence and policy implications for taxes and subsidies. Milbank Q 2009, 87(1):229-257.
32. Epstein LH, Dearing KK, Roba LG, Finkelstein E: The influence of taxes and subsidies on energy purchased in an experimental purchasing study. Psychol Sci 2010, 21(3):406-414.
33. Bell AC, Simmons A, Sanigorski AM, Kremer PJ, Swinburn BA: Preventing childhood obesity: the sentinel site for obesity prevention in Victoria, Australia. Health Promot Int 2008, 23(4):328-336.
34. Swinburn BA, de Silva-Sanigorski AM: Where to from here for preventing childhood obesity: an international perspective. Obesity (Silver Spring, Md) 2010, 18(Suppl 1):S4-S7.
35. Ebbeling CB, Pawlak DB, Ludwig DS: Childhood obesity: public-health crisis, common sense cure. Lancet 2002, 360(9331):473-482.
36. [http:/ / webarchives.cdlib.org/ wayback.public/ UERS_ag_1/ 20110914164016/ http:/ / ers.usda.gov/ publications/ tb1904/ tb1904.pdf] Seale J, Regmi A, Bernstein J: International Evidence on Food Consumption Patterns. 2003 []

CHAPTER 14

THE COSTS AND COST-EFFECTIVENESS OF A SCHOOL-BASED COMPREHENSIVE INTERVENTION STUDY ON CHILDHOOD OBESITY IN CHINA

LIPING MENG, HAIQUAN XU, AILING LIU, JOOP VAN RAAIJ, WANDA BEMELMANS, XIAOQI HU, QIAN ZHANG, SONGMING DU, HONGYUN FANG, JUN MA, GUIFA XU, YING LI, HONGWEI GUO, LIN DU, AND GUANSHENG MA

14.1 INTRODUCTION

During the past couple of decades, China has experienced rapid socio-economic and nutritional transitions [1-4]. Along with these life style changes, the prevalence of overweight and obesity among Chinese children has more than tripled, from 1.7% in 1982 to 5.3% in 2002 for 7-12 years of age [5]. The dramatic rise of overweight among children has led policy makers to rank it as a critical public health threat for several reasons. Firstly, childhood obesity are more likely to persist into adulthood [6,7]. Secondly, obesity in adults is one of the main risk factors for some chronic diseases [8]. Finally, the obesity epidemic greatly affects the social economic de-

The Costs and Cost-Effectiveness of a School-Based Comprehensive Intervention Study on Childhood Obesity in China. © *Meng et al.* PLoS ONE **8**,10 *(2013), doi:10.1371/journal.pone.0077971. Licensed under Creative Commons Attribution License.*

velopment. The indirect effects of obesity and obesity-related dietary and physical activity patterns reached 3.4% of gross national product (GNP) in 2000 and was projected to reach 8.7% in 2025 [9].

Schools have been identified as a key setting for public health strategies to prevent childhood obesity [10]. Research has shown that well-designed, well-implemented school obesity prevention programmes were effective in reduction of body mass index (BMI) and/or percent of body fat (PBF) [11]. However, some systematic reviews show that some short-term interventions (< 12 month) focused on combining dietary and physical activity approaches did not significantly decrease BMI [12,13]. In China, a few studies indicated that school based comprehensive intervention combined with nutrition and physical activity programs were effective [14,15]. However, whether it would be successful when expanded to a larger scale (from more regions to national-wide) still remains unclear.

As public health resources are limited, policy makers have to focus on how to set priorities among numerous public health issues. Therefore, interventions must not only be effective but also be cost-effective. Unfortunately, little information on the cost-effectiveness of different interventions is available in China. Under this background, this study was developed by National Institute for Nutrition and Food Safety (NINFS), Chinese Center for Disease Control and Prevention (China CDC), and funded by Ministry of Science and Technology of the People's Republic of China. The objective of this study is to evaluate the effects and the cost-effectiveness of a comprehensive intervention program for childhood obesity which combined nutrition education and physical activity interventions vs. control. We hypothesized the integrated intervention is both more effective in improving children's BMI and also more cost-effective than the same intensity of single nutrition education intervention or physical activity intervention.

14.2 METHODS

14.2.1 STUDY DESIGN

This study is a multi-center randomized controlled trial. Six centers included Beijing, Shanghai, Chongqing, Guangzhou, Jinan and Harbin were recruited. Two-step cluster sampling was used for subject selection. In the first step, 9 schools in Beijing were selected and assigned randomly to nutrition intervention (3 schools), physical activity (PA) intervention (3 schools) or control condition (3 schools). In other five cities, 6 schools in each city were selected randomly assigned to either combined with nutrition education and PA intervention (3 schools) or control condition (3 schools). Thus, there are a total of 15 schools in combined intervention and 15 schools in the control group in other 5 cities. In the second step, 2 classes from each grade in each school were chosen randomly. No intervention was taken place in the control schools.

14.2.2 SAMPLE SIZE CALCULATIONS

According to the study protocol, we calculated the sample size on the basis of cluster randomization trial design. "BMI changes" was used as the variable to calculate sample size. Based on the data from the 2002 China National Nutrition and Health Survey (CNNHS), a 0.7 kg/m^2 of BMI reduction could gain 2 percent reduction of overweight and obesity prevalence. A school-based obesity intervention strategy which gain 2 percent obesity prevalence reduction was considered as an effective strategy by World Health Organization [16,17]. We assumed that the intervention would be effective if a difference of 0.7 kg/m^2 of BMI changes between the intervention and control groups was detected. The intra-class correlation was assumed to be 0.05 and the power to detect the difference was set at 0.9. Statistical significance was set at 5% (two-sided). Thus the minimum number required would be 6 schools (3 for intervention and 3 for control) in each center with 250 students in each school. With consideration of loss of follow-up, the sample size of 9750 would be adequate.

14.2.3 PARTICIPANTS

The schools which meet the inclusion criteria (1. non-boarding school; 2. the students' overweight & obesity rate is over 10%; 3. school feeding, and more than 50% of the student eat lunch at school) were randomly chosen into the trial by a random number table. All of the students in the selected classes were enrolled in the trial, expect that: 1. the student who suffer from serious illnesses, such as congenital heart disease, the body carried out fixation or joint replacement surgery, and so on, can not withstand severe physical activity and diet control, not to participate in this study; 2. participated in the past one year or plan to participate in other similar intervention projects within one year.

14.2.4 ETHICS STATEMENT

This study was approved by the Ethical Review Committee of NINFS, China CDC. All participant students and their parents signed informed consent voluntarily.

14.2.5 INTERVENTION

The program was implemented for 2 semesters during one academic year (May 2009 to May 2010). Three means of intervention were included in the present study: nutrition education, physical activity intervention and comprehensive intervention.

14.2.5.1 NUTRITION EDUCATION INTERVENTION

The nutrition education handbook [18] was developed by the Department of Student Nutrition, NINFS, China CDC. Cartoon pamphlets were distributed to each student in the intervention schools. Class on nutrition and health were given 6 times for the students, 2 times for the parents and 4 times for teachers and health workers. The menu for students of school lunch cafeteria was evaluated periodically and specific nutrition improvement was suggested accordingly.

14.2.5.2 PA INTERVENTION

A classroom-based physical activity program for elementary students named "Happy 10" [19] was used in PA intervention. In each school day, the students were conducted "Happy 10" led by teachers to do a 10-minute segment moderate intensity, age- and space-appropriate exercises. The form of exercises was game, dance or rhythmic gymnastics. Students were also encouraged to develop more forms of exercises they like. Furthermore, education about physical activity was provided to students, parents, health workers and teachers. Each student attended the "Happy 10" 10 minutes for once, twice a day or 20 minutes for each time, once a day.

14.2.5.3 COMPREHENSIVE INTERVENTION

The comprehensive intervention was a combination of nutrition and PA interventions. Detailed information on the interventions can be found in previous published article [20].

14.2.6 OUTCOME MEASURES

Measurements were collected at baseline as well as at the end of the intervention. Consistent assessment methods were used throughout the study. Height was measured to an accuracy of 0.1 cm with a freestanding stadiometer mounted on a rigid tripod. Fasting body weight was measured to the nearest 0.1 kg on a digital scale. BMI was calculated as weight in kilograms divided by the square of height in meter (kg/m2). Overweight was defined as BMI between the 85th and the 95th percentiles, whereas obesity was defined as BMI ≥ 95th percentile, using age- and sex-specific BMI cutoff points developed by the Working Group for Obesity in China (WGOC) [21].

14.2.6.1 COSTS COLLECTION AND CALCULATION

The cost was collected and assessed from the social perspective. The project coordinator in each center was asked to recall all the costs related to the program. There are two components of the total costs in this paper. One is the 'Money costs' and the other one is the labor costs. Money costs means the direct currency investment during the program implementing. Labor costs was the transform of labor time investment. Three aspects data concerning costs were collected: a) Intervention costs in intervention schools; b) Evaluation cost for the pre- and post-intervention; and c) The development cost on structuring the program before intervention.

To estimate the intervention costs, we considered all costs associated with implementing the program during the intervention period, including expenses for materials, training, communication, transportation and accommodation, and monitoring. Material expenses included the cost of education material printing (Program Handbooks, nutrition and physical activity education book, pamphlet and foldout, dietary guideline manual), food pagoda model, "Happy 10" CD and poster. Training costs included meeting room, food, accommodation and training supplies as well as honorarium of instructors participating in the preprogram training. Communication costs included all the costs of communication meetings in which people shared the experiences and the limitations and would improve further in the future on the intervention during the intervention period. Transportation costs included traveling tickets for training and communication, the charge for taxi and compensation for transportation administrators. Monitoring costs included all the costs related to monitoring in each level, such as traveling and accommodation during the process of going to the intervention schools supervising, meetings for intervention and compensation of instructors participating in the monitoring.

To estimate the evaluation costs, we collected all the costs related to baseline and post-intervention survey implement and assessment, including questionnaire printing, instruments and tools for physical examination, expendables and allowance for blood samples taking, reagent and tests cost for biochemistry indices determination and related transportation cost.

Labor investment included the time been taken for preparing, implementing and evaluating the program. We collected the information on the salary of staff who implemented the program at each level and their working days for the program, based on which we calculated the labor cost. Subsidy for students and short-term personnel was also considered as a part of labor costs. Labor costs was also classified as intervention cost, development cost and evaluation cost. The labor costs for development included designing the program, developing the protocol used for intervention evaluation and implement, drafting the intervention materials, organizing start-up meeting and mobilizing the staff in collaboration centers as well as in schools. Labor costs for evaluation included time investment in training, implementing two times survey, data input computer and statistical analysis, reporting, blood samples collection, transport and biochemistry index tests. Labor costs for intervention included time investment in implementing the intervention in intervention schools, staff in collaboration centers monitoring, communication meeting with staff in NINFS, in collaboration centers and in intervention schools.

All the costs were collected on the population level because all the cash investment and labor time investment were based on the population level. Cost per capita in each group was calculated by total intervention cost divided by total participants in each group.

14.2.6.2 COST-EFFECTIVENESS ANALYSIS

The cost-effectiveness analysis was performed based on the results by comparing the changes between post-intervention and baseline in control schools with those in intervention schools. The effectiveness of the intervention was measured as BMI, BMI z-score (BAZ) reduction and cases of overweight & obesity prevented compared with the control condition. Cases of overweight & obesity prevented was calculated by the reduction of overweight & obesity prevalence multiply the participant numbers in intervention groups. Cost per capita was calculated with the number of the children who participated the baseline survey as the denominator. For BMI and BAZ, Cost-effectiveness ratio (CER) was calculated by cost per capita divided by reduction. While for case of overweight & obesity prevented, CER was calculated by total intervention cost divided by the overweight & obesity cases prevented.

TABLE 1: Characteristics of the subjects at baseline by group.

	Beijing						Other 5 centers			
	Control		Nutrition intervention		PA intervention		Control		Nutrition & PA intervention	
	N	%	N	%	N	%	N	%	N	%
Total	460	100.0	615	100	590	100	3280	100	3356	100
Sex										
Male	266	57.8[a]	300	48.8[b]	302	51.2[b]	1644	50.1	1695	50.5
Female	194	42.4	315	51.2	288	48.8	1636	49.9	1661	49.5
Age										
6-9.9	314	68.3	427	69.4	420	71.2	2357	71.9	2381	70.9
10-13.9	146	31.7	188	30.6	170	28.8	923	28.1	975	29.1
	%				%					
Income capita per month (yuan, RMB)										
<750	14.2		10.9		16.7		11.8		10.4	
750-2500	67.1		66.8		64.2		60.5		59.2	
≥2501	18.7		22.4		19.1		27.7		30.5	
P[c]			0.34		0.70				0.08	
Leisure time activity per day										
<1h	24.0		17.6		15.8		40.5		39.5	
1~1.9h	15.1		28.2		33.1		21.6		21.4	
2~2.9h	19.6		23.2		22.0		14.3		17.4	
≥3h	41.3		30.9		29.0		23.6		21.7	
P[c]			0.02		<0.001				0.21	
Sedentary activity per day										
<1h	62.2		61.8		63.9		51.6		52.8	
1~1.9h	33.8		33.5		33.7		38.2		37.2	
≥2h	4.0		4.7		2.3		10.1		10.1	
P[c]			0.86		0.20				0.44	
Average energy intake per day (Kcal), Mean (std)										
	1077.6(428.4)[a]		1036.4(403.1)[a]		929.4(388.9)[b]		1467.2(713.8)		1356.1(569.1)*	

a b: Percentage shared the different letter means significant difference at baseline among groups in Beijing, $p<0.05$. * Significant difference ($p<0.05$) between control and Nutrition & PA intervention group. c statistical analysis and compare between intervention group with it's control group. No superscript means no significant difference among groups.

14.2.7 STATISTICAL METHODS

Results of the continuous variables were expressed as mean and standard error. Calculation and comparison of the means and the changes of continuous variables among intervention and control groups were used covariance analysis with General Linear Model (GLM) adjusted for age, gender, daily energy intake and leisure time physical activity per day (for comparing changes, the baseline index was as a additional adjusted variable). For comparison of the means between post-intervention with baseline within each group a paired t test was used. Overweight & obesity prevalence and its' OR were compared using Generalized Linear Mixed Model (GLMM). Procedure GLMM was used to achieve it with center as random variable. The fixed variables included sex, age, baseline BMI and intervention types.

Statistical significance was set at $P<0.05$. SAS package version 9.1 (SAS Institute Inc, Cary, NC) was used for analyses.

14.3 RESULTS

A total of 9750 primary school students (aged 6-13 years) participated in the survey at baseline. Totally, 114 of the 5250 participants in intervention group and 309 of the 4500 participants in control group declined to participate. A total of 123 students were lost to follow-up because of school transfer or moving and 156 students accepted discontinued intervention because of illness and dropout in intervention group. According to the study protocol, the trial ended in May, 2010, after one academic year's intervention. As a result, a total of 8301 students followed full term (mean duration was 8.9 ± 0.1 months) intervention with logical general information and anthropometric index. Totally, 615 and 590 students completed the nutrition intervention and PA intervention in Beijing, respectively while 3356 participants completed the combined intervention in other 5 centers.

The percentage of males in the control group in Beijing was significantly higher than that in the two single intervention groups, however, no significant differences were found between the combined intervention and the control group in the other 5 centers. The distribution of age among control and intervention groups in Beijing was consistent, which was also seen between the control and the combined intervention group in other 5 centers. No significant differences were found in income, leisure time activity, sedentary activity and energy intake between combined intervention group and its' control group at baseline. However, children in combined intervention were less active and lower energy intake compared with its' control counterparts (Table 1).

Table 2 showed anthropometric characteristics at baseline, after intervention and the changes between post-intervention and baseline. No significant differences were found in height, weight and BMI between the nutrition intervention group and its' control group at baseline. Height, weight and BMI in each group in Beijing were significant higher in post intervention than those of at baseline. In the combined intervention group in the other 5 centers, height increasing was significantly more (6.82 cm vs. 6.59 cm) while weight, BMI and BAZ increasing were significantly less than those in its' control group (4.75 kg vs. 4.95 kg, 0.65 kg/m^2 vs. 0.84 kg/m^2, 0.12 vs 0.20, respectively). No significant differences were found in BMI change (after and before intervention) between the PA intervention group and its' control group in Beijing, the same case is for nutrition intervention group in Beijing. No significant differences were found in the changes of the overweight and obesity prevalence among nutrition intervention group, PA intervention group and their control group. However, the increment of the overweight and obesity prevalence in combined intervention group in other 5 centers was 87% less than that in control group, with a borderline significant difference (OR and 95% CI: 0.9 (0.7, 1.0)), see details in Table 2.

The costs of development and evaluation of the program was shown in Table 3. The total development costs in combined intervention group was RMB 26619 ($3915) for 5 collaboration centers. The development costs in nutrition intervention and PA intervention group was the same amount, RMB 4769 ($701). The development costs in each control group was zero. The total evaluation costs was RMB 173513 ($25517), RMB 141873 ($20864) and RMB 978614 ($143914) in nutrition intervention, PA intervention and combined intervention group, respectively.

Cost-Effectiveness of a Comprehensive Intervention Study on Obesity

TABLE 2: Anthropometric characteristics and obesity prevalence at baseline, after intervention and changes in different groups^.

	Beijing			Other centers	
	Control	Nutrition intervention	PA intervention	Control	Nutrition & PA intervention
Height (cm)					
N	460	615	590	3280	3356
Baseline	135.76±.00a	136.75±0.98a	136.20±0.97a	137.64±0.45	137.80±9.0.46
Post-intervention	141.36±1.05*	142.65±1.03*	141.91±1.02*	144.36±0.49*	144.77±0.49*
Change	5.60±0.27c	5.90±0.26d	5.71±0.26cd	6.59±0.14	6.82±0.14##
Weight (kg)					
N	460	615	590	3280	3356
Baseline	30.66±1.11a	31.57±1.09ab	31.90±1.08b	32.81±0.52	32.76±0.53
Post-intervention	34.77±1.33*	35.95±1.31*	36.22±1.30*	37.86±0.63*	37.62±0.64*
Change	4.10±0.38c	4.38±0.37c	4.33±0.37c	4.95±0.19	4.75±0.20#
BMI (kg/m^2)					
Baseline	16.42±0.43a	16.66±0.42ab	16.95±0.42b	17.07±0.20	17.01±0.20
Post-intervention	17.14±0.48*	17.40±0.67*	17.72±0.46*	17.91±0.23*	17.68±0.23*
Change	0.72±0.15c	0.74±0.15c	0.76±0.15c	0.84±0.09	0.65±0.09##
BAZ (BMI Z-score)					
Baseline	-0.17±0.19a	-0.05±0.18ab	0.06±0.18b	0.05±0.09	0.03±0.09
Post-intervention	0.07±0.19*	0.20±0.19*	0.31±0.18*	0.25±0.10*	0.15±0.11*
Change	0.25±0.07c	0.25±0.06c	0.26±0.06c	0.20±0.04	0.12±0.05##
Overweight and Obesity, n (%)					
Baseline	51 (11.1)	88 (14.3)	95 (16.1)	746 (22.7)	792 (23.6)
Post-intervention	81 (17.6)	122 (19.8)	129 (21.9)	795 (24.2)	798 (23.8)
Changes	30 (6.5)	34(5.5)	34(5.8)	49 (1.5)	6 (0.2)
P		0.24	0.17		0.06
OR (95% CI) †	1.0	0.8(0.0, 18.8)	0.94 (0.0, 20.8)	1.0	0.9(0.7, 1.0)

^ *Continuous variables were expressed as mean±standard error.*

a, b: Means shared the different letter means significant difference at baseline among groups in Beijing, p<0.05.
c, d : Means shared the different letter means significant difference of changes (post-intervention vs. baseline) among groups in Beijing, p<0.05.
* Comparison the mean between post-intervention and baseline in each group, p< 0.05.
# Comparison means between combined intervention group and control group at baseline as well as for changes (post-intervention vs. baseline), #p<0.05; ##p<0.01.
† OR and 95% CI for overweight & obesity prevalence using generalized linear mixed model, no significantly difference of OR between nutrition or PA individual intervention group with their control group, but a borderline difference between combined intervention group with its control group (p=0.06).

TABLE 3: The costs of development and evaluation of the program (RMB (US dollars)*).

Categories	Beijing			Other centers	
	Control	Nutrition intervention	PA intervention	Control	Nutrition & PA intervention
Development Costs					
Money costs	0 (0)	1817 (267)	1817 (267)	0 (0)	2425 (357)
Labor costs	0 (0)	2952 (434)	2952 (434)	0 (0)	24194 (3558)
Total	0 (0)	4769(701)	4769(701)	0 (0)	26619(3915)
Evaluation Costs					
Money costs subtotal	137510 (20222)	153010 (22501)	108310 (15928)	745904 (109692)	738978 (108673)
Materials	92592 (13616)	103792 (15264)	59592 (8764)	537372 (79025)	539311 (79310)
Training	2546 (374)	729 (107)	729 (107)	22718 (3341)	14656 (2155)
Personnel allowance	12489 (1837)	15589 (2293)	15089 (2219)	119693 (17602)	119429 (17563)
Transport and accommodation	31800 (4676)	33000 (4853)	33000 (4853)	47057 (6920)	39217 (5767)
Collaborate fee	0 (0)	0 (0)	0 (0)	29250 (4301)	34126 (5019)
Labor costs	25691 (3778)	20503 (3015)	33563 (4936)	22801 (3353)	239636 (35241)
Total evaluation costs	163201 (24000)	173513 (25517)	141873 (20864)	768705 (113045)	978614 (143914)

*US dollars was calculated by Jan, 2010 exchange rate (6.8).

TABLE 4: Cost of intervention in the intervention schools (RMB (US dollars))

	Nutrition intervention	PA intervention	Nutrition & PA intervention					Subtotal
			Jinan	Guangzhou	Shanghai	Harbin	Chongqing	
Money Costs								
Materials	4414 (649.1)	2593 (381.3)	6544 (962.4)	6372 (937.1)	5774 (849.1)	5959 (876.3)	4204 (618.2)	28853 (4243.1)
Training	3074 (452.1)	3074 (452.1)	3426 (503.8)	6914 (1016.8)	5427 (798.1)	4351 (639.9)	5410 (795.6)	25528 (3754.1)
Communication	1453 (213.7)	1453 (213.7)	3309 (486.6)	5350 (786.8)	4480 (658.8)	3850 (566.2)	4470 (657.4)	21459 (3155.7)
Transportation and accommodation	7800 (1147.1)	7800 (1147.1)	1700 (250.0)	1080 (158.8)	5220 (767.6)	1300 (191.2)	3900 (573.5)	13200 (1941.2)
Monitoring	8300 (1220.6)	8300 (1220.6)	5100 (750.0)	800 (117.6)	1440 (211.8)	500 (73.5)	2000 (294.1)	9840 (1447.1)
Subtotal	25041 (3682.5)	23220 (3414.7)	20079 (2952.8)	20516 (3017.1)	22341 (3285.4)	15960 (2347.1)	19084 (2938.8)	98880 (14541.2)
Labor costs								
School Intervention	10088 (1483.5)	10661 (1567.8)	95756 (14081.8)	87060 (12802.9)	235721 (34664.9)	66932 (9842.9)	4542 (667.9)	490011 (72060.4)
Center monitoring	5964 (877.1)	5964 (877.1)	27108 (3986.5)	15108 (2221.8)	41335 (6078.7)	8175 (1202.2)	23904 (3515.3)	115630 (17004.4)
National Communications§	638 (93.8)	638 (93.8)	638 (93.8)	638 (93.8)	638 (93.8)	638 (93.8)	638 (93.8)	3190 (469.1)

TABLE 4: *Cont.*

	Nutrition intervention	PA intervention	Nutrition & PA intervention				
			Jinan	Guangzhou	Shanghai	Harbin	Chongqing	Subtotal
Subtotal	16690 (2454.4)	17263 (2538.7)	123502 (18162.1)	102806 (15118.5)	277694 (40837.4)	75745 (11139.0)	29084 (4277.1)	608831 (89534.0)
Total costs‖	41731 (6136.9)	40483 (5953.4)	143581 (21114.9)	123322 (18135.6)	300035 (44122.8)	91705 (13486.0)	49068 (7215.9)	707711 (104075.1)
N	790 (116.2)	774 (113.8)	693 (101.9)	1008 (148.2)	749 (110.1)	722 (106.2)	707 (104.0)	3879 (570.4)
Money costs per capita	31,7 (4.7)	30,0 (4.4)	29,0 (4.3)	20,4 (3.0)	29,8 (4.4)	22,1 (3.3)	28,3 (4.2)	25,5 (3.8)
Total costs per capita	52,8 (7.8)	52,3 (7.7)	207,2 (30.5)	122,3 (18.0)	400,6 (58.9)	127,0 (18.7)	69,4 (10.2)	182,4 (26.8)

§*National communication costs in national lever was divided into each center in each intervention group.*
‖*Total costs means the sum of money costs and labor costs.*

The intervention costs was shown in Table 4. The intervention costs per child in combined intervention group was RMB182.4 ($26.8), which was 2.4 times higher than that in the nutrition intervention (RMB52.8, $7.8) or in the PA intervention (RMB52.3, $7.7). The money costs per child in combined intervention was 25.5 RMB ($3.8), which is lower then that in the individual intervention group ($4.7 for nutrition intervention and $4.4 for PA intervention). However, the labor costs per child was much higher in combined intervention ($23.0) compared with individual intervention and accounted for 86% of total costs. Guangzhou, Shanghai and Jinan in combined intervention group had the highest labor costs.

The cost-effectiveness results by center were shown in Table 5. Chongqing (one of the centers in combined intervention) as well as Beijing where the two individual interventions implanted were excluded in cost-effective analysis because that no consistent significant effect was found in these cities. We calculated the cost-effectiveness ratio separately in four cities (Jinan, Guangzhou, Shanghai and Harbin) in the combined intervention group, compared with controls, there was a 0.27 kg/m², 0.29 kg/m², 0.17 kg/m² and 0.61 kg/m² reduction of BMI attributing to the integrative intervention in Jinan, Guangzhou, Shanghai and Harbin, respectively. The cost for achieving 1 kg/m² BMI reduction, CER was $113.0, $62.1, $346.5 and $30.7, respectively, in Jinan, Guangzhou, Shanghai and Harbin, The cost for avoided one overweight and obesity case was $1308.9.

TABLE 5: Cost-effectiveness ratio (CER) by city in the nutrition & PA combined intervention group.

Index	Jinan		Guangzhou		Shanghai		Harbin		Total[d]	
	Effect[a]	CER[b]	Effect	CER	Effect	CER	Effect	CER	Effect	CER
BMI (kg/m²)	0.27	113.0	0.29	62.1	0.17	346.5	0.61	30.7	0.29	120.3
BAZ	0.09	338.9	0.15	120.0	0.09	654.4	0.29	64.5	0.14	249.3
One case of O & B[c] prevented	21	1005.5	19	954.5	22	2005.6	12	1123.8	74	1308.9

a For BMI, BAZ and overweight & obesity prevalence, the 'effect' means BMI, BAZ and overweight & obesity prevalence reduction (post intervention vs before intervention) in intervention group compared with that of in the control group, respectively. b ALL CER was presented in US dollars. c O & B means overweight & obesity. d Total' means the average effect of four intervention centers (Jinan, Guangzhou, Harbin, Shanghai), Chongqing was excluded here because the intervention in this city was not effective (p>0.05).

14.4 DISCUSSION

14.4.1 THE COSTS OF THE INTERVENTION

The intervention costs in this study were lower compared with other similar intervention studies [10,22]. A study of a 3-year, after-school program to prevent obesity among elementary school students [10] reported the net intervention costs per capita was $317 and the achieved effectiveness was a 0.7% PBF reduction. Teaching materials both for PA activity and for nutrition education were simple and inexpensive in this study. Participates in the same class can share one set of material such as "Happy 10" video, tracking posters, and stickers, which was one of the measures to reduce costs. Furthermore, the space for taking PA activity intervention was in classroom or in the playground in school, which is costless.

The money intervention costs per capita in the combined intervention group was relatively low in this study. However, the labor costs account for 86% of the total costs in the combined intervention group and the proportion was much higher compared to the single one. This may be due to the difference distance from the site national project office located to the intervention sites. As we known, the two single intervention groups was performed in Beijing, where the national working group located. So the traveling cost and time investment for training and supervision was saved largely. Meanwhile, the combined intervention was implemented in five centers separately. The organization, management and supervision were more difficult and needs more labor investment. There was also a variety of labor costs among the five combined intervention cities and the nonidentity of the salary income for the instructors and staff in collaboration centers maybe one of the reasons. For example, based on the questionnaire survey of labor cost, staff in Shanghai and Guangzhou subcenters have higher salary than those in other centers. Data from Statistical Bulletin for National Economic and Social Development showed that annual per capita disposable income in 2010 was RMB 34345 in Shanghai and RMB 34328 in Guangzhou, which was the two highest income levels in China.

14.4.2 THE EFFECTIVENESS OF THE INTERVENTION

Up to now, there are not generalizable conclusion about the effects of child obesity interventions [11-13]. There was a borderline significant difference in change of the overweight & obesity prevalence (OR and 95% CI: 0.8(0.7, 1.0)) between the combined intervention and the control group. The increment in BMI was significantly lower in the combined intervention than that in the control group. It indicates that the combined intervention improves in obesity prevention. More effective function of combined intervention in obesity prevention was found in long-term intervention studies [14,23]. In the both two 3-year nutrition education & PA combined intervention studies, one [24] found a significant 1.1 kg/m^2 reduction of BMI and another [14] found a significant 1.8 kg/m^2 reduction of BMI. However, inconsistent results were also presented in other studies [24,25]. One 2-year combined intervention found no impact on obesity [25], in which the author suggested that compensation in both energy intake and physical activity outside of school may be responsible for the lack of difference between the intervention group and the control group.

However, there was no effect found in BMI reduction in single intervention (PA or nutrition). Similar results were also found in other studies [26,27]. One possibility of this was that the "dose" of physical activity achieved in these studies was insufficient to improve BMI. A short term (10 months) but high intensity physical activity intervention was reported effectiveness and the reason for success, brought forward by the author, is partly the exercise 'dose' The average daily energy cost of the program is more than twice the magnitude of the proposed energy surplus associated with childhood obesity [28]. As similar with PA intervention, low intensity nutrition education intervention was also proved no effect neither in this study nor in others [29].

14.4.3 THE COST-EFFECTIVENESS OF THE INTERVENTION

Most reports about the cost-effectiveness analysis of school-based child obesity intervention usually were based on per QALY (quality-adjusted life year) or DALY (disability-adjusted life-year) saved and studies based on BMI improvement was limited. We can't convert BMI reduction into more meaningful measures such as QALYs or DALYs saved in this study due to the following reasons: 1) The information of the life quality of the subjects was in absence in this study and the quality weight was not available; 2) The effects in this study was not in strong evidence. Though there was a significant BMI reduction in combined intervention group, the reduction of overweight and obesity prevalence was not in statistical significance. Furthermore, the individual intervention group was not shown a significant effect compared with control group.

The cost-effectiveness analysis results showed that CER for BMI in combined intervention was $120.3, which was much lower than that in one study implemented in Australia. In that study, the cost for achieving 1 kg/m2 BMI reduction was AUD 11236 after 12 weeks consultation intervention targeting change in nutrition, physical activity, and sedentary behavior based on family [30]. One score of BAZ reduction cost $249.3 and this was markedly lower than that in a family-based 12-month treatment for children obesity in Canada [31]. There was a large variation of the CER among combined intervention cities. Achieving one unit of BMI or BAZ reduction or one case of overweight & obesity prevented was quite expensive in Shanghai with the reason of high intervention cost and low effects. On the contrary to the high income in Shanghai, the annual per capita disposable income was the lowest (RMB 16292) in Harbin. As a result of low intervention cost ($18.7 per capita) and relative high effects, Harbin had the lowest CER for BMI and BAZ.

This study has several limitations. Firstly, the long-term effects and cost-effectiveness of the intervention can not be assessed. Secondly, although the intervention implemented for 2 semesters during one academic year, the actual implemented duration is 8.9 months because it was interrupted by the two regular holidays (one month summer holiday and two months winter holiday), which would reduce the expectable effects. Thirdly, the combined intervention was not implemented in the same center with the individual intervention. Although all the involved centers are located in large city, there are still differences in economical level, salary income and expenditure level among them and this make it less comparable in the cost (especially for the part of labor cost) and the cost-effectiveness among intervention groups. Finally, the sample size in single intervention group in Beijing is small and is not sufficient enough to detect the difference of changes.

This study also had important strengths. Firstly, the program was standardized through the development (training of the instructors), intervention (uniform intervention materials) and evaluation (uniform measures and instruments for outcomes). Secondly, physical activity in style of "Happy 10" was a recreational and non-competitive. It was well acceptable and can avoid the danger of hurt during implementing. Thirdly, the parents, instructors, health workers, school canteen managers, operators were fully mobilized both in the nutrition education intervention and in the PA intervention, which played an important role on obesity prevention for students. Fourth, follow-up rates were high (85%) and similar rates among children in the control schools. This may be because parents knew in advance that biochemical results would be given shortly after the health examination at the end of the project, together with appropriate advice if any parameter was abnormal.

A good design and full implementation are the keys to accomplish an intervention program. The methodology of an intervention program, such as duration, intensity, and the criteria of control selection, needs to be further studied. Evaluation the background level of the children's physical activity and nutrition knowledge in both control schools and intervention schools are necessary. Future study needs to be conducted to identify whether the effects and the cost-effectiveness is sustainable in a long term, and a suitable model, such as QALYs, should be used to assess the cost-effectiveness for a long-term.

In conclusion, the school-based integrated intervention was cost-effectiveness to improve BMI in school children and had a potential effect on childhood obesity prevention in urban China. However, the long-term effects and cost-effectiveness needs to be evaluated in the further study.

REFERENCES

1. National Bureau of Statistics of China (2000). China Statistic Year Book 2000. Beijing: China: Statistic Press.

2. Zhai F, He Y, Ma G, Li Y, Wang Z et al. (2005) Study on the current status of food consumption among Chinese population. Zhong Hua Liu Xing Bing Xue Zhi 26(7): 485-488.
3. Liu Y, Zhai F, Popkin BM (2006) Trends in eating behaviors among Chinese children (1991-1997). Asia Pac J Clin Nutr 15(1): 72-80. PubMed: 16500881.
4. Tudor-Locke C, Ainsworth BE, Adair LS, Du S, Popkin BM (2003) Physical activity and inactivity in Chinese school-aged youth: the China Health and Nutrition Survey. Int J Obes Relat Metab Disord 27(9): 1093-1099. doi:10.1038/sj.ijo.0802377. PubMed: 12917716.
5. Li Y, Schouten EG, Hu X, Cui Z, Luan D et al. (2008) Obesity prevalence and time trend among youngsters in China, 1982-2002. Asia Pac J Clin Nutr 17(1): 131-137. PubMed: 18364338.
6. Whitaker RC, Wright JA, Pepe MS, Seidel KD, Dietz WH (1997) Predicting obesity in young adulthood from childhood and parental obesity. N Engl J Med 337: 869-873. doi:10.1056/NEJM199709253371301. PubMed: 9302300.
7. Guo SS, Roche AF, Chumlea WC, Gardner JD, Siervogel RM (1994) The predictive value of childhood body mass index values for overweight at age 35 y. Am J Clin Nutr 59: 810-819. PubMed: 8147324.
8. Pi-Sunyer FX (1993) Medical hazards of obesity. Ann Intern Med 119: 655-660. doi:10.7326/0003-4819-119-7_Part_2-199310011-00006. PubMed: 8363192.
9. Popkin BM, Kim S, Rusev ER, Du S, Zizza C (2006) Measuring the full economic costs of diet, physical activity and obesity-related chronic diseases. Obes Rev 7: 271-293. doi:10.1111/j.1467-789X.2006.00230.x. PubMed: 16866975.
10. Wang LY, Gutin B, Barbeau P, Moore JB, Hanes J et al. (2008) Cost-Effectiveness of a School-Based Obesity Prevention Program. J Sch Health 78: 619-624. doi:10.1111/j.1746-1561.2008.00357.x. PubMed: 19000237.
11. Doak CM, Visscher TS, Renders CM, Seidell JC (2006) The prevention of overweight and obesity in children and adolescents: a review of interventions and programmes. Obes Rev 7: 111–136. doi:10.1111/j.1467-789X.2006.00234.x. PubMed: 16436107.
12. Summerbell CD, Waters E, Edmunds LD, Kelly S, Brown T et al. (2005) Interventions for preventing obesity in children. Cochrane Database Syst Rev 3: 1-70. doi: 10.1002/14651858.cd001871.pub2
13. Campbell K, Waters E, O'Meara S, Summerbell C (2001) Interventions for preventing obesity in childhood. A systematic review. Obes Rev 2(3): 149–157. doi:10.1046/j.1467-789x.2001.00035.x. PubMed: 12120100.
14. Jiang J, Xia X, Greiner T, Wu G, Lian G et al. (2007) The effects of a 3-year obesity intervention in schoolchildren in Beijing. Child Care Health Dev 33(5): 641-647. doi:10.1111/j.1365-2214.2007.00738.x. PubMed: 17725789.
15. Wu X, Wang J, Dong H, Geng Y, Zhang X et al. (2010) Childhood obesity intervention study in Xuzhou. Modern. Prev Med 37(12): 2225-2230.
16. Primary Health Division, Ministry of Health, Singapore (1993) Annual Report 1993, school health service. Singapore: Ministry of Health.
17. Ministry of Health, Singapore (2001) State of health report 2000-the report of the director of medical services. Singapore: Ministry of Health.
18. Ma G, Hu X (2009) Healthy School. Beijing. China: Population Publisher.

19. Liu A, Hu X, Ma G, Cui Z, Pan Y et al. (2008) Evaluation of a classroom-based physical activity promoting programme. Obes Rev 9(Suppl 1): 130-134. doi:10.1111/j.1467-789X.2007.00454.x. PubMed: 18307715.
20. Li Y, Hu X, Zhang Q, Liu A, Fang H et al. (2010) The nutrition-based comprehensive intervention study on childhood obesity in China (NISCOC): a randomized cluster controlled trial. BMC Public Health 10: 229. doi:10.1186/1471-2458-10-229. PubMed: 20433766.
21. Group of China Obesity Task Force (2004) Body mass index reference norm for screening overweight and obesity in Chinese children and adolescents; Xing Zhong Hua Liu Bing Xue Za Zhi 25:97-102.
22. Carter R, Moodie M, Markwick A, Magnus A, Vos T et al. (2009) Assessing Cost-Effectiveness in Obesity (ACE-Obesity): an overview of the ACE approach, economic methods and cost results. BMC Public Health 9(419): 1-11. PubMed: 19922625.
23. Yannis M, Joanna M, Christos H, Kafatos A (1999) Evaluation of a Health and Nutrition Education Program in Primary School Children of Crete over a Three-Year Period. Prev Med 28: 149–159. doi:10.1006/pmed.1998.0388. PubMed: 10048106.
24. Gortmaker SL, Peterson K, Wiecha J, Sobol AM, Dixit S et al. (1999) Reducing obesity via a school-based interdisciplinary intervention among youth: Planet Health. Arch Pediatr Aolesc Med 153: 409–418. doi:10.1001/archpedi.153.4.409.
25. Donnelly JE, Jacobsen DJ, Whatley JE, Hill JO, Swift LL et al. (1996) Nutrition and physical activity programme to attenuate obesity and promote physical and metabolic fitness in elementary. school children. Obes Res 64 (3): 229–243. doi: 10.1002/j.1550-8528.1996.tb00541.x
26. Harris KC, Kuramoto LK, Schulzer M, Retallack JE (2009) Effect of school-based physical activity interventions on body mass index in children: a meta-analysis. CMAJ 180(7): 719-726. doi:10.1503/cmaj.080966. PubMed: 19332753.
27. Summerbell CD, Waters E, Edmunds LD, Kelly S, Brown T et al. (2005) Interventions for preventing obesity in children. Cochrane Database Syst Rev Volumes 3:CD001871. doi: 10.1002/14651858.cd001871.pub2
28. Howe CA, Harris RA, Gutin B (2011) A 10-Month Physical Activity Intervention Improves Body Composition in Young Black Boys. J Obes. doi:10.1155/2011/358581.
29. Simonetti DAA, Tarsitani G, Cairella M, Siani V, Filippis SD et al. (1986) Prevention of obesity in elementary and nursery school children. Public Health 100: 166–171. doi:10.1016/S0033-3506(86)80030-0. PubMed: 3737864.
30. Wake M, Baur LA, Gerner B, Gibbons K, Gold L et al. (2009) Outcomes and costs of primary care surveillance and intervention for overweight or obese children: the LEAP 2 randomised controlled trial. BMJ 339: b3308. doi:10.1136/bmj.b3308. PubMed: 19729418.
31. Goldfield GS, Epstein LH, Kilanowski CK, Paluch RA, Kogut-Bossler B (2001) Cost-effectiveness of group and mixed family-based treatment for childhood obesity. Int J Obes Relat Metab Disord 25(12): 1843-1849. doi:10.1038/sj.ijo.0801838. PubMed: 11781766.

AUTHOR NOTES

CHAPTER 1

Acknowledgments

All data were analyzed at the secure CDC National Center for Health Statistics (NCHS) Research Data Center at Atlanta. Approval for this study was obtained from NCHS. We thank Stephanie Robinson and Ajay Yesupriya at CDC Atlanta Research Data Center for their assistance with our access to the geocoded NSCH 2007. We appreciate the comments of 2 anonymous reviewers, which helped us improve the manuscript. We received no financial assistance for this study.

CHAPTER 2

Competing Interests

The authors declare that they have no competing interests.

Author Contributions

MW performed the literature research, wrote the first draft of the manuscript, and completed the final version. AM wrote sections of the manuscript, created figures and formatted the manuscript. KKH wrote sections of the manuscript and created figures. All authors read and approved the final manuscript.

Acknowledgments

This work was supported by grants of the German Federal Ministry for Education and Research (BMBF, project funding reference number 01GI1120A), and is integrated in the Competence Network Obesity (CNO).

CHAPTER 3

Acknowledgments

Funding for this project was made possible by cooperative agreement no. 3U58DP002626-01S1 from the Centers for Disease Control and Prevention, US Department of Health and Human Services; and Get Healthy Philly. We acknowledge the School District of Philadelphia for providing the data necessary for this analysis, and we thank Tracey Williams, Bettyann Creighton, Tonya Wolford, and the School District's Office of Research and Evaluation and Office of Accountability and Assessment.

CHAPTER 4

Competing Interests

The authors declare that they have no competing interests.

Author Contributions

This paper is based on research conducted by AD as part of his PhD, supervised by RJ and KRF. AD collected the data, performed the statistical analysis, and drafted the manuscript. All authors have contributed to the conception, design of the study and in writing the paper. All authors approved the final manuscript.

Acknowledgments

The authors would like to thank Silvan Zammit from the National Statistics Office for the assistance given in the selection of the sample, Mary Rose Debono (National Statistics Office – NSO) and Prof. Liberato Camilleri (University of Malta) for their advice on the measurement of socioeconomic status, the research assistants, the school administrators and the teachers, and finally the students that participated in this study. The authors would also like to thank the Directorate for Educational Services, the Directorate for Quality and Standards in Education, the Health Promotion and Disease Prevention Directorate, and the Parliamentary Secretariat for Youth and Sport for their support. This project was funded by the University of Malta.

CHAPTER 5

Mr Folkvord conceptualized and designed the study, collected the data, carried out the analyses, and drafted the initial manuscript; Drs Anschütz, Nederkoorn, and Westerik, and Prof Dr Buijzen conceptualized and designed the study and critically reviewed the manuscript; and all authors approved the final manuscript as submitted. This trial has been registered with the Australian New Zealand Clinical Trials Registry (identifier ACTRN12613000035729).

Financial Disclosure
The authors have indicated they have no financial relationships relevant to this article to disclose.

Funding
This research was granted by the Behavioural Science Institute, Radboud University Nijmegen.

Conflict of Interest
The authors have indicated they have no potential conflicts of interest to disclose.

CHAPTER 6

Funding
RCR is funded by the Wellcome Trust 4-year studentship (Grant Code: WT083431MF). NJT, GDS, and GM work within the Integrative Epidemiology Unit (IEU), which is supported by the MRC (MC_UU_12013/1 and MC_UU_12013/3) and the University of Bristol. ARN works within the NIHR Biomedical Research Unit at the University of Bristol and the University Hospitals Bristol NHS Foundation Trust in Nutrition, Diet and Lifestyle. The UK Medical Research Council and the Wellcome Trust (Grant ref: 092731) and the University of Bristol provide core support for ALSPAC. The funders had no role in study design, data collection and analysis, decision to publish, or preparation of the manuscript.

Competing Interests
GDS is a member of the Editorial Board of PLOS Medicine. All other authors have declared that no competing interests exist.

Acknowledgments
We are extremely grateful to all the families who took part in this study, the midwives for their help in recruiting participants, and the whole ALSPAC team, which includes interviewers, computer and laboratory technicians, clerical workers, research scientists, volunteers, managers, receptionists, and nurses.

Author Contributions
Conceived and designed the experiments: RCR NJT GDS. Analyzed the data: RCR GM. Wrote the first draft of the manuscript: RCR. Contributed to the writing of the manuscript: RCR GDS ARN MdH GM NJT. ICMJE criteria for authorship read and met: RCR GDS ARN MdH GM NJT. Agree with manuscript results and conclusions: RCR GDS ARN MdH GM NJT.

CHAPTER 7

Acknowledgment
The SPEEDY study is funded by the National Prevention Research Initiative consisting of the following funding partners: British Heart Foundation; Cancer Research UK; Chief Scientist Office, Scottish Government Health Directorates; Department of Health; Diabetes UK; Economic and Social Research Council; Health and Social Care Research and Development Office for Northern Ireland; Medical Research Council; Welsh Assembly Government and World Cancer Research Fund. Additional funding for the collection, data acquisition, and analysis of the 4-day diet diaries was provided by Norwich Medical School. The work of E.M.F.v.S. and S.J.G. was supported by the Centre for Diet and Activity Research, a UKCRC Public Health Research: Centre of Excellence.

CHAPTER 9

Acknowledgment

This work was supported by grants from the Robert Wood Johnson Foundation through the National Policy and Legal Analysis Network to Prevent Childhood Obesity, a project of Public Health Law & Policy, and the Rudd Center for Food Policy and Obesity, and by the Rudd Foundation. The authors thank Professor Mark Aaronson for his insights on framing the manuscript. This article highlights ideas generated and conclusions reached at the Symposium on Ethical Issues in Interventions for Childhood Obesity, sponsored by the Robert Wood Johnson Foundation and Data for Solutions, Inc.

CHAPTER 10

Funding

The Provincial evaluation was funded through a contract with Alberta Health. The APPLE Schools program was funded through a donation to the School of Public Health at the University of Alberta. The research was funded by an operating grant by the Canadian Institutes for Health Research (FRN: 91061), Heart and Stroke Foundation of Canada and Canadian Population Health Initiative, and through Canadian Institutes for Health Research and Alberta Innovates Health Solutions (AIHS) postdoctoral fellowships to Dr. Bach Tran, and a Canada Research Chair in Population Health, an Alberta Research Chair in Nutrition and Disease Prevention and AIHS Health Scholarship to Dr. Paul J. Veugelers. Dr. J. A. Johnson is a Centennial Professor at the University of Alberta and a Senior Health Scholar with AIHS. All interpretations and opinions in the present study are those of the authors. The funders had no role in study design, data collection and analysis, decision to publish, or preparation of the manuscript.

Competing Interests

The authors have declared that no competing interests exist.

Acknowledgments
We thank all of the grade five students, parents and schools for their participation in the REAL Kids Alberta evaluation and APPLE Schools program, and the evaluation assistants, health promotion coordinators and school health facilitators for their contributions in data collection.

Author Contributions
Conceived and designed the experiments: PJV AO SK JAJ BXT. Performed the experiments: PJV AO BXT. Analyzed the data: BXT. Contributed reagents/materials/analysis tools: PJV AO SK JAJ BXT. Wrote the paper: PJV AO SK JAJ BXT.

CHAPTER 11

Author Contributions
Conceived and designed the experiments: LF OA TH. Performed the experiments: LF. Analyzed the data: LF OA. Contributed reagents/materials/analysis tools: LF OA TH. Wrote the paper: LF OA TH.

CHAPTER 12

Competing Interests
All authors (VM van de Gaar, W Jansen, A van Grieken, GJJM Borsboom, S Kremers and H Raat) declare that they have no competing interests.

Author Contributions
HR and WJ had the original idea for the study and its design, and were responsible for acquiring the study grant. VvdG further developed the study protocol and is responsible for data collection, data analysis and reporting the study results. GB assisted with the statistical analyses. HR and WJ supervise the study. WJ, AvG, SK and HR helped to refine the manuscript. All authors participated regularly in discussions regarding the design and protocols used in the study. All authors read and approved the final manuscript.

Acknowledgments

This study is funded by a grant from the major funding body ZonMw, the Netherlands Organization for Health Research and Development, project no. 50-50102-96-015.

This study is part of the Dutch project CIAO, which stands for Consortium Integrated Approach Overweight. Within CIAO, several studies are being conducted that investigate the different components of the EPODE approach. This study reflects on the component 'social marketing'. The publication of this study was supported by a grant of the Netherlands Organization for Scientific Research (NWO).

CHAPTER 13

Competing Interests

The authors declare that they have no competing interests.

Author Contributions

All authors (EP, EK, APH and TC) contributed to designing and facilitating the study. EP undertook data entry and both EP and TC contributed to the interpretation of results. All authors (EP, EK, APH and TC) contributed to writing, editing and approving the manuscript for submission.

Acknowledgments

The present study was funded by the Australian National Preventive Health Agency. (Project reference number: 17COM2011). Tracy Comans was also supported by the above grant. Erin Pitt was supported by a Griffith University Postgraduate Research Scheme scholarship. Elizabeth Kendall was supported by Griffith University and the Centre of National Research on Disability and Rehabilitation Medicine. Andrew Hills was supported by the Mater Medical Research Institute and Griffith University. Ethics approval for this research was obtained through the Griffith University Human Research Ethics Committee (HREC - MED/32/12/ HREC). The authors would like to acknowledge the contribution of the Brisbane Childhood Obesity Panel and appreciation must be shown to the project's chief investigators in guiding the formation of the overall research. The authors would also like to acknowledge Angela Simons as former project manager, and Nicole Moretto and Simone Braithwaite for their independent contribution through review of the manuscript prior to submission.

CHAPTER 14CC

Funding
This project has been funded by China Ministry of Science & Technology as "Key Projects in the National Science & Technology Pillar Program during the Eleventh Five-Year Plan Period", grant number 2008BAI58B0 5. The funders had no role in study design, data collection and analysis, decision to publish, or preparation of the manuscript.

Competing Interests
The authors have declared that no competing interests exist.

Acknowledgments
The authors thank all participating students and their parents. We are grateful to the local education and health staffs and all numbers of the study team. We thank Heidi Fransen and Richard Heijink in National Institute for Public Health and the Environment, The Netherlands, who gave help in the data analysis and economic explanation.

Author Contributions
Conceived and designed the experiments: GM. Performed the experiments: JM GX YL HG LD. Analyzed the data: LM HX. Contributed reagents/materials/analysis tools: XH QZ SD HF AL. Wrote the manuscript: LM. Provided the method of cost and cost-effectiveness: JvR WB.

INDEX

A

accelerometer, xxi, xxiv, 48–49, 51, 55, 63, 65–66, 87, 92, 106, 111
active living, xxv, 157–159, 161, 163, 165, 167, 169–171, 173
adipoinsular axis, 128, 134, 140
adiposity, xxiii–xxiv, 27, 83–93, 95–103, 105, 107, 109–111, 113, 115–117, 119–123, 125, 127–128, 130–134, 136–138, 140–141
advergames, xxii, 69–71, 73, 75–81
advertising, 71, 78–79, 81, 146–153, 155–156, 240
age, xxiii, 4–7, 9–10, 15–16, 22–25, 27, 31–32, 37, 41, 46, 48, 56, 64–65, 67, 73–77, 81, 86–88, 92, 94, 96–98, 100, 102, 107, 113–115, 121–122, 124, 129, 131, 133, 135–137, 139, 149, 159–161, 169–170, 172, 177, 179–180, 184, 191, 207, 220–221, 243–244, 249, 255, 259, 262–264, 274
Akaike information criterion, 10
alcohol, 140, 236
allele, 87–88, 91, 93, 97–98
amino acids, 129, 133
analyses of covariance (ANCOVA), 49, 58, 76
anthropometry, 22, 28, 48, 100, 111–112, 116, 190–191, 263–265
appetite, 69, 73, 81, 128, 137
attention deficit hyperactivity disorder (ADHD), 71, 81
Australia, xiii, xv, xvii, xxi, 23, 52, 54, 56, 235, 237, 251, 253, 272
availability, 79, 95, 230, 236, 245, 248

B

Barker hypothesis, 127
bioimpedance, 112
birth weight, 88, 92, 94, 96, 127, 129, 138, 140
blood pressure, 38, 105, 107, 139
body fat, 21–22, 25, 86, 94, 103–104, 109–110, 112, 114, 119, 256
  body fat distribution, 110
body mass index (BMI), xxi, xxiii–xxv, xxviii, 5, 19, 21–22, 24–28, 30–31, 34–36, 38–41, 48, 51, 55, 64–66, 72, 74–76, 80, 83–84, 86–88, 90, 92–101, 103–105, 109, 112–114, 116, 119–121, 124–125, 130–132, 135–139, 141, 148, 159–161, 169, 172, 184, 189, 191, 205, 213, 220, 226, 228–229, 235, 256–257, 259, 261, 263–265, 269, 271–275
  BMI growth, 135–137, 160–161
  BMI trajectories, xxv, 159–160
breakfast, xxiv, 40, 64, 110–112, 114–115, 118–120, 122–124, 148, 158
breastfeeding, 136–138, 141

C

calorie, xxiv, 145–146, 148–149, 154, 190. 241
  caloric intake, xxii, 70, 72, 74–79
Canada, xxv, 20, 45, 53, 57, 65, 157–159, 161–162, 168–169, 171–172, 272, 281

Canadian National Population Health Surveys (NPHS), 159–160, 170
cancer, 123, 157, 280
carbohydrate, 114, 116, 119–121, 123, 207
cardiovascular, 19, 38, 108–109, 113, 125, 128, 157
causal loop, 178, 180
cereals, 146–148, 150, 155, 240
Children's Food and Beverage Advertising Initiative (CFBAI), 150, 156
China, xxviii, 22–23, 65, 255–259, 270, 273–275, 284
cholesterol, 38, 121, 123
chronic disease, xix, 3, 29, 31, 80, 110, 127, 145, 203, 206, 208, 255, 274
coefficient of variation (CV), 11, 18
commercial, 69, 78–79, 148, 152, 238
community, xxv–xxvi, 3–6, 11–12, 15, 18–19, 25, 30, 62–63, 146–147, 149–150, 152–154, 158, 171–172, 207, 212–215, 226–228, 230–231, 253
computer, xxii, 47–48, 52–56, 65, 73, 96–97, 207, 261, 280
confidence interval (CI), xx, xxiii. xxvii, 7, 10–11, 18, 51–52, 93, 95–98, 100, 112, 131–132, 172, 223–224, 226, 264–266, 271
confounders, 85, 93, 113, 115, 221
consensus, xxvii, 235–237, 241, 243, 248–249, 251–253
consumption, xx, xxvi–xxvii, 25–26, 28, 64, 69–70, 73, 80–81, 110–112, 119, 123, 148–149, 155, 178, 208, 211, 213–217, 221, 223–230, 236–253, 274
cost, xix, xxv, xxviii, 4–5, 26, 28, 145, 157–158, 161–162, 168–173, 204–205, 209, 255–257, 259–261, 263–265, 266–275, 284
county, xx, 3–12, 9, 11, 14–15, 17–20, 86, 111, 125
cue reactivity theory, 69, 78

D

dairy, 148, 217, 250
diabetes, xxiv, 41, 80, 107, 125, 127–141, 157, 206, 229, 280
   type 2 diabetes (T2D), xxiv, 127–136, 138–141, 157, 229
diet, xxiii–xxiv, 28, 65, 80, 106, 109–111, 113–115, 117, 119, 121–125, 148, 183–184, 190, 228–229, 233, 243, 251–252, 258, 274, 279–280
   dietary behavior, 19, 28, 110
   dietary guidelines, 69, 241
   dietary intake, 88, 92–94, 96, 107, 111–112, 118, 120, 233, 249
   dieting, 179, 189–190
disability, xv, 272, 283

E

eating
   eating frequency (EF), xxiii–xxiv, 66, 104, 109–125, 208, 230
   eating habits, 157–158, 236
economic, xxv, xxvii, 6–7, 64, 106, 153, 160, 171–173, 175, 205, 212, 215, 255, 270, 274–275, 280, 284
education, xxviii, 39, 41, 62, 88, 92, 94, 96, 113–115, 118–120, 208, 213, 225, 232, 250, 256–260, 270–271, 273, 275, 277–278, 284
   nutrition education, xxviii, 39, 256–258, 270–271, 273, 275
   parental education, 113–114, 118–120

energy
- energy expenditure, 64, 108, 110, 113, 121, 125, 134, 249
- energy intake (EI), xxiv, 24–25, 74, 76, 81, 102, 110, 112, 115, 118–121, 123, 125, 226, 229, 244–245, 249, 251, 262–264, 271
- energy-dense food, 26, 69, 78
- estimated energy requirements (EERs), 112

Enjoy Being Fit (EBF), 214–215, 232
epidemiology, xiii–xviii, 28, 104–105, 209, 238, 279
epigenetics, 137
EPODE (together let's prevent childhood obesity), 212, 231, 283
ethnic, xxvi, 3, 6–7, 20, 28, 30–32, 36–39, 113, 122, 129, 135, 212, 214, 220–223, 226–228
ethnicity, xx, 4–7, 9–10, 15, 18, 31–35, 129, 131, 212
exercise, 67, 81, 106, 108, 189, 271

F

fast food, 155, 177, 207–208, 240, 244
fatness, 28, 84, 101, 103–104, 123–124
feasibility, xxvii, 157, 236, 251
fetus, 128, 133, 140
- fetal growth, 127–129

fiber, 114, 116, 120–121, 123, 148
First Amendment, 146, 151–152
food cues, xxii, 69, 77, 79–80
food
- food environment, 80, 236
- food groups, xxvii, 88, 93, 96, 121, 236–237, 241, 243, 250
- food industry, 80, 145–146, 150, 152, 154, 156, 244, 247–248
- food intake, xxii, 69, 71, 73, 75, 77–81, 122, 192–193, 244, 247, 250
- food purchasing, xxvii, 236
- food retailers, 145, 151
- obesogenic food, 146, 151–153

free fatty acids (FFA), 129, 133, 137
fruit, xxiv, xxvii, 80, 114, 116, 120–122, 148, 150, 208, 217, 240, 242–243, 247, 250

G

gardens, 158
gender, 47, 49–51, 53, 56, 62, 66–67, 73–77, 113–115, 118–120, 191, 220–222, 263
- boys, xxi, 22, 24, 31–33, 36–37, 46–47, 49–56, 58, 62–64, 66, 74–76, 81, 92–94, 98, 113, 159, 169, 275
- girls, xxi–xxii, 22, 24, 31–33, 36–37, 39, 46–47, 49–56, 60, 62–64, 66–67, 74, 76, 81, 92–94, 98, 113–115, 121, 124, 147, 159, 169

genetics, xvi, 132, 178
genome-wide association studies (GWAS), 86, 88, 90–91, 100 106–107
genotype, 84, 87–88, 90–91, 93, 102, 105–106
geographic, xx, 3, 5–6, 12, 14–15, 18
- geographic diversity, 5, 14

gestational age, 88, 92, 94, 96, 131
gestational weight gain (GWG), 128, 137–139
glucose, 129, 131, 133, 136–137, 140
- glucose tolerance, 133, 140

government, xxv, 28, 41, 145–146, 151–154, 214, 232, 235, 237, 280

local government, 145, 153, 214
grade, 30–35, 38, 41, 66, 159–161, 163–164, 166, 216–217, 220–222, 230, 257, 282
gross national product (GNP), 256
growth trajectories, 135–137, 141

H

health care systems, 18
heart disease, 4, 20, 105, 258
height, xx–xxi, xxiv, 5, 15, 21, 30–32, 36, 42, 46, 48, 65, 72, 74, 86–87, 94, 106, 109, 112–114, 116, 119–120, 123, 125, 127–128, 135, 170, 213, 220, 259, 264–265
heterozygosity, 87
hunger, 72–77, 80
hyperglycemia, 129, 140

I

impact factor, 182, 184, 187, 193, 195, 200–201
impulsivity, xxii, 69–71, 73–81
inactivity, 55, 83–84, 103, 232, 249, 274
income, 6–7, 10, 15–17, 26, 30, 38, 150, 171, 243, 262, 264, 270, 272
infant formula, xxvii, 240–241, 243
insulin, 38, 107–108, 121, 128–129, 133–134, 137–140
 insulin resistance, 108, 133–134, 140
International Obesity Task Force (IOTF), 48, 51, 64, 92, 220
Internet, xxiv, 47, 53, 146, 149, 153
intervention, xx, xxiv–xxviii, 18, 31, 38, 41, 49, 63, 84, 102–104, 110, 123, 125, 138, 154, 158–159, 161–162, 169–173, 175–179, 181–184, 186–188, 191–195, 197–205, 207–209, 211–217, 221–228, 230–232, 236, 251–252, 255–275, 281
intrauterine, xxiv, 127–129, 132–133, 135–137, 139–140

J

juice, 28, 150, 217, 226, 240, 242, 250

L

leptin, 128, 134, 139–140
lifestyle, 6–7, 10, 12, 15, 26, 46–47, 209, 212, 214, 230, 279

M

macrosomia, 129, 133, 137, 139
Malta, xxi, 47, 56, 64, 278
marketing, xxiv–xxvi, 145–156, 212, 214, 226–227, 231, 236, 242, 283
 social marketing, xxvi, 212, 214, 226–227, 231, 283
meal, 30–35, 110–112, 115–116, 118, 120–122, 124, 147, 151, 240
 meal frequency, 120, 124
meat, 240–241, 250
media, xxiv, 81, 145–147, 150, 153, 155
Mendelian randomization (MR), xxiii, 83–86, 88, 90–91, 95, 98, 100–102, 104–106, 229–230, 279
metabolic syndrome, 38, 128, 131, 140
morbidity, 109, 173, 205
mortality, 109, 172–173, 205
multilevel logistic models, 7, 9

Index

N

National Health and Nutrition Examination Survey (NHANES), 4, 14, 20, 22–23, 37–38, 108, 121, 124, 189–191, 207
National Survey of Children's Health (NSCH), xx, 4–7, 9, 11–12, 14–15, 17–18, 277
neighborhood, 6–7, 10, 14–15, 20, 67, 150, 206
nervous system, 134
nominal group technique, xxvii, 237–238, 241, 249, 252–253
nutrient, xxiv, 112, 116, 121–122, 133–134, 145–146, 148–149, 154, 241, 243–245, 248, 251
  nutrient density, 243, 248
nutrition, xxvii–xxviii, 4, 20, 22–23, 28, 37, 39–40, 80, 121, 124, 127, 138, 151, 155, 158, 176–177, 207–208, 211, 229–231, 237, 245, 250–252, 256–260, 262–267, 269–275, 279, 281
  overnutrition, 105, 127–139, 141

O

obesity
  obesity intervention, xxv, xxviii, 171, 179, 183, 187, 193, 195, 203, 230, 257, 271, 274
  obesity prevalence, xx, xxvi, 5, 7, 9–15, 17, 19, 22, 25–27, 36–37, 39, 160, 162, 169, 173, 177–178, 192–193, 195–203, 205, 257, 261, 263–266, 269, 271–272, 274
  obesity prevention, xx, xxvii, 3–4, 65, 110, 151, 156, 171–173, 177, 183–184, 187, 193–195, 203, 206–207, 230–231, 252–253, 256, 271, 273–274
  obesity rates, xx, 4, 21–23, 25–27, 109, 175, 177, 230, 236, 248, 250, 257
  obesity status, xxiv, 5–6, 45, 47, 49, 51, 53, 55, 57, 59, 61, 63, 65, 67, 110
  maternal obesity, 131, 135, 139–140
obesogenic, 138, 145–146, 151–154, 177, 203, 209, 212, 231, 236
overweight, xix, xxv–xxvii, 4, 19, 21–23, 26–28, 37–38, 40, 43, 46, 48, 51, 54–55, 58, 61, 63–65, 67, 72, 75, 80–81, 92, 101, 103, 107–108, 110, 114–115, 120–125, 127–128, 131, 136, 160–162, 164, 166, 169–173, 175–203, 205, 208–209, 211–212, 214–215, 220, 226, 229–232, 235–236, 251, 255, 257, 259, 261, 263–266, 269, 271–272, 274–275, 283

P

physical activity (PA), xx–xxi, xxiii, xxviii, 15, 19, 25–26, 28, 39–41, 45–55, 57, 59, 61–67, 83–85, 87, 89–108, 110–111, 113–116, 118–125, 138, 141, 158, 171, 173, 176–179, 183–184, 189–190, 193, 206, 208–209, 211, 214, 231, 256–260, 262–267, 269–275
  moderate to vigorous physical activity (MVPA), xxi–xxiii, 45, 48, 50–52, 54–56, 58–62, 64, 66, 87–88, 91–97, 100–101, 104
  physical inactivity, 55, 84, 249

pleiotropy, 90, 101–102
population, xx, xxv, xxvii, 5–7, 11–12, 18, 25, 28, 30–32, 34–37, 40–41, 47, 62, 66, 95, 101, 103, 105–107, 110–111, 120, 122–125, 129–131, 134–135, 140, 152, 159–160, 169, 171–172, 177, 180–181, 183, 203, 205, 207, 209, 222, 227, 243, 246–249, 252, 261, 274, 281
portion, 111, 124, 151, 240–241, 244–245, 247–248
pregnancy, 31–32, 88, 94, 96, 129–130, 133, 138–140
prevention, xx, xxvi–xxvii, 3–5, 9, 19–21, 23, 29–30, 34, 41, 65, 80, 110, 121, 123, 137, 151, 156, 158, 169–173, 175–179, 181–184, 187, 192–195, 200–203, 206–209, 215, 229–231, 236, 252–253, 256, 271, 273–275, 278, 280–281
price, 30–35, 107, 147, 236, 239, 241–243, 247, 250, 252
  price elasticity, 239, 250, 252
progression model, 169
protein, xxvii, 105, 114, 116, 240–241, 243
psychosocial, xix, 38, 179
puberty, 88, 96, 136, 138
public health, xx–xxi, xxiii–xxiv, xxvii, 4, 18–19, 26–29, 40, 45, 65–66, 101, 103, 108, 113, 121, 123–125, 127–128, 134–135, 146, 150, 152–156, 158, 171–173, 204, 206–207, 209, 229–233, 235–237, 249–253, 255–256, 275, 280–281, 284

Q

questionnaire, xxi–xxii, xxvi, 47, 64–65, 73–74, 81, 86, 110–111, 190, 207, 215–217, 220–222, 225–228, 260, 270

R

race, xx, 4–7, 9–10, 15–16, 18, 31–35, 129, 131
randomization, vii, xxiii, 74, 83–85, 95, 104–106, 227, 257
  randomized trial, 84, 104, 137, 229
reporting bias, 122
response, xxiii, 32, 36, 46, 70, 78–81, 83, 110, 156, 159, 222, 225, 227, 242, 246
  response bias, 225
restaurants, xxv, 15, 145, 147–148, 150–151, 153, 155, 250
reward, 70–75, 78, 149, 154
rewarding, xxii, 70, 76–78, 147
rural, 6–7, 10, 12, 15, 17, 20, 22, 122, 171

S

school, xx–xxii, xxv–xxviii, 14, 18, 22, 25, 27–42, 47–49, 51, 53, 55, 57, 62–67, 73, 84, 104, 107, 111, 113–114, 147, 150–153, 155, 157–163, 165–167, 169–173, 211–216, 220–230, 232–233, 255–259, 260–261, 263, 267, 270–271, 273–275, 278, 280–282
  school-based program, 157–258, 230
screen time (ST), xxi–xxii, 25, 45–49, 51–55, 57, 59, 61, 63–65, 67
sedentary, xxi, xxiii, 28, 45–46, 48–50, 54–55, 58–61, 63, 65–66, 87, 91, 93–98, 100–101, 104, 157, 262, 264, 272

Index

sensitivity analyses, xxvi, 90, 98, 178, 192, 195–196, 202
serving size, 240, 244, 247
sex, 4–7, 9–10, 15–16, 22, 31–36, 38–39, 87–88, 92–93, 96–98, 131, 133, 160, 162, 259, 262–263
siblings, 132
single nucleotide polymorphism (SNP), 87–88, 90–91, 97–98, 102, 106–107
small-area estimates (SAEs), xix–xx, 4, 7, 9, 11–12, 1418
smoking, 19, 88, 92, 94, 96, 136, 140, 244
snack, xxii, xxiv, 25, 39, 55, 70, 72, 74–80, 110–112, 114–116, 118, 120–125, 148, 155, 158, 236, 238, 240–241, 244–245
social
    social context, 62
    social influences, 176, 178, 202, 205
    social networks, xxv, 176, 206, 208–209
    social norms, 154, 176, 203
    social responsibility, 247
    social transmission, xxv–xxvi, 175, 177–185, 187, 189, 191–197, 199, 201–205, 207, 209
socio-demographic, 6, 216, 220–222, 224
socio-economic, 64, 212, 215, 255
    socioeconomic status, 12, 31, 37, 47, 49, 51, 58, 206, 278
soft drink, xx, 26, 148, 155, 217, 226, 229, 236, 240, 242, 245–246, 250
stadiometer, 48, 259
standard deviation, xxiii, 24, 216
stock and flow diagram, 181
sugar-sweetened beverages (SSB), xxvi–xxvii, 28, 148, 150–151, 211–217, 219–221, 223–231, 233, 240, 245–246, 248, 251
supermarkets, 80, 147, 151, 155, 246
system dynamics, xxv, 176–177, 204, 206–208

T

tax, 151, 236, 240, 243–245, 247, 252–253
    taxation, xxvii, 235–237, 239, 241–251, 253
television (TV), xx, xxii, xxiv, 25–26, 47, 52–56, 65–66, 81, 107, 146–148, 150, 153, 155–156
tobacco, 19, 236, 252
treatment, v, viii, xxvi, 80, 104, 121, 125, 137, 141, 175–179, 181, 183–184, 187–188, 190–195, 200–203, 206–209, 231, 252, 272, 275

U

underweight, 22, 72, 75, 160
urban, xxviii, 6–7, 10, 15, 17, 20, 22, 122, 273
    urbanization, 6–7, 10, 17

V

vegetables, xxiv, xxvii, 26, 116, 122, 148, 240, 243, 250

W

waist-to-height ratio, xxiv, 109, 113, 116, 120, 123, 125
water, xxvi–xxvii, 73, 113, 125, 211–215, 221, 224–229, 233

water campaign, xxvi–xxvii, 212–215, 221, 224, 227–228
weekend, xxii, 47–54, 59–60, 62–63, 66–67, 111, 158, 228
weight, xx–xxii, xxiv, xxvi, 5, 15, 21, 26, 30–33, 36, 40, 42, 45–49, 54–55, 58, 61, 63–65, 67, 72, 75, 81, 84, 86, 88, 91–92, 94, 96, 101, 103, 109–125, 127–130, 133, 135, 137–140, 158, 160–164, 166, 169–171, 173, 176–186, 189–191, 193–195, 203–204, 206–208, 211–213, 215, 220–222, 224, 226, 229–231, 259, 264–265, 272
   birth weight, 88, 92, 94, 96, 127, 129, 138, 140
   body weight, xxiv, 101, 103, 110, 120, 122–124, 158, 160–162, 169–170, 206–208, 229, 259
   excess weight, 173, 176, 207
   weight category, 63
   weight control, 103, 111, 121
   weight cycling, 177, 207
   weight gain, 26, 55, 81, 84, 103, 128, 137–139, 171, 206–208, 211, 215, 226, 229

weight loss, xxvi, 84, 121, 178, 181, 183, 185, 189–191, 193–195, 203–204, 212, 229
weight status, xxi, 33, 45–47, 49, 54, 58, 63, 65, 110, 120, 123–124, 158, 160–161, 163–164, 166, 169–170, 220–222, 224, 226, 229
World Health Organization (WHO), xxii, xxv–xxvi, 30, 32, 38–39, 48, 51, 63–65, 70–72, 75–80, 87, 92, 101, 111–113, 115, 120–123, 130, 132–133, 149, 158–159, 160–162, 166, 170, 190–191, 208, 211–212, 216–217, 220, 222, 225, 243, 247–248, 252, 257
excess weight, 173, 176, 207 258, 261, 280, 284

Y

Youth Risk Behavior Survey, (YRBS), 4, 9–11, 14–15, 19

Z

zip code, xx, 4–7, 10, 14–18

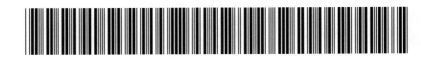